PEDIATRIC CARDIAC SURGERY

CURRENT ISSUES

Edited by

MARSHALL L. JACOBS, M.D.
Associate Professor of Surgery
University of Pennsylvania School of Medicine
Associate Surgeon
The Children's Hospital of Philadelphia

WILLIAM I. NORWOOD, M.D., PH.D.
Professor of Surgery
University of Pennsylvania School of Medicine
Chief, Division of Cardiothoracic Surgery
The Children's Hospital of Philadelphia

With 30 Contributing Authors

Butterworth–Heinemann
Boston London Oxford
Singapore Sydney Toronto Wellington

Every effort has been made to ensure that the drug dosage schedules within this text are accurate and conform to standards accepted at time of publication. However, as treatment recommendations vary in the light of continuing research and clinical experience, the reader is advised to verify drug dosage schedules herein with information found on product information sheets. This is especially true in cases of new or infrequently used drugs.

Recognizing the importance of preserving what has been written, it is the policy of Butterworth–Heinemann to have the books it publishes printed on acid-free paper, and we exert our best efforts to that end.

Library of Congress Cataloging-in-Publication Data

Pediatric cardiac surgery: current issues / edited by Marshall L. Jacobs, William I. Norwood : with 30 contributing authors.
p. cm.
Includes bibliographical references and index.
ISBN 0-7506-9061-5 (casebound: alk. paper)
1. Heart—Abnormalities—Surgery. 2. Pediatric cardiology. I. Jacobs, Marshall L. II. Norwood, William I.
[DNLM: 1. Heart Defects, Congenital—surgery. 2. Heart Surgery—in infancy & childhood. WS 290 C976]
RJ426.C64C85 1992
617.4′12059—dc20
DNLM/DLC
for Library of Congress 91-23318
CIP

British Library Cataloguing in Publication Data
Jacobs, Marshall L.
Pediatric cardiac surgery: current issues.
I. Title II. Norwood, William I.
618.9212

ISBN 0-7506-9061-5

Butterworth–Heinemann
80 Montvale Avenue
Stoneham, MA 02180

10 9 8 7 6 5 4 3 2 1

Printed in the United States of America

CONTRIBUTORS

Carl L. Backer, M.D.
Assistant Professor
Department of Surgery
Northwestern University Medical School
Attending Surgeon
Department of Cardiovascular and Thoracic Surgery
Children's Memorial Hospital
Chicago, Illinois

David Baum, M.D.
Department of Cardiovascular Surgery
Department of Pediatrics
Stanford University Medical Center
Stanford, California

Harvey W. Bender, Jr., M.D.
Professor of Surgery
Chairman, Department of Cardiac and Thoracic Surgery
Vanderbilt University Medical Center
Nashville, Tennessee

Daniel Bernstein, M.D.
Department of Cardiovascular Surgery
Department of Pediatrics
Stanford University Medical Center
Stanford, California

Edward L. Bove, M.D.
Professor of Surgery
University of Michigan Medical Center
Chief, Pediatric Cardiac Surgery
C. S. Mott's Children's Hospital, University of Michigan Medical Center
Ann Arbor, Michigan

Aldo R. Castaneda, M.D., Ph.D.
William E. Ladd Professor of Surgery
Harvard Medical School
Surgeon-in-Chief, Cardiovascular Surgery
The Children's Hospital
Boston, Massachusetts

David R. Clarke, M.D.
Associate Professor of Cardiovascular Surgery
University of Colorado Health Sciences Center
Chief, Cardiothoracic Surgery
University of Colorado Health Sciences Center and The Children's Hospital
Denver, Colorado

Daniel M. Cohen, M.D.
Assistant Professor of Surgery
Chief of Pediatric Cardiothoracic Surgery
East Carolina School of Medicine
Greenville, North Carolina

Davis C. Drinkwater, Jr., M.D.
Assistant Professor of Surgery
University of California at Los Angeles
Los Angeles, California

Ronald C. Elkins, M.D.
Professor of Surgery
University of Oklahoma College of Medicine
Chief, Section of Thoracic and Cardiovascular Surgery
Oklahoma City, Oklahoma

Patricia L. Gamberg, R.N., C.C.T.C.
Nurse Educator, Cardiothoracic Surgery
Stanford University
Stanford, California

Michael A. Greene, M.D.
Resident, General Surgery
Cardiovascular Surgery Research Fellow
Price Institute of Surgical Research
University of Louisville
Louisville, Kentucky

John W. Hammon, Jr., M.D.
Chairman of Cardiothoracic Surgery
Bowman Gray School of Medicine
North Carolina Baptist Hospital
Winston-Salem, North Carolina

Dolly D. Hansen, M.D.
Assistant Professor of Anesthesia (Pediatrics)
Harvard Medical School
Senior Associate in Anesthesia
The Children's Hospital
Boston, Massachusetts

Paul R. Hickey, M.D.
Associate Professor of Anaesthesia
Harvard Medical School
Director, Cardiac Anesthesia Service
The Children's Hospital
Boston, Massachusetts

Mark D. Iannettoni, M.D.
Research Fellow in Surgery
Section of Thoracic Surgery
University of Michigan Medical Center
Ann Arbor, Michigan

Farouk S. Idriss, M.D.
Professor of Surgery Emeritus
Northwestern University Medical School
Professor of Surgery Emeritus
Department of Cardiovascular and Thoracic Surgery
Children's Memorial Hospital
Chicago, Illinois

Richard A. Jonas, M.D.
Associate Professor of Surgery
Harvard Medical School
Associate in Cardiac Surgery
The Children's Hospital
Boston, Massachusetts

John F. Keane, M.D.
Associate Professor of Pediatrics
Harvard Medical School
Pediatric Cardiologist
The Children's Hospital
Boston, Massachusetts

Hillel Laks, M.D.
Professor and Chief, Cardiothoracic Surgery
UCLA Medical Center
Los Angeles, California

James E. Lock, M.D.
Associate Professor of Pediatrics
Harvard Medical School
Senior Associate and Director of Cardiac Catheterization Laboratory
The Children's Hospital
Boston, Massachusetts

Constantine Mavroudis, M.D.
Professor of Surgery
Northwestern University Medical School
Evanston, Illinois
A. C. Buehler Professor of Surgery
Chief, Division of Cardiothoracic Surgery
Children's Memorial Hospital
Chicago, Illinois

John E. Mayer, Jr., M.D.
Associate Professor of Surgery
Harvard Medical School
Senior Associate, Cardiac Surgery
The Children's Hospital
Boston, Massachusetts

Frank M. Midgley, M.D.
Professor of Surgery and Pediatrics
George Washington University Medical School
Chairman, Pediatric Cardiovascular Surgery
Children's National Medical Center
Washington, D.C.

Joan L. Miller, R.N.
Clinical Transplant Coordinator
Heart-Lung Adult and Pediatric Transplant Program
Department of Cardiovascular and Thoracic Surgery
Stanford University Medical Center
Stanford, California

Stanton B. Perry, M.D.
Assistant Professor of Pediatrics
Harvard Medical School
Boston, Massachusetts

Robert M. Sade, M.D.
Professor of Surgery
Department of Surgery
Medical University of South Carolina
Chief, Pediatric Cardiac Surgery
Department of Surgery
MUSC Medical Center
Charleston, South Carolina

Norman E. Shumway, M.D.
Frances and Charles D. Field Professor and Chairman
Department of Cardiothoracic Surgery
Stanford University School of Medicine
Stanford, California

Vaughn A. Starnes, M.D.
Assistant Professor
Cardiovascular Surgery
Chief, Pediatric Cardiac Surgery
Stanford University School of Medicine
Stanford, California

William G. Williams, M.D.
Professor of Surgery
University of Toronto
Head, Cardiovascular Surgery
Hospital for Sick Children
Toronto, Ontario, Canada

Benjamin Zeevi, M.D.
Instructor in Pediatrics
Harvard Medical School
Assistant in Cardiology
The Children's Hospital
Boston, Massachusetts

CONTENTS

PREFACE

The management of complex congenital cardiac malformations is a rapidly changing, rapidly evolving field. As practitioners in this field, we have learned that informal communication with our colleagues at other centers, and even visits to those other centers to experience firsthand the "ways that it is being done," are among the most important methods of keeping abreast of the rapid progress that is taking place in the fields of pediatric cardiology and congenital heart surgery. Thus, we have attempted to compile in this book that type of information which we can glean from candid and informal exchanges of information with our colleagues. The authors have been asked to share with us and our readers very timely information regarding their approaches to selected problems in congenital heart surgery, primarily in areas where rapid growth has occurred over the past several years, and in fact continues to take place. Our colleagues have been kind enough to respond by producing the seventeen chapters that make up this edition. We are grateful for the enthusiasm with which our colleagues brought their expertise to this endeavor. Finally, we are grateful to Butterworth–Heinemann for the opportunity to collaborate on a project that embraces the concept of open and up-to-the-minute communication between practitioners in a rapidly evolving field, and for their constant support of ourselves and our author-colleagues, which ensured the timely completion of this edition.

Marshall L. Jacobs
William I. Norwood
Philadelphia, PA

INTRODUCTION

Over the last two decades, the management of congenital heart disease has continued to evolve. New operations for seemingly unmanageable structural abnormalities of the cardiovascular system were devised. New techniques were introduced to improve long-term functional results for a number of congenital cardiac defects. Old techniques were modified and adapted to the management of a wide range of congenital cardiac defects, and, most importantly, the overall strategy of minimal palliation and early reparative surgery has begun to prove feasible and efficacious. At the very foundations of this modern era of congenital cardiac surgery were the reintroduction of deep hypothermia and circulatory arrest, the introduction and increased understanding of myocardial preservation in the young, commercial availability of prostaglandins, and the appreciation and improved understanding of the management of the dynamic pulmonary vascular resistance in the young.

In 1958, Senning introduced an atrial inversion operation for the definitive management of transposition of the great arteries [S,D,D]. Four years later, Mustard's modification of Senning's operation made atrial inversion surgery central to the management of simple and complex forms of transposition of the great arteries. While the mortality rate for atrial inversion repair of transposition of the great arteries decreased during the 1960s, the late development of systemic and pulmonary venous obstruction, supraventricular arrhythmias, and occasional right ventricular failure were complications of this surgical approach. In 1975, Jatene reintroduced anatomic correction of transposition of the great arteries by arterial switch, including transplantation of the coronary arteries. Although the mortality rate in the early experience of arterial switch surgery was higher than with atrial inversion operations, Jatene's efforts were accepted principally because of concerns of late right ventricular failure and sinus arrhythmias following atrial inversion surgery—complications that are avoided by anatomic repair. Many of the patient deaths during this period have been attributed to patient selection. The left ventricle, working against the low pulmonary vascular resistance of the older infant with transposition of the great arteries, may not be prepared for the higher resistance of the systemic circulation following arterial switch. By preparing the left ventricle with a pulmonary artery band prior to repair, Yacoub sought to increase the applicability of this operation in those without a coexisting large ventricular septal defect or patent ductus. In the last decade, the feasibility and efficacy of anatomic repair in the first month of life, when the left ventricle is still managing the higher resistance of the immature lung, has been established. Significant long-term follow-up and comparison with atrial inversion surgery will define the ultimate role of arterial switch surgery in the management of transposition of the great arteries, as well as other forms of complex congenital cardiac disease. To date, intermediate term results stress the need to consider the impact of highly variable coronary artery anatomy in transposition of the great arteries as well as hypothetical considerations of late supravalvar great artery obstruction and semilunar valve function.

In the early 1970s, Fontan and Kreutzer independently introduced treatment for tricuspid atresia that produced nearly normal oxygen saturation of the systemic arterial circulation and normal volume work for the systemic ventricle. Since its initial introduction, the principles of this surgery have been adapted to virtually all forms of single-ventricle complexes as well as other complex congenital cardiac malformations. The longest survivors of the original Fontan operation continued to have remarkably good function following a Glenn shunt, placement of a prosthetic valve in the inferior vena cava, and a valved conduit interposed between the right atrium and pulmonary artery for separation of the systemic and pulmonary circulations in tricuspid atresia. However, there is increasing evidence that low pulmonary vascular resistance and a large unobstructed anastomosis between the systemic venous return and pulmonary arterial vasculature are the most important elements of a good outcome.

Hypoplastic left heart syndrome is an extreme form of left ventricular outflow tract obstruction. This is the most common form of single ventricle, and it is universally fatal without surgical intervention, usually within the first days to week after birth. Stimulated by the potential applicability of Fontan's operation to this common form of single ventricle, palliative surgery was developed and evolved over the early 1980s to allow for stable systemic circulation and normal maturation of the pulmonary vasculature in preparation for a modified Fontan procedure. Management of these neonates has greatly increased our understanding not only of hypoplastic left heart syndrome but also of other complex congenital cardiac diseases presenting in the newborn.

While heart transplantation had been established as effective therapy for end-stage heart disease in the adult, the application of heart transplantation to the treatment of hypoplastic left heart syndrome was associated with a rapid development of the use of heart transplantation in children with cardiomyopathy and complex structural heart disease. With the introduction of new technology and materials, invasive catheter techniques, extracardiac valved conduits, valve autografts, and allografts have been added to the armamentarium of the pediatric cardiac surgeon. Such advances in diagnostic and surgical techniques and post-operative management have made possible repair or significant palliation of virtually all congenital cardiac malformations. While the possibilities are increasingly apparent, our treatment of congenital cardiac defects which were corrected with open heart surgery at the very beginnings of cardiac surgery continue to evolve.

Recognition of long-term sequelae of reparative techniques, restructuring of such developmental abnormalities, and revision of initial management strategies and techniques will continue to make our speciality a dynamic one. Contained in the chapters of this book written by some of the contributors to this evolution are many examples of this exciting and developing phase of congenital cardiac surgery.

William I. Norwood
Marshall L. Jacobs
Philadelphia, PA

1

Simple Transposition of the Great Arteries: The Arterial Switch Operation in Neonates

Aldo R. Castaneda

The natural history of transposition of the great arteries (TGA) reveals that close to 95% of patients die within the first year of life (Liebman et al. 1969). The early pioneering surgical contributions to the treatment of this serious condition by Blalock and Hanlon (1950), Albert (1954), Senning (1959), and Mustard (1964) have dramatically changed the fate of these children. However, despite the impressive decreases in hospital mortality of the atrial switch operations, long-term follow-up has revealed disturbing incidences of arrhythmias (Hayes and Gersony 1986; Vetter et al. 1987) and ventricular dysfunction (Graham et al. 1975; Borow et al. 1981). Many of these complications seem inherent to the intraatrial repair, such as the need for extensive atrial incisions and suture lines and dependence on the right ventricle (RV) and tricuspid valve as the systemic ventricle and atrioventricular valve, respectively.

A number of theoretical considerations support the notion that the left ventricle (LV) is more suitable than the RV to serve the systemic circulation. The left ventricle with its cylindrical shape and its concentric contraction pattern seems more adapted to pressure work, whereas the RV with its crescent-shaped cavity, its large internal surface area-to-volume ratio, and its bellows-like contraction pattern seems better suited to serve as a volume pump.

In 1975, Jatene described the first successful arterial switch operation (ASO) in a patient with TGA and a large ventricular septal defect (VSD) (Jatene et al. 1975; Jatene et al. 1982). Jatene recognized the need for an LV capable of supporting the systemic circulation and therefore initially limited this operation to patients with complex TGA, that is, TGA with a VSD (TGA/VSD), a large patent ductus arteriosus, or left ventricular outflow tract obstruction. The early high operative mortality of the ASO was at least in part related to these selection criteria.

Furthermore, only 20% of patients with TGA have complex TGA. Thus, the application of the ASO principle to the largest subset of patients with TGA, that is, patients with TGA and an intact ventricular septum (TGA/IVS), remained a surgical challenge. Aside from sporadic reports of successful primary ASO in infants, the majority of early attempts at this approach failed mostly because of LV dysfunction. To "prepare" the LV for systemic pressure work, Yacoub in 1977 introduced the two-stage approach for TGA/IVS by first banding the pulmonary artery, with or without a systemic pulmonary artery shunt, to stimulate the development of left ventricular hypertrophy, followed by an ASO many months later (Yacoub et al. 1977). The principle of performing the ASO as a primary repair in neonates with TGA/IVS, while the LV is still capable of pressure work, was successfully introduced at the Boston Children's Hospital in 1983 (Castaneda et al. 1984). Primary ASO for TGA/IVS in neonates has now become the operation of choice in many centers.

PHYSIOLOGIC AND ANATOMIC CONSIDERATIONS

In the fetus with TGA/IVS, the left and right ventricular pressures are equal. Consequently, LV wall thickness is normal at birth. However, after birth, the rapidly decreasing pulmonary vascular resistance is accompanied by a parallel decline in peak LV pressure, which in turn decreases the stimulus for the development of left ventricular muscle mass. For example, at 1 month of age, the peak LV to RV pressure ratio in patients with TGA/IVS commonly has fallen to 0.5 or less (Bano-Rodriguez et al. 1980). Because of the significant concomitant increase in pulmonary blood flow and hence left ventricular volume overload, the LV tends also to dilate progressively. All these factors combine in creating an urgency to perform the ASO during the neonatal period while the LV is still capable of supporting the systemic circulation. Theoretically, and borne out by our clinical experience, the repair is ideally performed within the first few weeks of life (Castaneda et al. 1988). It is our present policy to carry out the ASO in all patients within the first 2 weeks of life regardless of preoperative LV-to-RV pressure measurements. Beyond 2 weeks of life, we have arbitrarily selected an LV-to-RV ratio of 0.6 as the lower limit of acceptable LV pressure. Echocardiographic parameters of LV suitability for ASO include ventricular septal position, LV wall thickness, and LV muscle mass to volume ratio. However, the validity of these parameters as predictors of outcome following arterial switch operations have not yet been definitely established.

An infant with TGA/IVS who presents beyond the neonatal period or who has an LV to RV pressure ratio of less than 0.6 is subjected to a preliminary pulmonary artery banding and a systemic artery to pulmonary artery shunt (modified Blalock-Taussig shunt) in preparation for an ASO (Jonas et al. 1989). This operation is then followed within 7 to 10 days by removal of the pulmonary artery band, division of the aortopulmonary shunt, and an ASO. Thus far, all 21 infants treated

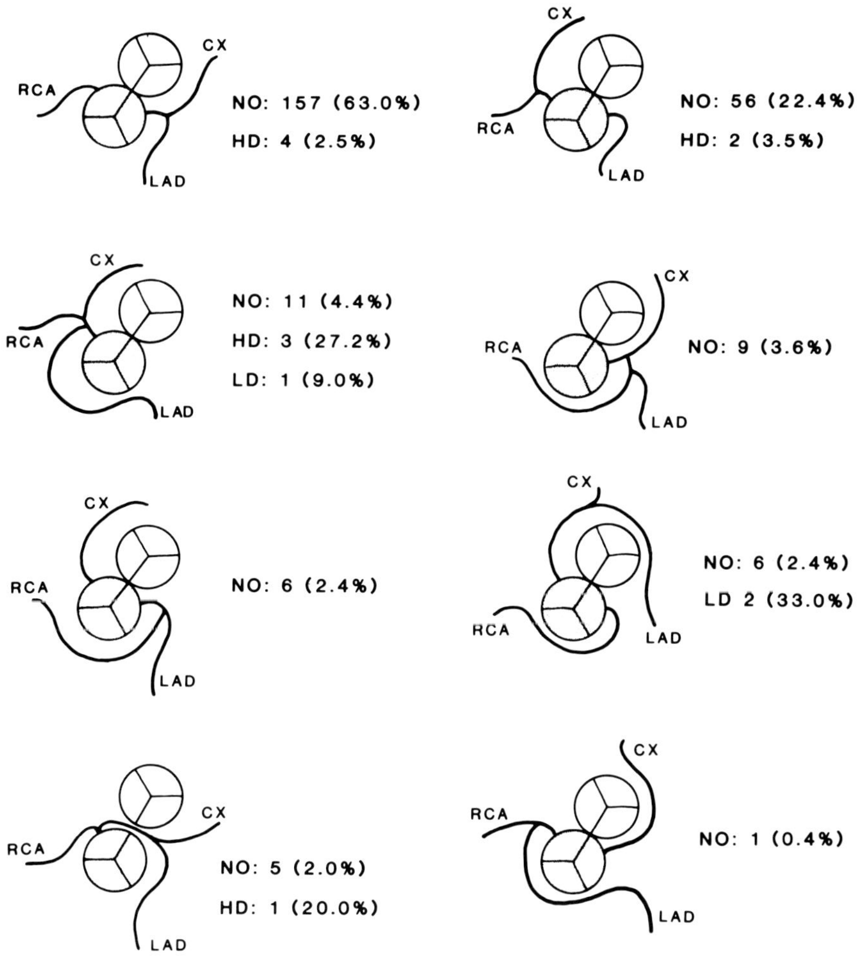

Figure 1.1 Coronary artery patterns in 251 patients with TGA, including patients with TGA and VSD.

by this "rapid switch" protocol have survived both the initial banding and subsequent ASO.

The outcome of an ASO in a properly selected neonate is also dependent upon successful transfer of the coronary arteries. Gittenberger-DeGroot and her colleagues introduced a descriptive terminology that includes naming the three aortic sinuses as left, right, and nonfacing (Gittenberger-DeGroot et al. 1983). Coronary arteries in TGA almost always originate from the facing sinuses and supply three major coronary branches: the left anterior descending, the left circumflex, and the right coronary artery. The most common types of coronary anatomy in TGA are illustrated in Figure 1.1. Most coronary arterial patterns lend themselves to an ASO; however, in our experience a single right coronary artery and a left coronary artery with an intramural course, and its ostium located within the right facing sinus, immediately adjacent to the posterior commissure, carry a higher early and late risk.

Left ventricular outflow tract obstruction (LVOTO) is present in approximately 15% of patients with TGA/IVS. The LVOTO is usually dynamic, caused by leftward displacement of the ventricular septum, often accentuated by abnormal systolic motion of the anterior mitral leaflet. Only rarely is the obstruction organic, caused either by a fibrous ring or an excrescence of endocardial cushion tissue or by pure valvar stenosis. Functional LVOTO is not a contraindication for an ASO; in fact, preoperatively measured gradients tend to disappear after the ASO and after reestablishing a normal LV-to-RV pressure ratio. In fact, the only contraindication in our experience is a long tunnel-type LVOTO or any significant degree of organic pulmonary valve pathology (Mayer et al. 1988).

PREOPERATIVE, OPERATIVE, AND POSTOPERATIVE MANAGEMENT

All neonates are evaluated preoperatively by 2D-echocardiography, cardiac catheterization, and angiography, including an aortic root injection to define coronary anatomy. A balloon atrial septostomy (BAS) during cardiac catheterization is generally recommended unless the ASO can be performed immediately after the catheterization. In critically ill neonates, a BAS can be accomplished at the patient's bedside under 2D-echocardiographic guidance. If severe hypoxia and metabolic acidosis are present, prostaglandin E_1 (PGE_1) may be added to maintain ductal patency and improve oxygenation in association with BAS.

Through a midline sternotomy, a generous segment of pericardium is harvested and prepared with 0.6% glutaraldehyde solution. After administering 2 mg/kg of body weight of heparin, the ascending aorta is cannulated as far distally as possible to allow adequate length for the aortic anastomosis (Mayer et al. 1986). A single venous cannula is placed within the right atrium, and cooling to profound hypothermia (18°C rectal temperature) is initiated. Immediately after commencing cardiopulmonary bypass, the commonly large ductus arteriosus is divided. The left and right pulmonary arteries are then dissected peripherally until the first pulmonary artery branches are clearly identified. This maneuver is essential to minimize tension on the pulmonary artery anastomosis. At 18°C rectal temperature, the distal aorta is clamped and cold cardioplegic solution (Plegisol, 20 ml/kg) is injected into the proximal ascending aorta. The operation is performed either under total circulatory arrest or under continuous deep hypothermic low-flow perfusion (30 to 50 ml/kg/min) with a period of circulatory arrest to close the atrial or ventricular septal defects. To secure optimal cardiac decompression during continuous deep hypothermic perfusion, we find it most convenient to position the tip of the atrial cannula close to the superior vena cava/right atrial junction.

The ascending aorta is divided approximately 1 centimeter distal to the origin of the coronary arteries (Figure 1.2A). The ostia of the coronary arteries within the facing sinuses are then inspected. Next, the pulmonary artery is divided proximal to its bifurcation, and the native pulmonary valve is inspected. Only then are the left and right coronary ostia explanted along with as large a segment of surrounding aortic wall as possible (Figure 1.2B). Only minimal dissection of the proximal segments of the coronary arteries is necessary. Occasionally small conal branches encountered during this dissection may have to be sacrificed to gain additional length. An equivalent U-shaped segment of pulmonary arterial wall is removed from both the left and the right anterior aspects of the native pulmonary artery. The coronary flaps are then sewn into these incisions with continuous 7–0 absorbable monofilament suture (Figure 1.2C). When the circumflex coronary artery arises from the right coronary artery, the sight of right coronary implantation must be kept slightly higher to avoid kinking of the circumflex coronary artery. If the two coronary arteries originate from the same sinus, they can be included in the same aortic flap. In the case that both the right and the left coronary arteries originate from the right facing sinus, the left coronary artery courses either intramurally or extramurally between the ascending aorta and pulmonary artery, and the ostium of the left coronary artery is usually located immediately adjacent to the posterior valve commissure (Figure 1.3). Therefore, the upper portion of this commissure must be included as part of the left coronary artery flap.

The distal pulmonary artery is then brought anterior to the aorta (Lecompte maneuver) and the distal aorta is anastomosed to the proximal neo-aorta with a 6–0 continuous absorbable monofilament suture (Figure 1.2D). Portions of the excess coronary flaps may be incorporated into this anastomosis to compensate for discrepancies in size. At this point, the right atrial communication, usually enlarged preoperatively by BAS, is closed through the right atrium. If the operation is carried out under continuous deep hypothermic perfusion, a short period of circulatory arrest is necessary at this point. If a VSD is present, this is also closed either through the right atrium or preferentially through the anterior semilunar valve. After closure of the right atriotomy, the venous cannula is reinserted and cardiopulmonary bypass is restarted. The aortic cross clamp can be removed at this point, provided that the left side of the heart is adequately vented through a stab incision in the ascending aorta.

The coronary donor sites in the neo-pulmonary artery are then filled with a single segment of pretreated autologous pericardium, which is also used to bridge the gap between the proximal and distal pulmonary artery (Figure 1.4). Discrepancies in caliber between the two stomas can also be easily reconciled with this pericardial flap technique. The anastomosis can be made larger by extending the incision into either the left or the right pulmonary arteries.

Rewarming, generally initiated when the aortic clamp is released, is completed on bypass to a rectal temperature of 36°C. Immediately after release of the aortic

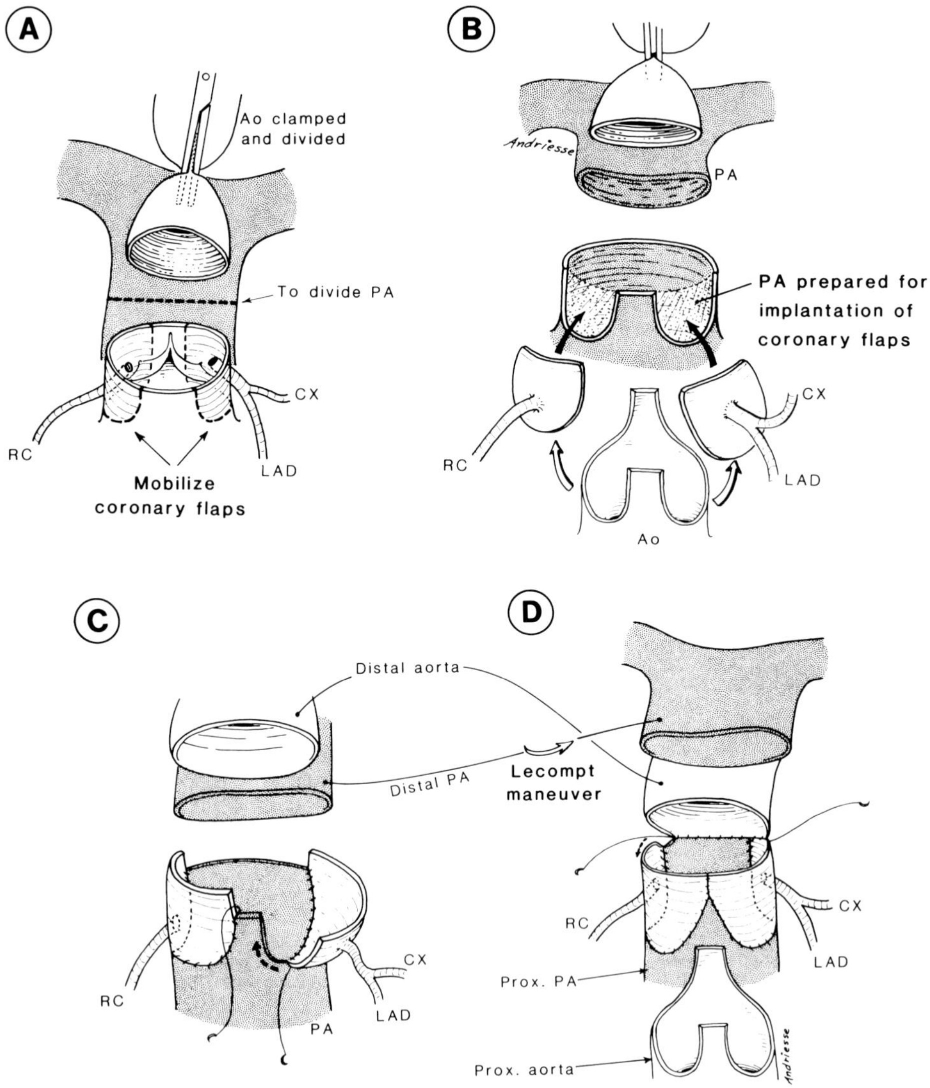

Figure 1.2 (A) Ascending aorta is divided approximately 1 centimeter distal to the origin of the coronary arteries. (B) The pulmonary artery is divided proximal to its bifurcation. The left and right coronary arteries are explanted with a large segment of aortic wall. An equivalent U-shaped segment of pulmonary arterial wall is excised from both left and right anterior aspects of pulmonary artery. (C) The coronary flaps are sewn into the prepared pulmonary artery wall with continuous 7–0 absorbable monofilament sutures. (D) The distal pulmonary artery is brought anterior to the aorta (Lecompte maneuver), and the distal aorta is anastomosed to the proximal neo-aorta.

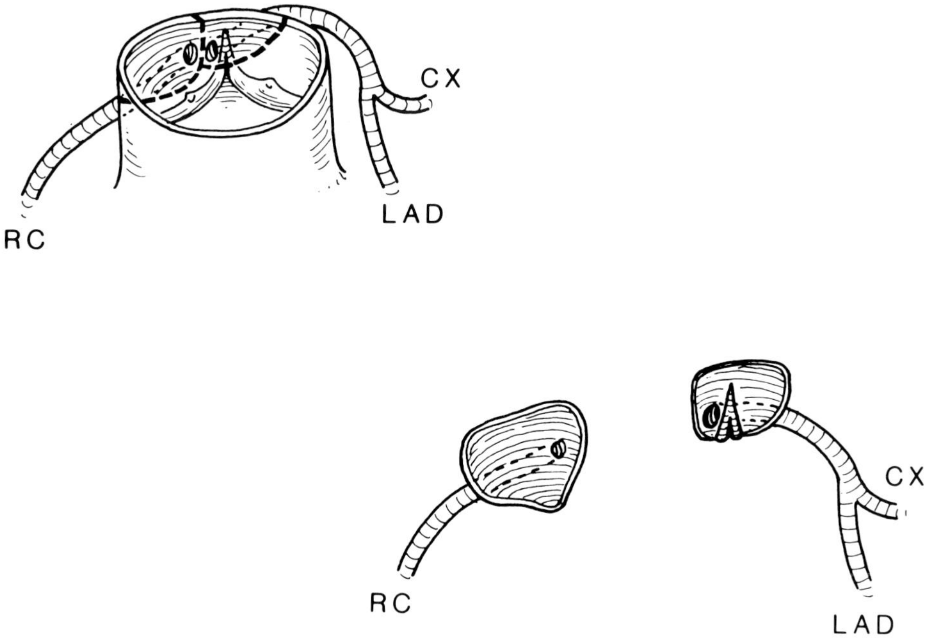

Figure 1.3 Both right and left coronary arteries originate from the right facing sinus. The left coronary artery courses between the aorta and pulmonary artery. The ostium of the left coronary artery is located adjacent to the posterior commissure. The upper portion of the posterior commissure is included as part of the left coronary flap.

cross clamp, one must evaluate the adequacy of the coronary anastomoses. Blood should rapidly fill both the left and right coronary arteries, and the myocardium should "pink up." During weaning from cardiopulmonary bypass, close monitoring of heart rate, systemic blood pressure, and left atrial pressure is employed. Systemic blood pressure is maintained above 60 mmHg, adding calcium and inotropic agents, usually dopamine if necessary. Abnormalities of cardiac rhythm or of myocardial performance are strongly suggestive of coronary perfusion problems. Should this be the case, the cause must be rapidly identified and aggressively corrected. After removal of the venous and arterial cannulae, right and left atrial and pulmonary artery lines are placed for postoperative monitoring and venous access.

Postoperative management is similar to that of neonates undergoing repair of other complex cardiac lesions (Castaneda et al. 1989). Mechanical ventilation, sedation, and moderate inotropic support are customarily maintained during the first 24 to 48 hours, or until hemodynamic stability is achieved.

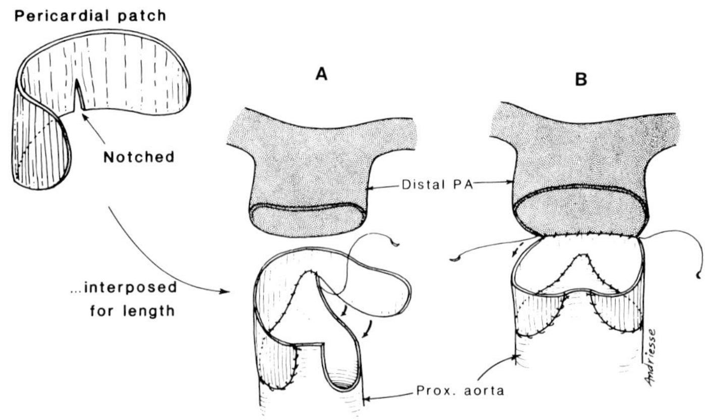

Figure 1.4 (A) The coronary donor sites in the neo-pulmonary artery are filled with a single segment of autologous pericardium. (B) The pericardial segment also serves to bridge the gap between the proximal and distal pulmonary arteries. If necessary, the anastomosis can be made wider by incising both the left and the right pulmonary arteries.

RESULTS

From January of 1983 through May of 1989, 321 children have undergone an ASO at The Children's Hospital in Boston: 190 for TGA/IVS and 110 for TGA/VSD or double outlet RV with subpulmonary VSD. Twenty-one patients with TGA/IVS have undergone a "rapid" two-stage pulmonary artery banding and ASO.

□ Hospital Mortality

The hospital mortality for simple transposition (TGA/IVS) after ASO was 5.7% (11/190 patients). Since July of 1985, the mortality has decreased to 2.5%. Five of the deaths related to coronary artery transfer. Patients with a single right coronary artery and those who had both the right and left coronary artery originating from the right facing sinus were at highest risk.

□ Follow-up Clinical Data

There was one late death among 179 hospital survivors. The majority of the survivors have no cardiac symptoms. None of the patients are on cardiac medications, and all are following a normal growth pattern.

□ Follow-up Hemodynamic Data

Supravalvar pulmonary stenosis (SPS) with RV to pulmonary artery gradients in excess of 40 mmHg occurred in seven patients, five of whom had successful relief of the obstruction at reoperation. The SPS was caused by (1) tension on the anastomosis with anterior-posterior flattening of the pulmonary artery and (2) less frequently (two patients), circumferential narrowing of the anastomosis itself. These complications, which occurred early in our experience, prompted modifications of the technique used to reconstruct the pulmonary artery (Figure 1.4).

Only one patient had a gradient of greater than 40 mmHg across the aortic anastomosis. Mild pulmonary regurgitation was found in two patients, whereas trivial aortic regurgitation was observed in 15 patients.

□ Late Occlusion of Coronary Arteries

Occlusion of the left coronary artery has occurred in three patients, one with the usual pattern of coronary anatomy and two with the circumflex coronary arising from the right coronary artery and a small anterior descending coronary artery originating from the left facing sinus. All three patients had adequate retrograde perfusion through collaterals and had no left ventricular dysfunction at either 2D-echocardiography or cardiac catheterization.

□ Postoperative Left Ventricular Function

Left ventricular function is normal in all the patients studied after primary ASO for TGA/IVS. Echocardiographically, the relationship between mean velocity of fiber shortening (VCFC) and end systolic wall stress (an afterload-adjusted, pre-loaded-independent index of contractility) and the relationship between percent fiber shortening (%FS) and end systolic wall stress (an afterload-adjusted, preload-dependent index of contractility) have been within the normal range in all patients. Segmental regional wall motion, both in short and long axis dimensions, was also normal. Indices of diastolic function, such as peak rate of filling and peak rate of wall thinning, showed normal values in all patients as late as 50 months after the ASO (Wernovsky et al. 1988).

□ Electrocardiographic and Electrophysiologic Postoperative Data

Normal sinus rhythm was present in 98% of patients up to 55 months after ASO. Only one patient has late sinus node dysfunction. On Holter monitoring, there was occasional uniform ventricular ectopic activity in 29% of the patients. However, none has multiform ventricular ectopic activity. Postoperative electrophysiologic studies reveal that 98% of patients had normal sinus node and atrioventricular node recovery times, and 100% of the patients had normal AH and AHV intervals.

DISCUSSION

In a multicenter study conducted in the United States, the 1-year predicted survival rate of a patient with TGA/IVS and a weight of 3.4 kg currently entered into an atrial or arterial switch protocol is 92%. Using hazard function analysis, the ASO presents a single phase of rapidly declining risk, whereas the atrial repair (Mustard or Senning) shows a constant hazard phase extending indefinitely, in addition to an early phase of declining risk. A more recent analysis revealed that old age (at repair) and earlier date of operation, that is, before 1985, proved to be incremental risk factors for death after the ASO. Although not directly relevant to this discussion, it is of interest that a hemodynamically important VSD does not increase the risk for ASO at this time.

Although coronary translocation has been possible in all of the described branching patterns, some coronary artery patterns are distinctively more difficult to deal with and carry a higher operative mortality. Patients with a single right coronary artery were initially at higher risk mostly because of unrecognized kinking of the circumflex coronary artery. We therefore modified the technique, implanting the single coronary artery slightly more superior to avoid kinking of the circumflex coronary artery. Perhaps the technically most demanding coronary pattern is the origin of both left and right coronary arteries from the right facing sinus. Echocardiography has proved accurate and reliable in displaying the coronary variants. We have lately evolved the concept that the upper third of the posterior commissure has to be included in the aortic wall flap. This also facilitates inclusion of an intramural segment of the left coronary artery. This technique has helped significantly in improving our results with this subset of patients. In fact, four of five patients with this coronary anatomy have survived the ASO.

The intermediate results after the ASO, including echocardiographic and hemodynamic analysis of left ventricular function and electrocardiographic and electrophysiologic data, are most encouraging, particularly since patients treated with ASO are at risk for myocardial injury because of (1) ischemia during the surgical procedure itself, (2) acute imposition of a systemic arterial pressure load to the left ventricle, and (3) the potential for coronary insufficiency after coronary reimplantation. In light of these potential hazards, the data on normal systolic and diastolic LV function are even more reassuring. In contrast, systemic ventricular dysfunction (anatomic RV) has been documented after atrial switch operations.

Borow and associates, using afterload augmentation to determine end systolic pressure dimension relationships in patients 1 to 5 years after either a Mustard or a Senning operation, found depressed contractility in approximately 25% of these patients (Borow et al. 1981). In that study, a strong correlation between age at repair and ventricular contractility was also demonstrated.

The high incidence of normal sinus rhythm and the virtual absence of Lown >1 ventricular ectopic activity also compares most favorably with results after atrial switch operations. Evidently, by eliminating the need for extensive intraatrial manipulations, including excision of atrial septum and long suture lines, damage to the sinoatrial node is minimized.

Similar to our experience with early repair of tetralogy of Fallot (Walsh et al. 1988), it is our contention that primary repair in the neonate or during early infancy leads to improved myocardial performance and increased electrical stability, which would explain the reduced incidence of ventricular ectopic activity after the ASO.

The use of deep hypothermic low-flow (50 mm/kg/min) cardiopulmonary bypass has resulted in shorter periods of circulatory arrest. Although shorter periods of circulatory arrest may be beneficial to later central nervous system function, studies of neurologic sequelae following prolonged continuous low-flow cardiopulmonary bypass are lacking, and the issue of circulatory arrest and long-term neurologic outcome remains largely unresolved. We have now initiated a formal assessment of developmental, cognitive, and neurologic sequelae of circulatory arrest and cardiopulmonary bypass in our institution.

Clearly, a longer period of follow-up is necessary before the absolute superiority of the ASO over the atrial switch operation for TGA/IVS is demonstrated. Also, the potential hazard of late coronary insufficiency and aortic valve (anatomic pulmonary valve) dysfunction requires continued monitoring of these patients.

REFERENCES

Albert HM. Surgical correction of transposition of the great vessels. Surg Forum 1954;5:74.

Bano-Rodrigo A, Quero-Jiminez M, Moreno-Granado F, Gamallo-Amat C. Wall thickness of ventricular chambers in transposition of the great arteries. Surgical implications. J Thorac Cardiovasc Surg 1980;79:592.

Blalock A, Hanlon CR. The surgical treatment of complete transposition of the aorta and the pulmonary artery. Surg Gynecol Obstet 1950;90:1.

Borow KM, Keane JF, Castaneda AR, Freed MD. Systemic ventricular function in patients with tetralogy of Fallot, ventricular septal defect and transposition of the great arteries repaired during infancy. Circulation 1981;64:878.

Castaneda AR, Mayer JE Jr, Jonas RA, et al. The neonate with critical congenital heart disease: A surgical challenge. J Thorac Cardiovasc Surg 1989;98:869.

Castaneda AR, Norwood WJ, Lang P, Sanders SP. Transposition of the great arteries and intact ventricular septum: Anatomical repair in the neonate. Ann Thorac Surg 1984;38:438.

Castaneda AR, Trusler GA, Paul MH, Blackstone EH, Kirklin JW, and the Congenital Heart Surgeons Society. The early results of treatment of simple transposition in the current era. J Thorac Cardiovasc Surg 1988;95:14.

Gittenberger-DeGrott AC, Sauer U, Oppenheimer-Dekker A, Quaegebeur J. Coronary arterial anatomy in transposition of the great arteries: A morphologic study. Ped Cardiol 1983;4 (suppl I):15.

Graham TP, Atwood GF, Boucek RJ, Boerth RC, Bender HW. Abnormalities of right ventricular function following Mustard's operation for transposition of the great arteries. Circulation 1975;52:678.

Hayes CJ, Gersony WM. Arrhythmias after the Mustard operation for transposition of the great arteries: A long-term study. J Am Coll Cardiol 1986;7:133.

Jatene AD, Fontes VF, Paulista PP, et al. Successful anatomic correction of transposition of the great vessels. A preliminary report. Arq Braz Cardiol 1975;28:461.

Jatene AD, Fontes VF, Souza LCB, et al. Anatomic correction of transposition of the great vessels. J Thorac Cardiovasc Surg 1982;83:20.

Jonas RA, Giglia TM, Sanders SP, et al. Rapid two stage arterial switch for transposition of the great arteries and intact ventricular septum beyond the neonatal period. Circulation (in press).

Liebman J, Cullum L, Belloc NB. Natural history of transposition of the great arteries. Anatomy and birth and death characteristics. Circulation 1969;40:237.

Mayer JE, Jonas RA, Castaneda AR. Arterial switch operation for transposition of the great arteries with intact ventricular septum. J Cardiol Surg 1986;1:97.

Mayer JE, Wernovsky G, Jonas RA, et al. Arterial switch operation for transposition of the great arteries with abnormal left ventricular outflow tract (abstract). Circulation 1988;78(suppl II):4:292.

Mustard WT. Successful two-stage correction of transposition of the great vessels. Surgery 1964;55:469.

Senning A. Surgical correction of transposition of the great vessels. Surgery 1959;45:966.

Vetter VL, Tanner CS, Horowitz LN. Electrophysiologic consequences of the Mustard repair of d-transposition of the great arteries. J Am Coll Cardiol 1987;10:1265.

Walsh EP, Rockenmacher S, Keane JF, et al. Late results in patients with tetralogy of Fallot repaired during infancy. Circulation 1988;77:1062.

Wernovsky G, Hougen TJ, Walsh EP, et al. Midterm results after the arterial switch operation for transposition of the great arteries with intact ventricular septum: Clinical, hemodynamic, echocardiographic and electrophysiologic data. Circulation 1988;77:1333.

Yacoub MH, Radley-Smith R, MacLaurin R. Two-stage operation for anatomical correction of transposition of the great arteries with intact interventricular septum. Lancet 1977;1:1275.

2

Arterial Switch Operations in Infants and Children with Complex Forms of Transposition of the Great Arteries

Daniel M. Cohen and William G. Williams

When complete transposition of the great arteries (TGA) occurs in association with other major cardiovascular defects, it is termed *complex* transposition (van Praagh et al. 1977). The associated defects are important in determining the natural history of this group of patients as well as in defining the most appropriate surgical approach for repair. The incidence of complex TGA varies depending on the mean age of the patients selected. At the Hospital for Sick Children in Toronto, of the total group of patients undergoing repair for TGA, 42% had complex TGA (Williams et al. 1983). In the Congenital Heart Surgeons Society (CHSS) cooperative study of TGA, of 889 neonates (age 0 to 14 days), 74% had simple TGA; 21%, TGA and ventricular septal defect (VSD); 5%, TGA, VSD, and pulmonic stenosis (PS); and 0.7%, intact ventricular septum and PS. More complex lesions, such as univentricular heart and transposition, were not included (CHSS, 1989).

VENTRICULAR SEPTAL DEFECTS

The combination of TGA and VSD constitutes the largest subset of patients with complex TGA. Five anatomic types of VSD may be encountered: conoventricular (perimembranous), muscular, atrioventricular (AV) canal type (inlet septum), conotruncal (supracristal), and conoseptal malalignment. The importance of understanding these different anatomic types pertains to the surgical approach adopted in repairing these defects. The first three types of VSD may be closed readily through the right atrium; visualization of the latter two types may be difficult with this approach and necessitate a right ventriculotomy or closure through one of the ventriculoarterial valves.

Interest in arterial repair for TGA and VSD was prompted by the operative mortality and late results of atrial repairs in these patients (Arciniegas et al. 1981; Penkoske et al. 1983; Turina et al. 1989). At the Hospital for Sick Children, results with the Mustard procedure in complex transposition demonstrated an operative mortality of 22% with 16% late deaths compared with a 1.2% operative mortality and 3.7% late deaths, respectively, for simple transposition (Trusler and Freedom 1985). Similar results have been observed with the Senning operation (Turina et al. 1988). Nevertheless, the risk of the arterial switch operation for complex transposition has been substantial and less than ideal. In the September 1989 CHSS report, the mortality for neonates undergoing arterial repair and VSD closure, between January 1, 1985, and March 1, 1989, was 21% (that is, 25 deaths in 123 patients) compared with 17% (63 deaths in 370 patients) for isolated TGA (CHSS, 1989).

Because patients with TGA and large VSD have systemic pressure in the left ventricle (LV), there is no need to prepare the LV for arterial switch operation, and there has been a tendency to delay repair. Neither younger nor older age is a risk factor for death; however, efforts to delay surgery may result in severe congestive heart failure and poor growth of the infant. In addition, the risk of early development of pulmonary vascular disease in untreated patients, even as early as 3 months of age, is well established (Viles et al. 1969). Previously, pulmonary artery banding and elective repair at some later date has been practiced; however, this approach may complicate the arterial switch operation because of adhesions or great vessel or valve distortion. The CHSS report has shown a higher mortality for the two-stage repair.

Presently, the surgical approach in neonates with TGA and isolated, large VSD differs little from those with intact ventricular septum. These patients should undergo early cardiac catheterization and balloon atrial septostomy (BAS). Repair is then undertaken within the first month of life, using hypothermic cardiopulmonary bypass or circulatory arrest. Initially, the VSD is closed through the right atrium, and the arterial repair is accomplished using standard techniques. Information from the CHSS cooperative study has shown the following incremental risk factors for death after arterial switch operation for TGA and VSD: staged repair and shorter experience interval of the institution (unpublished data). The operative mortality for arterial repair in patients with TGA and large VSD has been reported to be as low as 0 to 6.7% (Planche et al. 1988; Bove et al. 1988). This, however, has not been the experience of others (Quagebeur et al. 1986). Data from the Hospital for Sick Children have revealed an operative mortality of 21% (unpublished data).

LEFT VENTRICULAR OUTFLOW TRACT OBSTRUCTION

Left ventricular outflow tract obstruction (LVOTO) may be present to some degree in one-third of patients with TGA (Sansa et al. 1979). A precise diagnosis of the severity and type of obstruction as well as the existence of associated lesions such as VSD is imperative to provide optimal surgical management. Axial biplane cineangiography and 2D-echocardiography with color-flow Doppler capability are essential for the accurate assessment of the left ventricular outflow tract.

□ Intact Ventricular Septum

Approximately 20% of older infants with TGA and intact ventricular septum have LVOTO (Chin et al. 1984). The majority of these obstructions are of a "dynamic" nature because of the leftward shift of the muscular ventricular septum as a result of the elevated right ventricular pressures (Shaher et al. 1967a). The muscular septum impinges on the anterior mitral leaflet, and, in combination with a large pulmonary-to-systemic flow ratio, a pressure gradient in the left ventricular outflow tract may be present (Shaher et al. 1967b). Often this dynamic obstruction may become worse following BAS as better interatrial mixing is produced. The dynamic LVOTO is usually relieved by the arterial switch operation performed in the early neonatal period. As the LV assumes its "new" role as a systemic pumping chamber, septal orientation is reversed along with the leftward shift of the muscular septum. Stark and de Leval, however, have reported a few infants in their personal series who have developed LVOTO after successful neonatal switch operation (personal communication). In fact, should LVOTO become severe, a ridge of endocardial thickening may be evident on the septum at its point of contact with the mitral leaflet. We would concur that LVOTO is frequently an acquired lesion. In a review of 115 consecutive neonates with isolated TGA, two had LVOTO at birth, representing 1.7% of the patient population. At the time of preoperative evaluation before the Mustard procedure, however, nine of 104 infants had LVOTO, or 8.7% (Williams et al. 1988).

Less commonly, LVOTO may be due to a discrete fibrous diaphragm below the pulmonary valve cusps or fibrous tissue tags arising from mitral valve apparatus or membranous septum (Chin et al. 1984). Direct resection of subpulmonary fibrous ridges, tissue tags, or diaphragm may be readily accomplished through the pulmonary valve following transection of the main pulmonary artery during the course of an arterial switch procedure.

Isolated pulmonary valvar stenosis is a rare cause of LVOTO in TGA. In the CHSS cooperative study, only 0.7% of neonates had isolated pulmonary valvar stenosis (CHSS, 1989). Usually it can be managed quite easily by a simple valvotomy. However, it may preclude an arterial switch operation, especially if the valve is severely dysplastic or significant incompetence is likely to ensue.

□ Ventricular Septal Defect

LVOTO was encountered in approximately 21% of patients with TGA and VSD enrolled in the CHSS cooperative study (CHSS, 1989). The obstruction is usually more severe and complex than is seen in patients with TGA and intact ventricular septum. Ventricular septal defect occurs as a result of posterior conoseptal malalignment and the LVOTO is subvalvular, most frequently due to a long, subpulmonary fibromuscular tunnel (Sansa et al. 1979). The posterior wall of the tunnel is usually formed by fibrous tissue of the anterior leaflet of the mitral valve, but in a few cases was formed by muscular tissue due to persistence of the subpulmonary conus creating fibrous discontinuity between the anterior leaflet of the mitral valve and the pulmonary valve leaflet. Almost 30% of these patients have additional ventricular septal defects within the trabecular septum that are usually quite small and likely to close spontaneously.

The Rastelli operation was conceived because of the excessively high mortality associated with previous attempts at direct resection of the left ventricular outflow tract, although Idriss et al. have demonstrated that this can be accomplished with reasonable results in selected cases (Idriss et al. 1977). Following the Rastelli operation, the left ventricular outflow is redirected through the VSD and out the aorta beneath an intracardiac baffle. The proximal main pulmonary artery is oversewn and an external valved conduit is used to establish continuity between the right ventricle and the distal pulmonary artery (Rastelli 1969; Rastelli et al. 1969). The advantages of this procedure are several. First, it provides satisfactory relief of the LVOTO, which would be difficult to achieve by direct means for a variety of anatomic reasons. Second, it restores the normal ventriculoarterial connections allowing the LV to function as the systemic pumping chamber. Third, troublesome arrhythmias associated with atrial repair may be avoided.

The disadvantages of the Rastelli operation are several also. First, the long-term fate of the external valved conduit commits the patient to certain reoperation. By performing the operation when the child is between 3 and 5 years of age, an adult-sized conduit can be used, minimizing the risk of outgrowing the prosthesis. Even though cryopreserved homografts are now used and reported to be more durable, all these conduits fail eventually, resulting in stenosis, insufficiency, or both, necessitating replacement at some stage. Second, if the VSD is small and potentially restrictive, it should be enlarged. Usually this can be accomplished without interfering with myocardial function or producing complete heart block. Occasionally, a muscular bar or the tricuspid valve apparatus may be obstructive, rendering the performance of this operation inadvisable. In such circumstances, the surgical options are less ideal, and usually an atrial repair combined with a

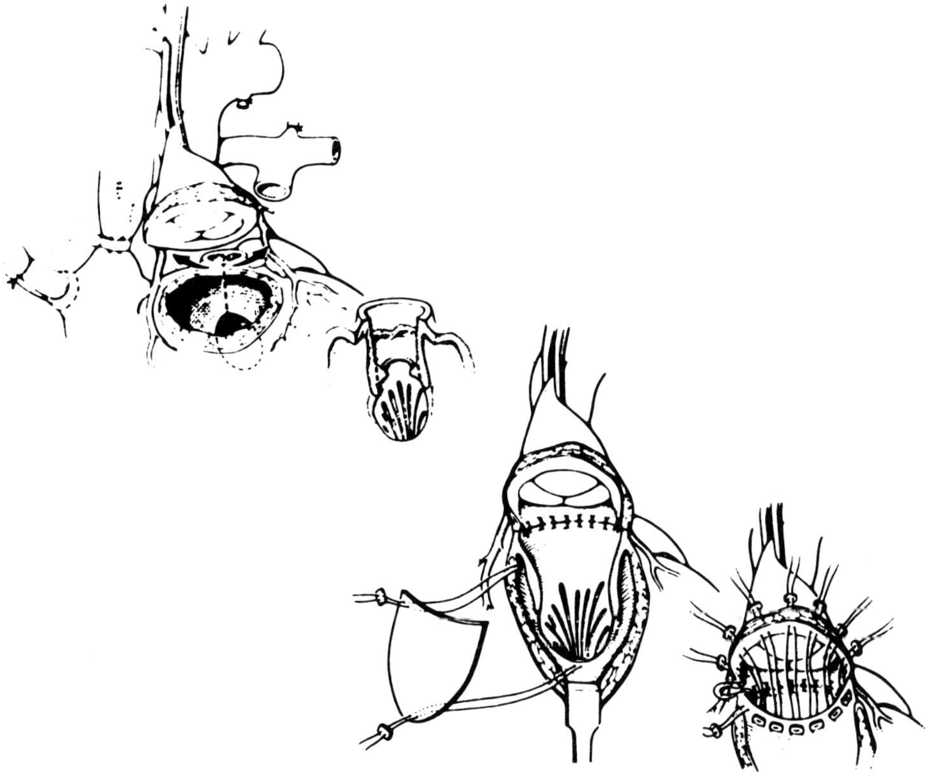

Figure 2.1 Nikaidoh operation. The aortic root is mobilized and the main pulmonary artery transected. The left ventricular outflow tract is opened and subpulmonary stenosis relieved. The aortic root is repositioned and the VSD closed with a patch. (Nikaidoh H. Aortic translocation and biventricular outflow tract reconstruction. A new surgical repair for transposition of the great arteries associated with ventricular septal defect and pulmonary stenosis. J Thorac Cardiovasc Surg 1984;88:365. By permission).

valved conduit from the apex of the LV to the pulmonary artery is the next best alternative (Marceletti et al. 1976; McGoon 1976).

Nikaidoh, prompted by the work of Bex and Konno, has described an elaborate repair for TGA and LVOTO (Konno et al. 1975; Bex et al. 1980; Nikaidoh 1984). This procedure uses aortic root mobilization and transfer, combined with techniques to reconstruct the right and left ventricular outflow tracts. Aortic root, tethered by its attached coronary arteries, is completely mobilized. The main pulmonary artery is transected above the valve commissures. Next, the LVOTO is opened anteriorly by making an incision in the annulus and carrying it through the infundibular septum into the VSD. the subpulmonic obstruction is then re-

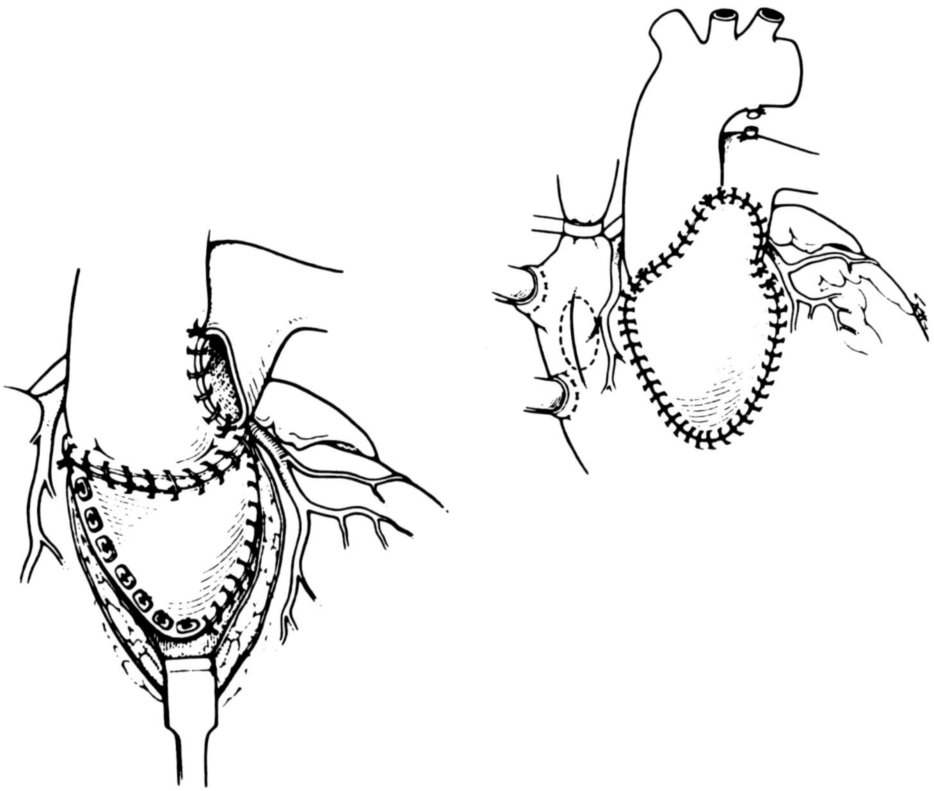

Figure 2.2 Nikaidoh operation. Distal segment of the main pulmonary artery is transfixed to the aorta, and the right ventricular outflow tract is reconstructed with a pericardial gusset. (Nikaidoh H. Aortic translocation and biventricular outflow tract reconstruction. A new surgical repair for transposition of the great arteries associated with ventricular septal defect and pulmonary stenosis. J Thorac Cardiovasc Surg 1984;88:365. By permission).

sected, and the aortic root is moved posteriorly, partially suturing it to the left ventricular outflow tract before closing the VSD. The left ventricular outflow repair is then completed by suturing the remainder of the aortic root to the ventricle, and the right ventricular outflow tract is reconstructed with a pericardial gusset (Figures 2.1 and 2.2). This technique, which has been used in only two cases, provides an anatomic repair preserving the LV as the systemic pumping chamber. To determine the durability of this procedure, long-term follow-up is necessary.

The current operative mortality with the Rastelli operation is less than 10% with excellent long-term survival, in spite of the late complications with valve conduits (Marcelletti et al. 1976). Presently, it remains the procedure of choice for TGA, VSD, and LVOTO.

RIGHT VENTRICULAR OUTFLOW TRACT OBSTRUCTION

In contrast to LVOTO, right ventricular outflow tract obstruction (RVOTO) is encountered much less frequently in patients with TGA. In an extensive pathologic study, RVOTO has been identified in 27% of specimens associated with a VSD and in only 3% with intact ventricular septum (Moene et al. 1983). In clinical practice, significant RVOTO is present in less than 10% of patients with TGA (Schneeweiss et al. 1981).

The pathogenesis of RVOTO appears to be secondary to anterior conoseptal malalignment, resulting in a reduction of the distance between the subaortic conus and the anterior, free, right ventricular wall. This narrowing is exacerbated by systemic pressure in the right ventricle (RV), which promotes hypertrophy of the muscle and progression of the obstruction. Although the VSD is usually of the malalignment type, perimembranous extension or additional trabecular defects may also be seen.

RVOTO results in subaortic stenosis. Valvular aortic stenosis is quite usual, but obstructive anomalies of the aortic arch, including severe coarctation of the aorta or interruption, are not an infrequent concomitant finding (Vogel et al. 1984). Occasionally, tricuspid insufficiency and hemodynamic deterioration may be observed as a consequence of the elevated right ventricular pressure (Huhta et al. 1982).

An atrial repair will not relieve the increased hemodynamic burden on an already overloaded RV, and anatomic correction at the arterial level is the treatment of choice. When subaortic stenosis is not severe, normalization of right ventricular pressure following an arterial switch operation may prevent progression of right ventricular hypertrophy, and surgical relief of the infundibular narrowing is not required. In contrast, with severe RVOTO, an arterial switch operation may have to be combined with infundibular resection, and generally resection of the RVOTO in TGA is readily accomplished.

In certain circumstances, in which infundibular resection is deemed unsuitable or coronary artery anatomy is unfavorable for an arterial switch, a Damus-Kaye-Stansel procedure provides a surgical option (Damus 1975; Stansel 1975; Kaye 1975; Alvarez et al. 1975; Damus et al. 1982). This operation has the advantage of restoring ventriculoarterial concordance without the need for coronary artery relocation but has the disadvantage of requiring the use of an external conduit between the RV and the pulmonary artery. In this procedure, the aorta is left in continuity with the RV, and the proximal pulmonary artery is anastomosed to the side of the ascending aorta. Because the aortic pressure remains higher than the right ventricular pressure throughout the cardiac cycle, the aortic valve remains closed. A vertical right ventriculotomy is made, and the VSD is closed through it with a prosthetic patch. A homograft valved conduit is then anastomosed to the

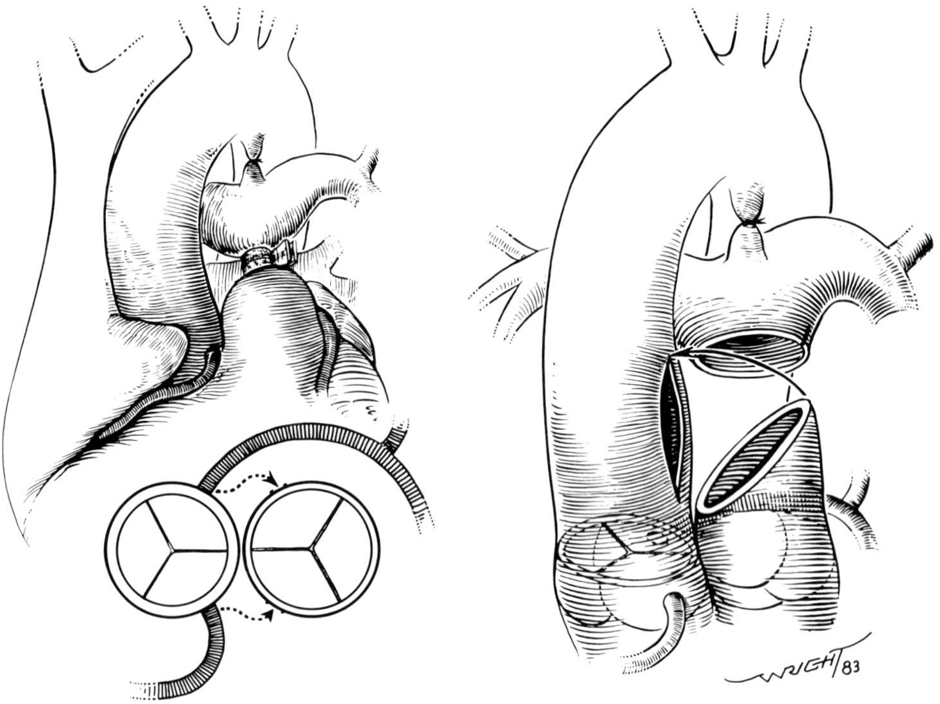

Figure 2.3 Damus-Kaye-Stansel operation. Main pulmonary artery is debanded and transected before performing an end-to-side anastomosis between the proximal main pulmonary artery and aorta.

distal pulmonary artery segment and the edges of the right ventriculotomy (Figures 2.3 and 2.4). The overall operative mortality for this procedure is quite high and has been reported to be 58% (Ceithaml et al. 1984). Causes of death have included low cardiac output, pulmonary vascular obstructive disease, technical problems, ventricular arrhythmias, and hemorrhage. Three risk factors have been identified: age less than 18 months, weight less than 10 kilograms, and an unprepared LV. Preoperative preparation of the LV, on a natural basis because of the large VSD or the result of pulmonary artery banding, has been associated with a lower operative mortality. Late results have demonstrated selective instances of right ventricular failure and problems relating to conduit stenosis or incompetence.

COARCTATION OF THE AORTA

Coarctation of the aorta in TGA may exist as a discrete lesion or may be due to distal arch hypoplasia, reflecting RVOTO, which would favor pulmonary blood

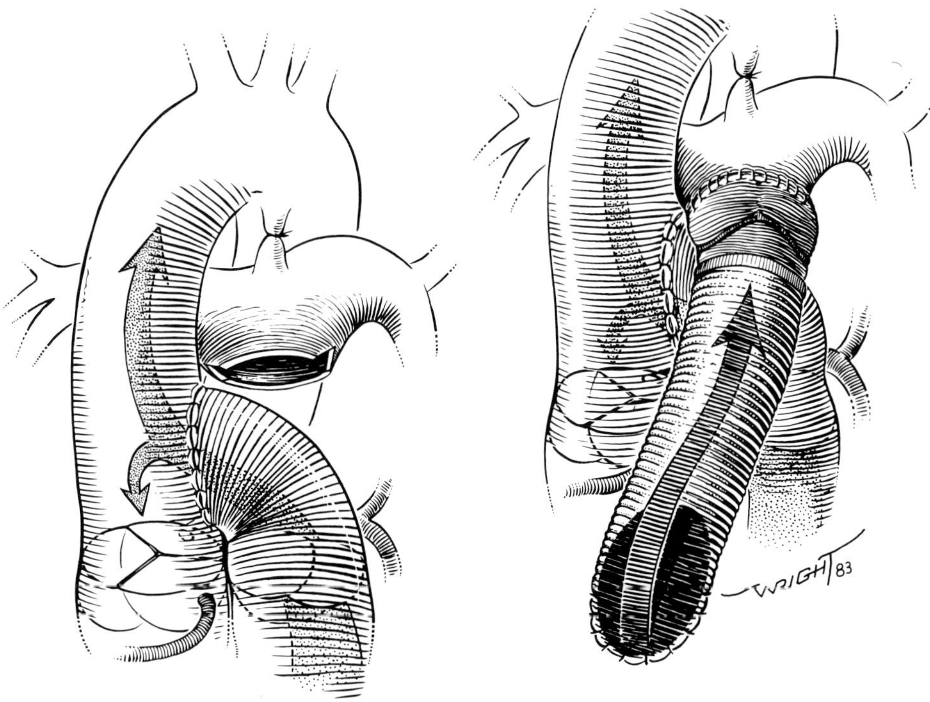

Figure 2.4 Damus-Kaye-Stansel operation. Aortopulmonary anastomosis is completed, and a valved conduit is led from the right ventricle to the distal main pulmonary artery.

flow at the expense of aortic blood flow. Data from the Hospital for Sick Children has indicated that 5% of patients with TGA have an associated coarctation of the aorta (Vogel et al. 1984). VSD is present in 72% of patients and is a result of anterior conoseptal malalignment in approximately one-half of the group. Hypoplasia of the sinus portion of the right ventricle and tricuspid annulus has also been observed (Riemenschneider et al. 1968).

The presence of an obstructive anomaly of the aortic arch has influenced survival adversely in the past. Vogel and associates found the probability of survival in this group of patients beyond the neonatal period to be 68% and the 5-year survival following Mustard operation to be only 57% (Vogel et al. 1984). By comparison, the probability of survival in patients with uncomplicated TGA is 98% beyond the neonatal period and 89% 5 years following the Mustard operation (Trusler et al. 1980). Early recognition of the problem, aided by the routine use of prostaglandins and improved surgical experience, should lead to better short-term and long-term survival in the future.

A discrete coarctation of the aorta in TGA may be corrected by a staged procedure in the newborn period, that is, subclavian flap angioplasty for the coarctation followed by an arterial switch operation within a short time frame (24 to 48 hours) or patch angioplasty and arterial switch through a median sternotomy as a simultaneous procedure. If the arch is hypoplastic, we favor the latter approach; otherwise, we would opt for the two-stage repair.

How hypoplasia of the aortic arch in association with subaortic stenosis and VSD is managed depends on a number of factors, especially the degree of subaortic obstruction in hypoplasia of the RV. Should the subaortic obstruction be mild and the RV of normal size, arterial switch operation with resection of infundibular obstruction and closure of the VSD can be carried out with the expectation of a satisfactory short-term and long-term result. Patients with marked subaortic obstruction associated with a VSD and hypoplastic RV may need to undergo pulmonary artery banding and a Blalock-Hanlon septectomy as an initial palliative procedure. This may be followed by a Damus-Kaye-Stansel operation or an arterial switch combined with a Fontan operation. We would emphasize that surgical palliation by means of pulmonary artery banding carries the risk of potentiating subaortic obstruction and consideration should be given to performing a "palliative" switch or Norwood stage I palliation in selected circumstances. This may be followed by complete repair or a modified Fontan operation later.

TRICUSPID VALVE ANOMALIES

Tricuspid valve anomalies are rarely found in TGA with intact ventricular septum but may be encountered in one-third of patients with TGA and VSD, although only 14% have surgical significance (Huhta et al. 1982). The abnormalities include abnormal chordal insertions, tricuspid valve straddling, prolapse of tricuspid valve tissue through the VSD with LVOTO, dysplasia, and hypoplasia of the tricuspid annulus.

Abnormal chordal insertions of single or multiple tricuspid valve chordae, about the circumference of the VSD, are the most frequent abnormalities seen in TGA and VSD. In about one-third of cases, these may be of surgical significance in that they interfere with the utilization of the VSD in a Rastelli procedure. Straddling of tricuspid valve with chordal attachments to the LV may prevent closure of the VSD and preclude a biventricular repair (Gale et al. 1979). Dysplasia of the valve is manifested by redundant tissue with valvular insufficiency, necessitating an annuloplasty or valve replacement. Prolapse of accessory valve tissue through the VSD may produce a windsock deformity with LVOTO. Relief may be obtained by simply closing the VSD and plicating the redundant valve tissue in the suture line. Hypoplasia of the tricuspid valve annulus is seen in combination with right ventricular hypoplasia and may be associated with severe subaortic stenosis (deVivie et al. 1989). This combination may mitigate against biventricular repair, and a modified Fontan procedure with proximal pulmonary artery to ascending aortic anastomosis may be necessary. Arterial repair may be possible if tricuspid valve diameter is within 2 standard deviations of normal.

RIGHT VENTRICULAR HYPOPLASIA

Hypoplasia of the RV has been noted in 17% of postmortem specimens associated with TGA (Riemenschneider et al. 1968). It occurs in combination with severe RVOTO and tricuspid valve hypoplasia. It is also associated with juxtaposition of the left atrial appendage (Wood et al. 1983). Modified Fontan operation is the corrective procedure of choice for severe hypoplasia of the RV.

MITRAL VALVE ANOMALIES

Mitral valve anomalies are present in approximately 20% of patients with TGA, mainly in association with a VSD (Layman and Edwards 1967; Moene and Oppenheimer-Dekker 1982). Four categories of anomalies may be recognized: (1) clefts in the anterior leaflet of the mitral valve, partial or complete, which can be associated with outflow tract obstruction; (2) mitral valve hypoplasia and clockwise rotation of the valve ring; (3) redundant tissue tags; and (4) deficient papillary muscles and chordae, including parachute mitral valve.

These anatomic variations may produce functional disturbances, and clinical recognition of mitral valve dysfunction is important when considering surgical options. First, BAS might fail to produce adequate mixing at the atrial level because obstruction to the left ventricular inflow produces a predominantly left to right shunt rather than bidirectional shunting. Second, the arterial switch procedure places a greater demand on the integrity of the mitral valve apparatus compared with atrial repair because the LV is now systemic and normal mitral valve function is of paramount importance if these patients are to survive this operation. Therefore, the presence of a significant mitral valve anomaly is a contraindication to the arterial switch operation.

UNIVENTRICULAR HEART

Subaortic obstruction may develop de novo or following pulmonary artery banding in certain univentricular heart complexes. This results in myocardial hypertrophy

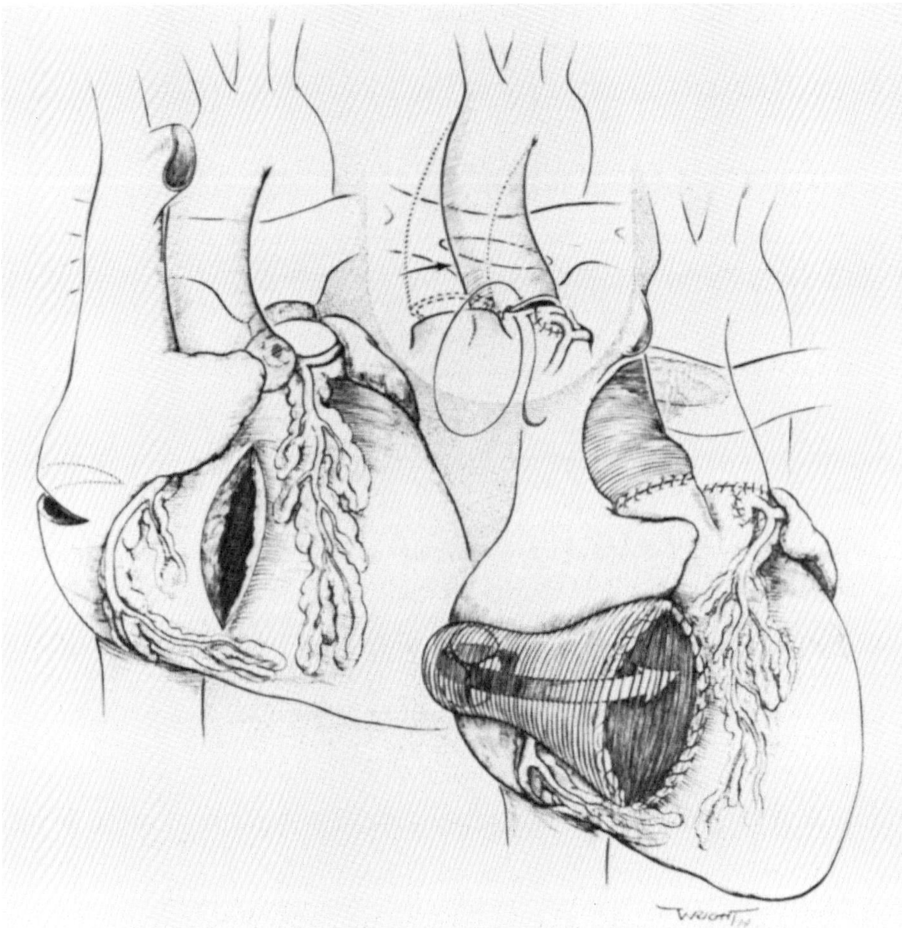

Figure 2.5 Fontan-arterial switch operation. Main pulmonary artery and aorta are transected. The coronary arteries are removed as buttons and reattached to the neo-aorta. The proximal main pulmonary artery is anastomosed to the distal pulmonary artery and a right atrial–right ventricular conduit is established. (Freedom R, et al. Tricuspid atresia, transposition of the great arteries, and banded pulmonary artery repair by arterial switch, coronary artery reimplantation, and right atrioventricular valved conduit. J Thorac Cardiovasc Surg 1980;80:621. By permission).

and ultimately leads to a stiffer, noncompliant, and ischemic ventricle with impaired diastolic function (Fifer et al. 1985). This bodes poorly for the successful performance of a Fontan operation later, leaving cardiac transplantation as the only therapeutic option.

Tricuspid atresia with VSD and TGA and single ventricle of the left ventricular type with a rudimentary RV and transposition are prime examples of this problem

(Freedom et al. 1977a). Previously, pulmonary artery banding has been employed to provide temporary relief of symptoms in these patients by limiting the torrential pulmonary blood flow. Frequently, these patients have small or potentially restrictive VSDs. The presence of a pulmonary artery band, by promoting myocardial hypertrophy, may accelerate the predilection for diminution or spontaneous closure of these defects, causing subaortic stenosis (Freedom et al. 1977b). Those patients at risk must be identified by selective angiography and 2D-echocardiography, and surgical alternatives must be provided in these instances.

A variety of surgical approaches have been used to treat subaortic obstruction in this group of patients, including LV to descending aortic conduit, enlargement of the VSD, or creation of an anterior-posterior window. The results have been disastrous frequently, and more recently efforts have concentrated on anastomosing the proximal main pulmonary trunk to the aortic root, creating a controlled, central systemic to pulmonary artery shunt (Norwood type approach) to palliate these patients, with plans to perform a modified Fontan operation later (Rothman et al. 1987).

Pulmonary artery banding may still have a place in the presence of a large, nonrestrictive VSD. Close scrutiny is necessary to avoid complications and provide appropriate surgical relief of subaortic obstruction should it occur before or at the time of the Fontan operation. These measures have included enlargement of the VSD, Damus-Kay-Stansel approach, or a Norwood operation. The combination of arterial switch with reimplantation of the coronaries and a Fontan procedure has been used successfully at the Hospital for Sick Children in three patients with tricuspid atresia and transposition who had previously undergone pulmonary artery banding (Freedom et al., 1977b) (Figure 2.5). This approach circumvents the potential problems of the VSD becoming restrictive and leading to impairment of ventricular function while making use of the small RV and normal pulmonary valve in the pulmonary circulation.

TAUSSIG-BING MALFORMATION

In 1949, Taussig and Bing described a complex congenital heart malformation in which the aorta arose entirely from the RV posterior to the pulmonary artery, which also exited from the RV and overrode a VSD (Taussig and Bing 1949). Because of the controversy that ensued, van Praagh analyzed the original specimen and defined this complex congenital heart malformation as consisting of four distinctive features: double outlet RV, side-by-side semilunar valves, bilateral conus without pulmonary-mitral continuity, and a large subpulmonary VSD (van Praagh, 1968). Over the years, numerous different surgical approaches to this lesion have been employed. The intraventricular repair for double outlet RV, described by Patrick and McGoon, whereby a patch is placed so as to direct left ventricular blood through the VSD beneath the patch and out of the aorta, has a definite place in the repair of certain cases of double-outlet RV or transposition, VSD, and pulmonary override (Patrick and McGoon, 1968) (Figure 2.6). Because of the side-by-side alignment of semilunar valves, the area between the tricuspid valve and the pulmonary annulus is the narrowest point of the LV to aortic tunnel, and such a patch would encroach on a right ventricular outflow tract if subaortic obstruction were to be avoided. Most acceptable methods of repair have been one of two approaches. First, the VSD is closed in such a way that left ventricular blood is baffled into the pulmonary artery, and this is combined with a Mustard or Senning operation (Hightower et al. 1969). Second, the pulmonary artery is closed after the left ventricular blood is baffled through the VSD out of the aorta, and an external valved conduit is placed between the RV and distal pulmonary artery (McGoon et al. 1973).

The operative mortality associated with these procedures, in the setting of Taussig-Bing malformation, has been as high as 32% (Stewart et al. 1979). Also, the long-term complications associated with atrial-type repairs has forced alternative approaches to be investigated (Harvey et al. 1977). In the absence of pulmonary stenosis, the Damus-Kaye-Stansel procedure may be considered (Damus et al. 1982). The long-term prognosis is dependent on the behavior of the external valved conduit, and reoperation with replacement is inevitable because of degeneration of the conduit. This is a significant drawback (Ceithaml et al. 1984).

Kawashima has devised an intraventricular repair that involves the resection of infundibular septum adjacent to the aorta and tunneling of the VSD such that blood from the LV passes beneath the patch out of the aorta, maintaining the LV as a systemic pumping chamber (Kawashima et al. 1971). It is a *posterior layout*, and blood from the RV passes over the patch out of the pulmonary artery (Figure 2.7). Although this procedure has its merits in that an external conduit is avoided, it also has limitations. Attachments of the tricuspid valve or its tension apparatus to the infundibular septum prevents its resection without causing significant tricuspid insufficiency. This repair necessitates a right ventriculotomy, and anomalous origin of the left anterior descending artery from the right coronary artery precludes its use. Again, the narrowest point between the left ventricular aortic tunnel is the distance between the tricuspid valve and the pulmonary annulus, and the patch may obstruct the right ventricular outflow tract.

The arterial switch operation with reimplantation of the coronary arteries has been applied successfully to the Taussig-Bing malformation, whether the great arteries are side-by-side or the aorta lies anterior to the pulmonary artery (Kanter et al. 1985). Should the great arteries lie side-by-side, the *Lecompte maneuver* may not be required. The aorta is transected as far distally as possible, and the pulmonary trunk is transected near the valve commissures. Continuity is established by direct suture of the pulmonary artery behind the aorta, avoiding the use of an interposed graft. Both coronary arteries are excised separately as buttons and are transferred to the neo-aorta. The defects are repaired with pericardial patches to avoid valve distortion.

The successful outcome of the switch operation is dependent on strict attention

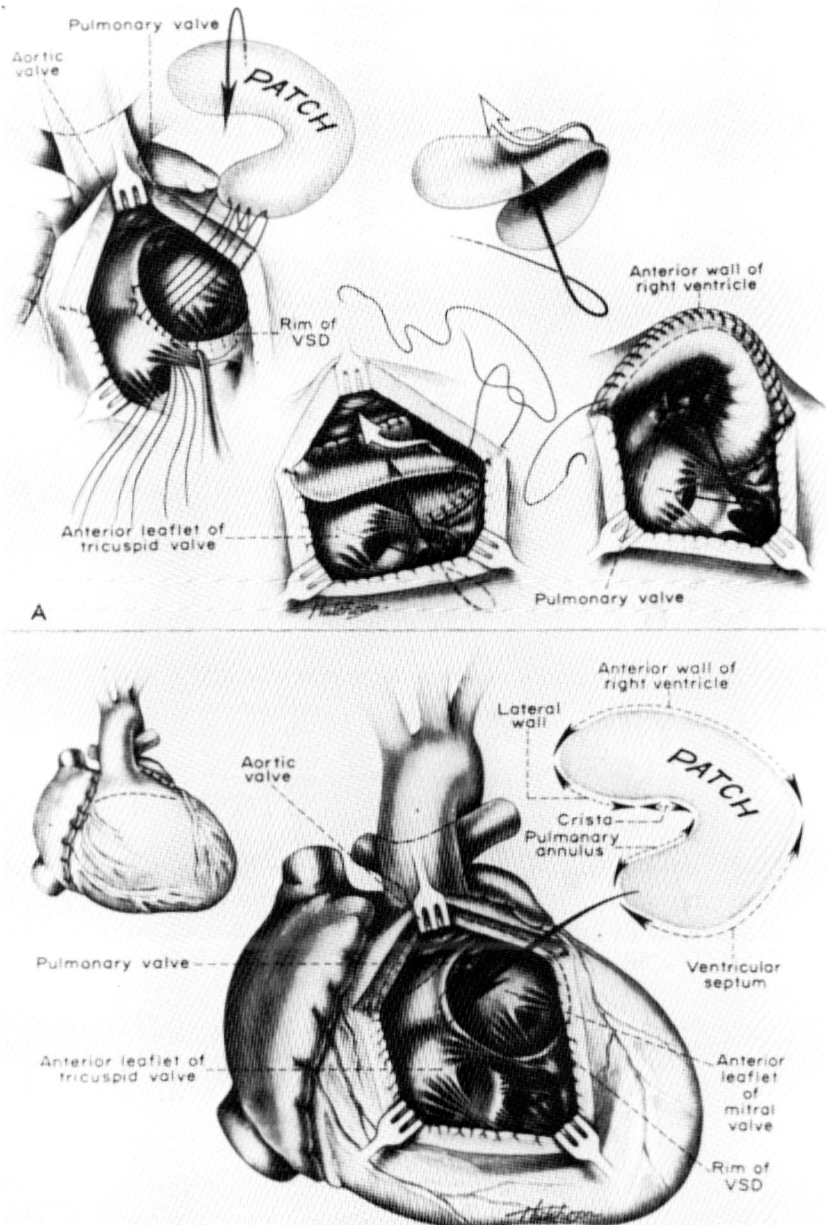

Figure 2.6 Intraventricular repair of TGA. Patch is sutured to the margins of the VSD, redirecting left ventricular blood through the VSD beneath the patch and out of the aorta. (McGoon D. J Thorac Cardiovasc Surg 1972;64:430. By permission).

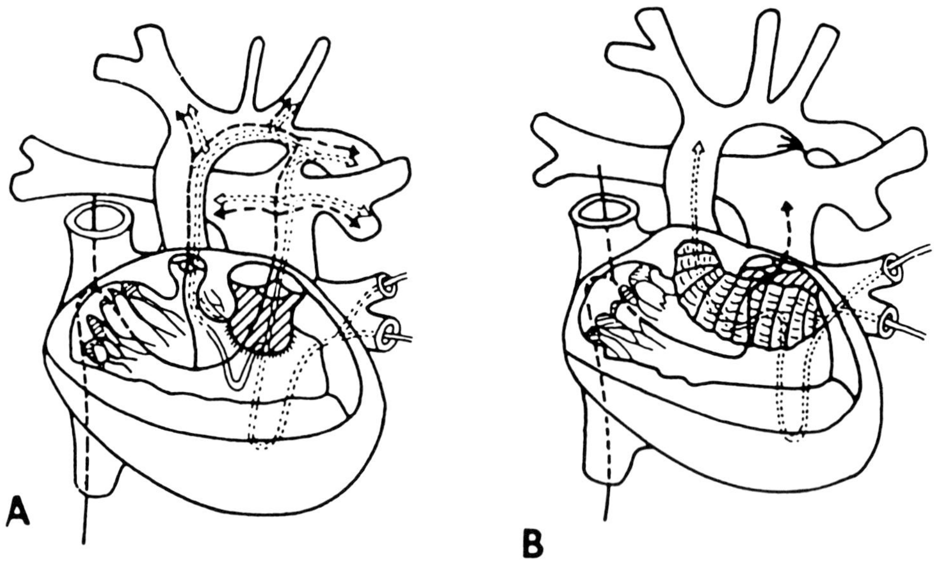

Figure 2.7 Kawashima operation. (A) Taussig-Bing malformation. (B) Resection of infundibular septum and attachment of patch to the margins of VSD, redirecting left ventricular blood through the VSD beneath the patch and out of the aorta. (Kawashima Y, et al. Intraventricular rerouting of blood for the correction of Taussig-Bing malformation. J Thorac Cardiovasc Surg 1971;62:825. By permission).

to the morphology and size of the mitral valve and LV, coronary artery anatomy, and the possible presence of subaortic obstruction. Mitral dysplasia or hypoplasia of the mitral valve and LV would contraindicate use of the arterial switch operation. Furthermore, a single coronary ostium may not make the arterial transfer feasible. At the completion of the repair, right ventricular and pulmonary artery pressures should be measured directly to determine the presence of any significant gradient that may require an infundibular resection or a right ventricular outflow tract patch.

Presently, one should aim to correct the Taussig-Bing anomaly primarily; however, this may not be possible in a critically ill infant. Surgical palliation by banding the pulmonary artery to protect against the development of pulmonary vascular disease may be combined with a Blalock-Hanlon septectomy to improve mixing. Complete repair is then carried out at 6 to 12 months of age, at which time the pulmonary artery band is removed and the arterial switch operation performed.

RIGHT VENTRICULAR DYSFUNCTION

Right ventricular dysfunction allowing atrial repair is encountered in up to 10% of patients within 10 years of operation (Trusler et al. 1980; Jurina et al. 1988; Williams et al. 1988). It appears to be more common in patients with TGA in whom a VSD has been closed. The clinical course is slowly progressive with increasing tricuspid insufficiency ultimately leading to right ventricular failure. Previously, the only treatment option available to these patients was orthotopic heart transplantation.

Mee has devised a two-stage operation whereby the LV is prepared initially by pulmonary artery banding (Mee 1986). This is followed, after an appropriate interval, by takedown of the atrial repair, pulmonary artery debanding, and an arterial switch operation. The appropriate timing of this operation remains a difficult judgment call. It appears that when right ventricular dysfunction has become so advanced that these patients are quite symptomatic and dependent on pharmacologic support, surgical intervention is warranted.

Current recommendations regarding how tight the band should be suggest that left ventricular pressure should attain levels of approximately 60% to 70% systemic arterial pressure once the band has been applied. These patients are maintained on inotropic support for several days postoperatively. During the ensuing weeks or months, they either "grow into their bands" or develop concentric left ventricular hypertrophy with rising pressures. The decision when to proceed to arterial switch operation is not clear-cut. Most of these patients have been restudied between 3 to 6 months postoperatively. At the time of cardiac catheterization, the left ventricular pressure should be systemic; however, there is no definite recommendation as to what LV-to-RV pressure ratio is safe or unsafe to allow the atrial switch operation to be performed. Indeed, it may be detrimental in that the incidence of aortic regurgitation (in anatomic pulmonary valve) was found to be consistently higher in Yacoub's two-stage repair because of dilatation of the pulmonary root in response to the pulmonary artery band (Yacoub et al. 1977).

Also, adhesions following pulmonary artery banding may add to the difficulty of an arterial switch by obscuring the coronary artery anatomy and distorting the pulmonary arteries so that a primary anastomosis without a patch may be difficult to perform. Jonas and associates have shown in young infants that the LV can be prepared in approximately 1 week after pulmonary banding (Jonas et al. 1989). It was demonstrated that a LV-to-RV pressure ratio of greater than 1 at cardiac catheterization, following banding, had occurred within this small time frame. In addition, the adhesions were less, and fibrinous and valve distortion was avoided. Whether this rapid two-stage arterial switch procedure can be applied to this older group of patients with right ventricular dysfunction remains to be seen. Echocardiographic studies of athletes in training have suggested that the mature, human myocardium also responds within days to an increase in workload (Ehsani et al.

1978). Perhaps echocardiographic evidence of increasing left ventricular wall thickness may be an appropriate parameter to follow.

The two-stage arterial switch procedure for right ventricular dysfunction has been performed in a small, select group of patients with initial, short-term success. With time, this procedure may need to be invoked more frequently as the cohort of patients who have undergone atrial repair developing right ventricular dysfunction increases.

PULMONARY VASCULAR DISEASE

Pulmonary vascular disease develops in a variety of different congenital heart defects. Its onset, however, is evident at an earlier age and is more rapidly progressive in patients with TGA, especially in the presence of an associated large VSD or patent ductus arteriosus (Ferguson et al. 1960; Ferencz 1966; Viles et al. 1969). Furthermore, even patients with TGA and intact ventricular septum have exhibited premature advanced pulmonary vascular disease.

Hemodynamic studies have demonstrated that almost all patients with TGA and VSD over 1 year of age have elevated pulmonary vascular resistance, the presence of which may be considered a contraindication to complete corrective surgery (Mair et al. 1971). These hemodynamic findings correlate well with histologic findings of advanced pulmonary vascular changes (Heath-Edwards grades 3, 4, or 5) in which the operative risk of corrective surgery is markedly increased, with death from right ventricular failure occurring in the postoperative period (Heath and Edwards 1958; Newfeld et al. 1974). Therefore, should corrective surgery be contemplated in children beyond 6 to 9 months of age, repeated cardiac catheterization is mandatory to rule out significantly elevated pulmonary vascular resistance (Lakier et al. 1975).

The prognosis of patients with TGA, VSD, and pulmonary vascular disease has been improved by the "palliative Mustard" operation, conceived by Lindesmith and colleagues, in which an atrial baffle is inserted but the VSD is left open (Lindesmith et al. 1972). This has produced increases in systemic oxygenation with an improvement in exercise tolerance and in the general condition of the patient. The long-term prognosis of these patients is dependent on the progression of the pulmonary vascular disease. Stark and associates have carried this procedure one step further by creating a VSD at the ventricular apex in patients with TGA and intact ventricular septum with pulmonary vascular disease. The oxygen saturations and an amelioration of symptoms have been observed in two reported cases (Stark et al. 1976).

A palliative arterial switch operation is likely to produce similar results to the palliative Mustard operation, but there is no obvious advantage to this approach.

REFERENCES

Alvarez F, Murtado E, DeLeon JP, et al. Tecnica de correcion anatomica de la transposicion completa de grandes vasos. Rev Esp Cardiol 1975; 28:255.

Arciniegas E, Farooki ZQ, Hakimi M, Perry BL, Green EW. Results of the Mustard operation for dextro-transposition of the great arteries. J Thorac Cardiovasc Surg 1981; 81:580.

Bex JP, Lecompte Y, Baillot F, Hazan E. Anatomical correction of transposition of the great arteries. Ann Thorac Surg 1980; 29:86.

Bove EL, Beckman RH, Snider AR, et al. Arterial repair for transposition of the great arteries and large ventricular septal defect in early infancy. Circulation 1988; 78(suppl III):26.

Ceithaml EL, Puga FJ, Danielson GK, McGoon DC, Ritter DG. Results of the Damus-Stansel-Kaye procedure for transposition of the great arteries and for double-outlet right ventricle with subpulmonary ventricular septal defect. Ann Thorac Surg 1984; 38:433.

Chin I, Anderson RH, Macartney FJ, DeLeval MR, Stark J. Morphologic features of an intact ventricular septum susceptible to subpulmonary obstruction in complete transposition. Am J Cardiol 1984; 53:1633.

Damus P. Letter to the editor. Ann Thorac Surg 1975; 20:724.

Damus P, Thomson WB, McLoughlin TG. Arterial repair without coronary relocation for complete transposition of the great vessels with ventricular septal defect. J Thorac Cardiovasc Surg 1982; 83:316.

deVivie R, van Praagh S, Bein G, et al. Transposition of the great arteries with straddling tricuspid valve. Report of two rare cases with acquired subaortic stenosis after main pulmonary artery banding. J Thorac Cardiovasc Surg 1989; 98:205.

Ehsani AA, Hagberg JM, Mickson RC. Rapid changes in left ventricular dimensions and mass in response to physical conditioning and deconditioning. Am J Cardiol 1978; 42:52.

Ferencz C. Transposition of the great vessels; pathophysiologic consideration based upon a study of the lungs. Circulation 1966; 33:232.

Ferguson DJ, Adams P, Watson D. Pulmonary arteriosclerosis in transposition of the great arteries. Am J Dis Child 1960; 99:653.

Fifer MA, Boron KM, Colan SD, Lorrell BH. Early diastolic left ventricular function in children and adults with aortic stenosis. J Am Coll Cardiol 1985; 5:1147.

Freedom RM, Dische MR, Rowe RD. Pathologic anatomy of subaortic stenosis and atresia in the first year of life. Am J Cardiol 1977a; 39:1035.

Freedom RM, Sondheimer H, Dische R, Rowe RD. Development of subaortic stenosis after pulmonary arterial banding for common ventricle. Am J Cardiol 1977b; 39:78.

Freedom RM, Williams WG, Fowler RS, Trusler GA, Rowe RD. Tricuspid atresia, transposition of the great arteries, and banded pulmonary artery repair by arterial switch, coronary artery reimplantation, and right atrioventricular valved conduit. J Thorac Cardiovasc Surg 1980; 80:621.

Gale AW, Danielson GK, McGoon DC, Mair DD. Modified Fontan operation for univentricular heart and complicated congenital lesions. J Thorac Cardiovasc Surg 1979; 78:831.

Harvey JC, Sondheimer HM, Williams WG, Olley PM, Trusler GA. Repair of double-outlet right ventricle. J Thorac Cardiovasc Surg 1977; 73:611.

Heath D, Edwards JE. The pathology of hypertensive pulmonary vascular disease: A description of six grades of structural changes in pulmonary arteries with special reference to congenital cardiac septal defects. Circulation 1958; 18:533.

Hightower BM, Barcia A, Bargeron LM Jr, Kirklin JW. Double-outlet right ventricle with transposed great arteries and subpulmonary ventricular septal defect. The Taussig-Bing malformation. Circulation 1969; 50(suppl I):207.

Huhta JC, Edwards WD, Danielson GK, Feldt RH. Abnormalities of the tricuspid valve in complete transposition of the great arteries with ventricular septal defect. J Thorac Cardiovasc Surg 1982; 83:569.

Idriss FS, DeLeon SY, Nikaidoh H, et al. Resection of the left ventricular outflow obstruction in d-transposition of the great arteries. J Thorac Cardiovasc Surg 1977; 74:343.

Jonas RA, Giglia TM, Sanders SP, et al. Rapid two-stage arterial switch for transposition of the great arteries and intact ventricular septum beyond the neonatal period. Circulation 1989; 80(suppl I):203.

Kanter KR, Anderson RH, Lincoln C, Rigby ML, Shinebourne EA. Anatomic correction for complete transposition and double-outlet right ventricle. J Thorac Cardiovasc Surg 1985; 90:690.

Kawashima Y, Fujita T, Miyamoto T, Manabe H. Intraventricular rerouting of blood for the correction of Taussig-Bing malformation. J Thorac Cardiovasc Surg 1971; 62:825.

Kaye MP. Anatomic correction of transposition of the great vessels. Mayo Clin Proc 1975; 50:638.

Konno S, Imai Y, Iida Y, Nakajima M, Tatsuno K. A new method of prosthetic valve replacement in congenital aortic stenosis associated with hypoplasia of the aortic valve ring. J Thorac Cardiovasc Surg 1975; 70:909.

Lakier JB, Stanger P, Heymann MA, Hoffman JIE, Rudolph AM. Early onset of pulmonary vascular obstruction in patients with aortopulmonary transposition and intact ventricular septum. Circulation 1975; 51:875.

Layman TE, Edwards JE. Anomalies of the cardiac valves associated with complete transposition of the great vessels. Am J Cardiol 1967; 19:247.

Lindesmith GG, Stiles QR, Tucker BL, et al. The Mustard operation as a palliative procedure. J Thorac Cardiovasc Surg 1972; 63:75.

Mair DD, Ritter DG, Ongley PA, Helmholz HF. Hemodynamics and evaluation for surgery of patients with complete transposition of the great arteries and ventricular septal defect. Am J Cardiol 1971; 28:632.

Marcelletti C, Mair DD, McGoon DC, Wallace RB, Danielson GK. The Rastelli operation for transposition of the great arteries. Early and late results. J Thorac Cardiovasc Surg 1976; 72:427.

McGoon DC. Left ventricular and biventricular extracardiac conduits. J Thorac Cardiovasc Surg 1976; 72:7.

McGoon DC, Wallace RB, Danielson GK. The Rastelli operation: Its indications and results. J Thorac Cardiovasc Surg 1973; 65:65

Mee RBB. Severe right ventricular failure after Mustard or Senning operation. Two-stage repair: Pulmonary artery banding and switch. J Thorac Cardiovasc Surg 1986; 92:385.

Moene RJ, Oppenheimer-Dekker A. Congenital mitral valve anomalies in transposition of the great arteries. Am J Cardiol 1982; 49:1972.

Moene RJ, Oppenheimer-Dekker A, Bartelings MM. Anatomic obstruction of the right ventricular outflow tract in transposition of the great arteries. Am J Cardiol 1983; 51:1701.

Newfeld EA, Paul MH, Muster AJ, Idriss FS. Pulmonary vascular disease in complete transposition of the great arteries: A study of 200 patients. Am J Cardiol 1974;34:75.

Nikaidoh H. Aortic translocation and biventricular outflow tract reconstruction. A new surgical repair for transposition of the great arteries associated with ventricular septal defect and pulmonary stenosis. J Thorac Cardiovasc Surg 1984; 88:365.

Patrick DL, McGoon DC. An operation for double outlet right ventricle with transposition of the great arteries. J Cardiovasc Surg 1968; 9:537.

Penkoske PA, Westerman GR, Marx GR, et al. Transposition of the great arteries and ventricular septal defect. Results with the Senning operation and closure of the ventricular septal defect in infants. Ann Thorac Surg 1983; 36:281.

Planche C, Bruniaux J, Lacour-Gayet F, et al. Switch operation for transposition of the great arteries in neonates. A study of 120 patients. J Thorac Cardiovasc Surg 1988; 96:354.

Quagebeur JM, Rohmer J, Ottenkamp J, et al. The arterial switch operation. An eight year experience. J Thorac Cardiovasc Surg 1986; 92:361.

Rastelli GC. A new approach to "anatomic" repair of transposition of the great arteries. Mayo Clin Proc 1969; 44:1.

Rastelli GC, Wallace RB, Ongley PA. Complete repair of transposition of the great arteries with pulmonary stenosis. A review and report of a case corrected by using a new surgical technique. Circulation 1969; 39:83.

Riemenschneider TA, Vincent WR, Ruttenburg HD, Desilets DT. Transposition of the great vessels with hypoplasia of the right ventricle. Circulation 1968; 38:386.

Rothman A, Lang P, Lock JE, et al. Surgical management of subaortic obstruction in single left ventricle and tricuspid atresia. J Am Coll Cardiol 1987; 10:421.

Sansa M, Tonkin IL, Bargeron LM Jr, Elliot LP. Left ventricular outflow tract obstruction in transposition of the great arteries. An angiographic study of 74 cases. Am J Cardiol 1979; 44:88.

Schneeweiss A, Motro M, Shem-Tov A, Neufeld HN. Subaortic stenosis: An unrecognized problem in transposition of the great arteries. Am J Cardiol 1981; 48:336.

Shaher RM, Moes CAF, Khoury GC. Radiologic and angiographic findings in complete transposition of the great vessels with left ventricular outflow tract obstruction. Radiology 1967a; 88:1092.

Shaher RM, Puddu GC, Khoury GC, Moes CAF, Mustard WT. Complete transpositon of the great vessels with anatomic obstruction of the outflow tract of the left ventricle. Surgical implications of anatomic findings. Am J Cardiol 1967b; 19:658.

Stansel HC Jr. A new operation for d-loop transposition of the great vessels. Ann Thorac Surg 1975; 19:565.

Stark J, DeLeval MR, Taylor JFN. Mustard operation and creation of ventricular septal defect in two patients with transposition of the great arteries, intact ventricular septum and pulmonary vascular disease. Am J Cardiol 1976; 38:524.

Stewart RW, Kirklin JW, Pacifico AD, Blackstone EM, Bargeron LM Jr. Repair of double-outlet right ventricle. An analysis of 62 cases. J Thorac Cardiovasc Surg 1979; 78:502.

Taussig HB, Bing RJ. Complete transposition of the aorta and levoposition of the pulmonary artery. Clinical, physiological and pathological findings. Am Heart J 1949; 37:551.

Trusler GA, Freedom RM. Complete transposition of the great arteries. In Pediatric Cardiac Surgery. Arciniegas E. ed. Chicago: Year Book, 1985; 257.

Trusler GA, Williams WG, Izukawa T, Olley PM. Current results with Mustard operation in isolated transposition of the great arteries. J Thorac Cardiovasc Surg 1980; 80:381.

Turina M, Siebenmann R, Nussbaumer P, Senning A. Long term outlook after atrial correction of transposition of the great arteries. J Thorac Cardiovasc Surg 1988; 95:828.

Turina MI, Siebenmann R, von Segesser L, Schonbeck M, Senning A. Late functional

deterioration after atrial correction for transposition of the great arteries. Circulation 1989; 80(supp I):162.
van Praagh R. What is the Taussig-Bing malformation? Circulation 1968; 38:445.
van Praagh R, Weinberg PM, Calder L, Buckley LFP, van Praagh S. The transposition complexes: How many are there? Davila JC, ed. Second Henry Ford Hospital International Symposium on Cardiac Surgery. New York: Appleton Century Crofts, 1977;207.
Viles PH, Ongley PA, Titus JL. The spectrum of pulmonary vascular disease in transposition of the great arteries. Circulation 1969; 40:31.
Vogel M, Freedom RM, Smallhorn JF, et al. Complete transposition of the great arteries and coarctation of the aorta. Am J Cardiol 1984; 53:1627.
Williams WG, Freedom RM, Duncan WJ, et al. Indications for arterial repair of complete transposition of the great arteries. Ped Cardiol 1983; 4(suppl I):93.
Williams WG, Trusler GA, Kirklin JW, et al. Early and late results of protocol for simple transposition leading to an atrial switch (Mustard) repair. J Thorac Cardiovasc Surg 1988; 95:717.
Wood AE, Freedom RM, Williams WG, Trusler GA. The Mustard procedure in juxtaposition of the great arteries associated with juxtaposition of the atrial appendages with and without dextrocardia. J Thorac Cardiovasc Surg 1983; 85:451.
Yacoub MH, Radley-Smith R, MacLaurin R. Two-stage operation for anatomical correction of transposition of the great arteries with intact ventricular septum. Lancet 1977; 1:1275.

3

Current Status of Atrial Switch Operations for Transposition of the Great Arteries

John W. Hammon and Harvey W. Bender

□

Interest in the atrial switch operation for transposition of the great arteries (TGA) dates to the 1950s, when Albert (1955) suggested an ingenious technique for baffling systemic venous return to the mitral valve and allowing pulmonary venous return to enter the right ventricle in an experimental model. The first successful intraatrial repair was performed by Senning in 1959 using autogenous flaps of atrial wall and septum. Kirklin and coworkers reported the use of this technique in 1961 with success but with a high mortality rate. In 1963, Mustard applied Albert's suggestions by using a patch or baffle of pericardium to partition and redirect the venous inflow to match the transposed arteries. The advantage of Mustard's approach at the time was a relatively simple technique, which could be reproduced safely.

The Mustard procedure was therefore used in large numbers of patients in the 1960s and early 1970s with a low operative mortality and generally good results. During this time most children undergoing these procedures had received a previous palliative Blalock-Hanlon septectomy and were 2 to 4 years of age before the final repair was performed. When balloon atrial septostomy (BAS) appeared (Rashkind and Miller 1968), the period of palliation before final repair decreased, and simultaneously Tynan (1971) pointed out a finite mortality in patients receiving palliative BAS before final repair.

Therefore, interest turned toward applying the Mustard procedure to neonates, thus avoiding early mortality. In smaller hearts, difficulties with baffle obstruction appeared, and despite reports of good results with the Mustard procedure in neonates (Turley et al. 1982), renewed interest in the Senning operation was evidenced after the publication of excellent results in neonatal transposition (Quaegebeur et al. 1977). Since that time the Senning procedure appears to be the most popular atrial switch operation and can be performed with very low operative mortality rates and with good long-term results. The Senning procedure can be applied to almost all patients with simple transposition with a low operative mortality and the possible advantage that autogenous atrial tissue comprising the repair will preserve atrial transport function.

On the basis of this past experience, we examine here the current acceptable methods of performing the Mustard and Senning procedures and review long-term follow-up in both groups of patients. We particularly focus our attention on difficulties with atrial flaps and baffles, atrial dysrhythmias, and right ventricular function.

MUSTARD PROCEDURE

In neonates weighing less than 5 kg, the Mustard procedure is performed using profound hypothermia and circulatory arrest with a nasopharyngeal temperature lowered to 18°C. In instances in which the operation is performed in older children, it is performed using cardiopulmonary bypass and direct caval cannulation employing small metal right angle cannulae. The patient is then cooled to 25°C, and short periods of low flow or circulatory arrest are used when the occasion dictates. A median sternotomy incision is performed, and the anterior aspect of the pericardial sac is cleared for a width of 5 to 6 cm, inferiorly to the diaphragm and superiorly to the reflection of the pericardium on the great arteries. The thymus gland is resected or reflected so as to maximize the amount of anterior pericardium that can be resected. This creates a patch with a rounded upper end, which is ideal for suturing around the circumference of the inferior vena cava, and a smaller lower end, which can be tailored to fit the circumference of the superior vena cava (Figure 3.1). In ideal circumstances, the patch is hollowed or made more narrow at the waist, because atrial tissue is quite compliant at this point and a narrower patch between the mitral valve and the pulmonary venous orifices minimizes the chance of pulmonary venous obstruction. Cardiopulmonary bypass is then instituted, and nasopharyngeal temperature is lowered to the appropriate level. A ductus arteriosus, if present, is ligated or divided during the cooling period. Cold cardioplegic solution is infused into the aortic root, and the aorta is cross clamped.

In the case of circulatory arrest, the venous cannula can be removed, thus facilitating the interatrial repair considerably. An oblique incision is made in the right atrium (Figure 3.2). Any remaining portion of atrial septum is excised. Great care is taken to preserve the artery to the sinoatrial node. This artery ordinarily lies in the very superior portion of the atrial septum, and thus the ridge of septum lying underneath the superior caval orifice is preserved to as much extent as possible. This excision is extended to include any septal remnant near the inferior vena cava. The coronary sinus is incised back into the left atrium for approximately

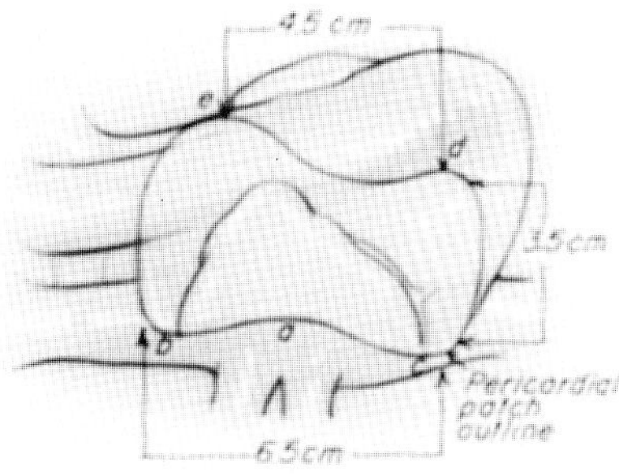

Figure 3.1
The size of the pericardial baffle superimposed on the heart of a 5-kg child giving the rough shape and dimensions. (Kirklin JW, Barrett-Boyes BG. Cardiac surgery. New York: Wiley, 1986:P1165. By permission.) © Churchill Livingstone.

1.5 cm, and any residual septum between the inferior vena cava and the coronary sinus is excised. The raw margins left by excising septum are oversewn with a 5–0 suture of prolene, and great care is taken to avoid a pursestring effect.

The atrial baffle is now sutured into the common atrium using a double-armed continuous 5–0 prolene suture interrupted at several points. The mesothelial surface of the pericardium is directed toward the pulmonary venous atrium. The suture line is begun in the midpoint of the lower edge of the baffle to the left of the left-sided pulmonary veins (Figure 3.3). Difficulties lie in constructing the suture line across the posterior portion of the superior vena cava without obliterating the artery to the sinoatrial node or making the superior vena caval orifice too small, so that later baffle contraction will narrow the superior vena caval orifice. If the eustachian valve is well formed and intact, the baffle can be sutured to this structure to enlarge the inferior vena caval orifice. The suture line is then continued across the junction of the valve with the coronary sinus, and superficial bites are taken at this point to avoid injuring the periphery of the atrioventricular node.

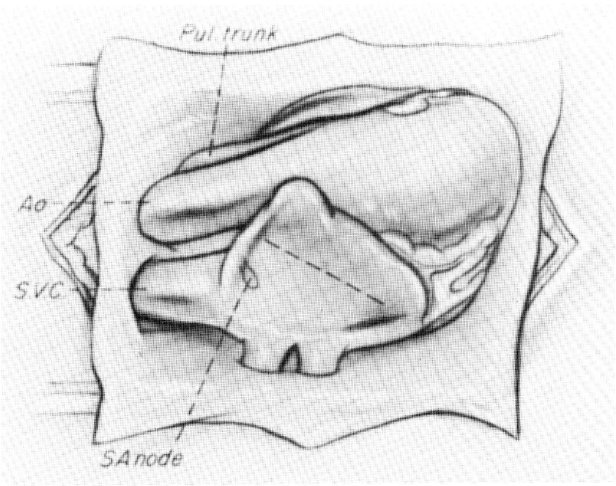

Figure 3.2
The location of the atrial incision for the Mustard repair in relation to the sinoatrial node. (Kirklin JW, Barrett-Boyes BG. Cardiac surgery. New York: Wiley, 1986:P1164. By permission.) © Churchill Livingstone.

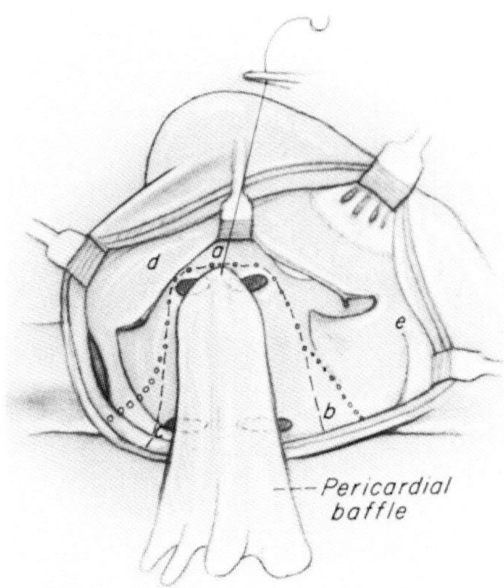

Figure 3.3
The starting point and two possible paths for suture lines (A,B, and C) in the Mustard operation. Also, the superior remnant of the atrial septum (D) and the eustachian valve (E). (Kirklin JW, Barrett-Boyes BG. Cardiac surgery. New York: Wiley, 1986:P1165. By permission.) © Churchill Livingstone.

It is again emphasized that the waist of the baffle covering the mitral valve should be tailored with smaller dimensions than the caval orifices to avoid ballooning of the baffle at this point and consequent obstruction of pulmonary venous return (Figure 3.4). If there is concern that the pulmonary venous atrium is too small, the remnants of pericardium left after trimming the patch can be used to enlarge the pulmonary venous atrium by enlarging the right atriotomy. After closing the right atrium, a venous cannula is then inserted into the right atrial appendage, and partial cardiopulmonary bypass is used for rewarming after circulatory arrest (Figure 3.5). Gentle ventilation of the lungs facilitates this procedure and helps remove air from the left-sided cardiac chambers.

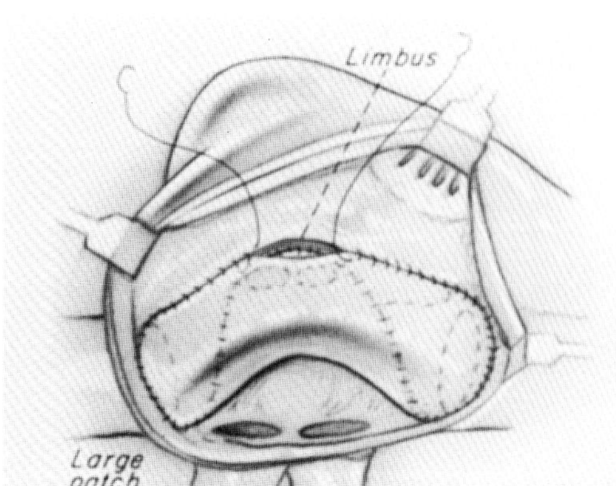

Figure 3.4
The completed baffle, demonstrating its relationship to the pulmonary veins and the limbus of the fossa ovalis. (Kirklin JW, Barrett-Boyes BG. Cardiac Surgery. New York: Wiley, 1986:P1165. By permission.) © Churchill Livingstone.

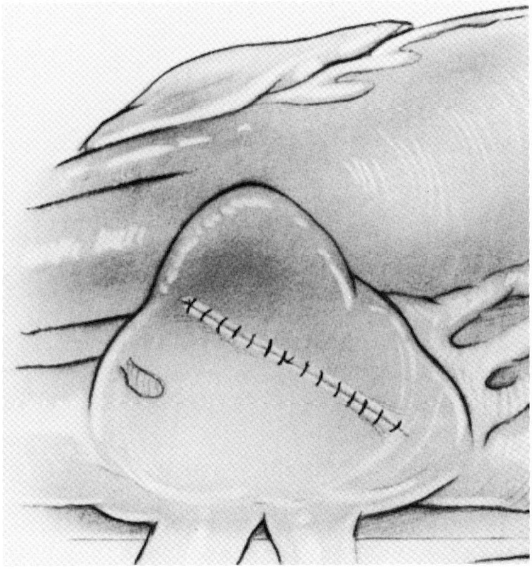

Figure 3.5
The completed repair. (Kirklin JW, Barrett-Boyes BG. Cardiac surgery. New York: Wiley, 1986:P1166. By permission). © Churchill Livingstone.

MUSTARD REPAIR IN CONJUNCTION WITH OTHER CARDIAC PROCEDURES

In patients with small ventricular septal defects (VSDs) complicating transposition, no attempt is made to close the VSD. When the VSD is large, however, repair can be undertaken through the tricuspid valve, should the defect be subpulmonary. Great care should be taken not to disturb the tricuspid apparatus, in that the tricuspid valve will be the new systemic atrioventricular valve, and surgically created tricuspid incompetence can spoil an otherwise adequate repair. In cases in which pulmonary vascular resistance is considerably elevated, the VSD can be left open with adequate palliation using a simple Mustard repair. In rare cases of simple transposition with high pulmonary vascular resistance, an apical VSD can be created (Byrne et al. 1978).

Left ventricular outflow obstruction in the localized form can be approached through the mitral valve or pulmonary artery. In rare occasions involving severe and fixed left ventricular outflow tract obstruction associated with simple transposition, a conduit from the left ventricle to the pulmonary artery is required as a part of the repair.

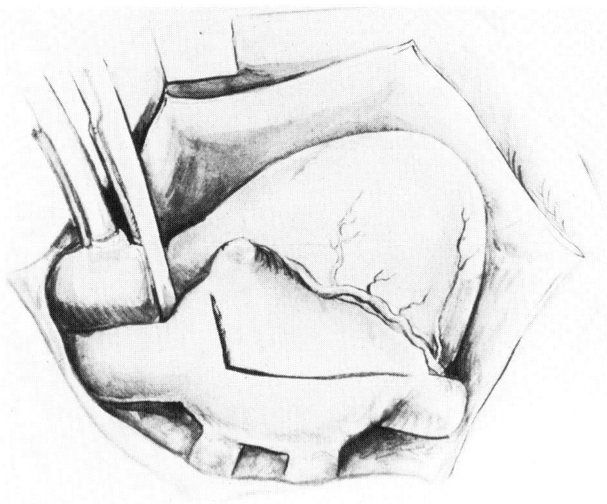

Figure 3.6
The incision used to begin the Senning operation.

THE SENNING PROCEDURE

Patients are operated on through a median sternotomy incision, and circulatory arrest is preferred in children less than 5 kg of body weight. A small portion of pericardium is prepared in the left free edge of the pericardium, after it has been divided in the midline. After cooling and cross clamping the aorta and the administration of cardioplegic solution, the venous cannula is removed, and an inverted hockey-stick incision is made with the small limb into the right atrial appendage (Figure 3.6). The inferior and long limb extends parallel to and just above the

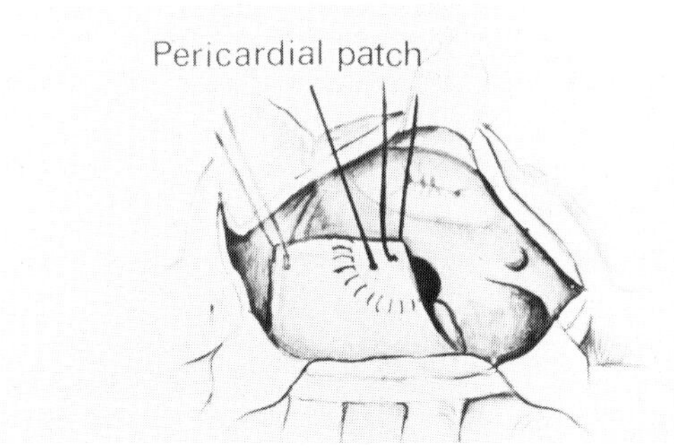

Figure 3.7
The septal flap after excising the superior, lateral, and inferior atrial septal edges and filling in the defect created by the fossa ovalis with pericardium.

Figure 3.8
Forming the roof of the new pulmonary venous atrium using the septal flap.

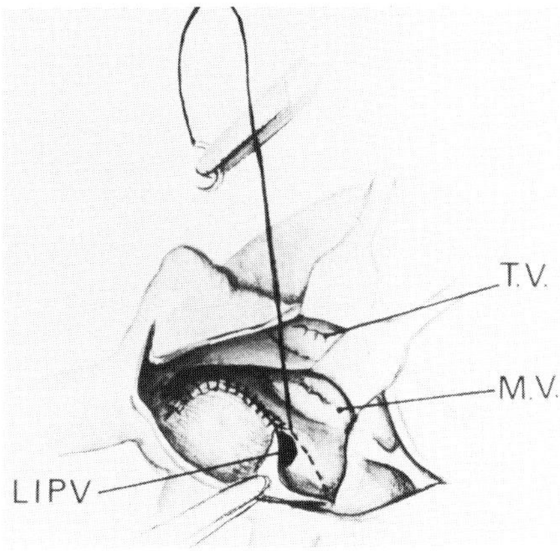

crista terminalis of the right atrium. The interior of the right atrium is inspected, and the atrial septal defect (ASD), if present, evaluated. If the ASD is small, it can be closed primarily. Most patients, however, will have had a BAS, which results in some damage to the fossa ovalis and the surrounding tissue.

It is usually possible to preserve the majority of the atrial septum and to fill in the area of the BAS with a small semicircular portion of pericardium using a running 7–0 prolene suture (Figure 3.7). This is performed after the atrial septum has been formed into a flap based on its attachment to the right atrial free wall just anterior to the right-sided pulmonary veins. The cut edges of atrium on the superior and inferior rim of the septum are approximated with running sutures of 5–0 prolene, with great care to avoid damage to the artery to the sinoatrial node and to avoid a pursestring effect. Using 5–0 prolene sutures, the atrial septal trapezoid is then anchored to the atrial wall just anterior to the left-sided pulmonary veins. A suture line is then carried out along the septal trapezoid that provides a roof for the new pulmonary venous atrium and is situated well below the mitral valve annulus (Figure 3.8).

In instances in which a large ASD is present or damage to the atrial septum by the balloon septostomy is severe, the entire atrial septum is excised, and a trapezoidal portion of pericardium in the appropriate shape is cut and used for the septal trapezoid. The interatrial groove is then dissected outside the heart just above the right-sided pulmonary veins (Figure 3.9). An incision is then made in the atrium just anterior to the right-sided pulmonary veins, and the posterior chamber is entered. This incision is carried to the superior and inferior extent of the pulmonary veins, and a T incision is made out into the confluence of the veins.

The lower portion of the right atrium is then used to construct the new systemic venous atrium (Figure 3.10). A suture is begun at the inferior extent of the atriotomy joining the cut edge of the right atrium to the eustachian valve, if present, or to atrial tissues anterior to the inferior vena caval orifice. This is carried along the eustachian valve and on the junction of the eustachian valve with the

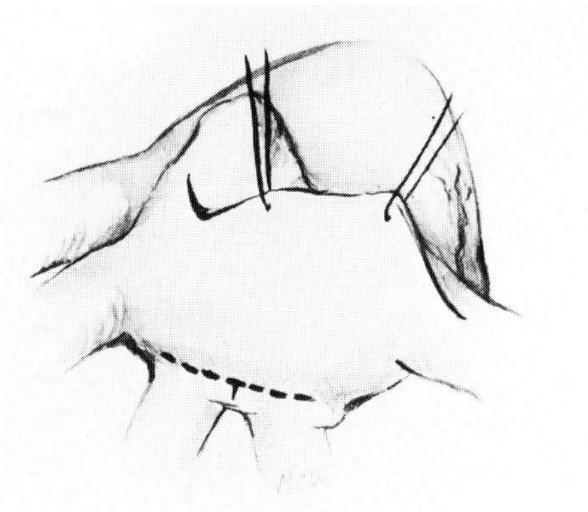

Figure 3.9
The incision in the interatrial groove to provide outlet for pulmonary venous blood.

coronary sinus, and superficial bites are taken, leaving the coronary sinus in the pulmonary venous atrium. Another suture is begun at the junction of the right atrium and the superior vena caval orifice, and a similar suture line is passed along the remnant of the atrial septum, creating a venous pathway from the superior and inferior vena cava to the mitral valve. The upper flap of right atrium is then used to reconstruct a new pulmonary venous atrium. A suture line is carried out along the anterior rim of the distal superior vena cava with the cut edge of the right atrium down to the confluence of the pulmonary veins. Great care is taken not to narrow the orifice to the pulmonary veins for fear of creating pulmonary venous obstruction. On the inferior vena caval side, the cut edge of atrium is attached to the free edge of the atrial wall down to the pulmonary venous ostium in a similar fashion (Figure 3.11). The atrial cannula is then reintroduced, and the patient is rewarmed on partial bypass as previously described.

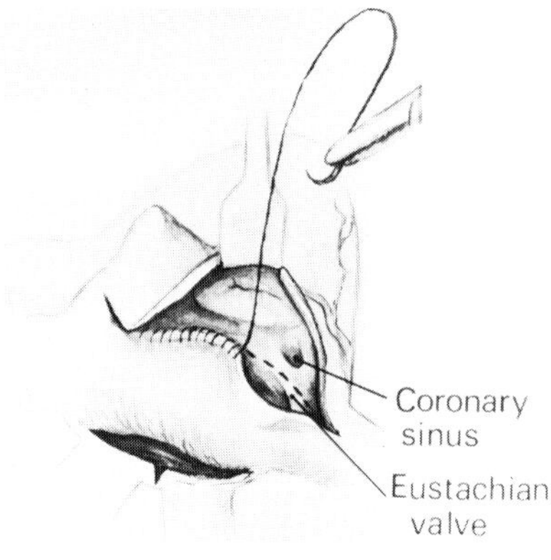

Figure 3.10
Constructing the systemic venous atrium with the lower right atrial flap.

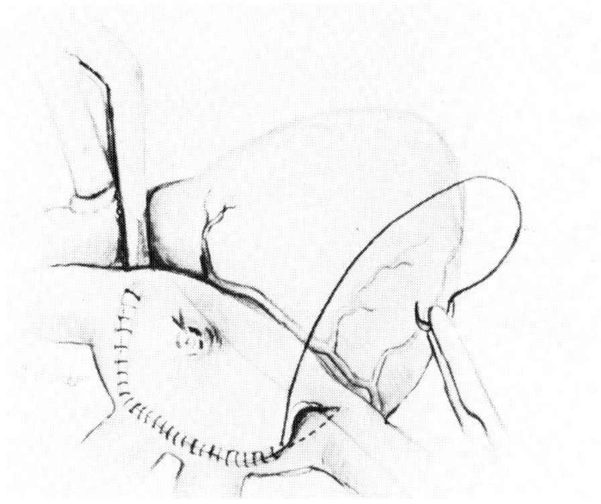

Figure 3.11
The new pulmonary venous atrium constructed using the upper right atrial flap.

POSTOPERATIVE CARE

Atrial filling through the relatively small superior venal caval orifice is facilitated by placing the patient in a slight head-up position. Positive end-expiratory pressure ventilation is avoided to facilitate ventricular filling. The pericardial baffles and atrial flaps tend to accumulate edema for the first 48 postoperative hours, and thus a higher than normal central venous pressure often has to be maintained to permit an adequate cardiac output. Infusions of isoproterenol or dopamine at low to moderate doses are often required for optimum postoperative cardiac performance. Temporary pacing wires are left on the atrium and ventricle, and it is often necessary to pace the atrium for a period of time postoperatively because of a slow atrial or junctional rhythm and digoxin is avoided. Prolonged elevation in central venous pressure often results in pleural effusions and occasionally in chylothorax. Communicating hydrocephalus has been reported on rare occasions.

EARLY RESULTS

In the modern era operative mortality from either form of atrial switch operation is remarkably low. In 239 patients with simple transposition, Trusler et al. (1987) reported only two deaths related to operation. In a smaller group of patients with associated anomalies such as VSD or left ventricular outflow tract obstruction, the operative mortality is higher, approximating 10%. Early results after the Senning procedure are equally good. At Vanderbilt Hospital, 93 consecutive infants with simple transposition operated in the 10 years preceding 1988 had an operative mortality of 5.4%. Hospital mortality in 146 patients from three institutions collected by Pacifico et al. (1983) was 2.7%.

The results of the Mustard and Senning procedures were compared in 123 consecutive patients with TGA and intact ventricular septum who had the atrial switch procedure performed between 1972 and 1980 at the Childrens' Hospital Medical Center in Boston (Marx et al. 1983). A Mustard operation was done in 66 patients at a mean age of 15.5 months with an operative mortality of 11% and an 8% late mortality. In 57 patients in whom a Senning operation was performed, there was 5% hospital mortality and a 4% late mortality during a follow-up period that extended 2 years. Almost uniformly the cause of early operative mortality is low cardiac output, which is often related to the preoperative condition of the infant. Poor preoperative condition can be related to a failed balloon septostomy or massive pulmonary blood flow and cardiac failure related to a large patent ductus arteriosus. These two conditions are incremental risk factors for early mortality (Kirklin and Barrett-Boyes 1988).

Another factor related to operative death is improper construction of the atrial baffle in the Mustard repair or errors in cutting or suturing the atrial flaps in the Senning operation. This is a technically demanding procedure, and inaccurate placement of the atrial baffle or atrial flaps can result in either systemic or pulmonary venous obstruction leading to improper loading of the ventricles and early death. In patients with combined VSD and atrial switch repair, causes of operative mortality are related both to myocardial protection and to increased pulmonary vascular resistance. The time of operation is necessarily longer and more complicated, and operative mortality is substantially higher.

LATE RESULTS

Three factors generally contribute to late death or disability following atrial switch procedures. Right ventricular (systemic ventricular) dysfunction is the most common cause of late death (Trusler and Freedom 1990). Dysrhythmias account for a significant incidence of late death and disability, and abnormalities of venous return related to construction of the baffles and atrial flaps contribute to late morbidity and mortality as well.

There has been concern for some time that placement of the right ventricle into the circulation as the systemic ventricle would result in late heart failure. The reasons for this particular situation are complicated but relate to abnormal right ventricular mass and geometry in transposition, greater difficulty in protecting the right ventricle at time of operation, and potential damage to the right atrioventricular valves, especially in repair of VSDs coexisting with transposition.

Trusler et al. (1987) reports that 11% of his series of nearly 500 patients with simple transposition following Mustard repair showed clinically significant right ventricular dysfunction. Benson et al. (1982) evaluated right ventricular function during bicycle exercise stress in 19 children following the Mustard operation and found over half had an abnormal response. Of great interest is the report of Graham et al. (1985) demonstrating that the Mustard procedure performed after 1975 at Vanderbilt University Hospital resulted in less right ventricular dysfunction than Mustard procedures that had been performed in an earlier era. They suggested that operations performed at an earlier age in the later series plus better myocardial protection during operation played a role in preventing ventricular dysfunction.

There have been few studies comparing ventricular function in survivors of both the Senning and the Mustard procedure. Bender et al. (1980) compared 16 consecutive patients with both the Senning and the Mustard procedure in the modern era. Right ventricular function was generally within normal limits or slightly below normal, and there was no significant difference between the two studied groups. In a larger group of patients following Senning repair of transposition (Bender et al. 1989), right ventricular ejection fraction at rest was normal in approximately 50% of patients; however, response to afterload stress was abnormal in 12 of 14 patients tested. This suggests subthreshold right ventricular dysfunction, although the majority of these patients were asymptomatic and in New York Heart Association class I.

Dysrhythmia is a relatively common complication following both types of atrial repair. It is generally accepted that most dysrhythmias are due to interference with a function of the sinoatrial node either from direct injury or interference with its blood supply during the repair. In Toronto, 92% of children with simple transposition who had a Mustard operation since 1973 were in sinus rhythm on discharge from the hospital (Trusler et al. 1987). Of these children, 71.7% were still in sinus rhythm by 1988 on follow-up ECG. In a smaller group of 126 patients studied with Holter monitoring after Mustard repair in Toronto, sinus rhythm was observed; however, the predominant cardiac rhythm was junctional bradycardia or atrial flutter (Trusler and Freedom 1990). In 11 of these patients, late death occurred suddenly and was thought to be due to dysrhythmia. At Vanderbilt Hospital, 72 of 80 patients following Senning operation showed sinus rhythm on surface ECG (Bender et al. 1989). Postoperative Holter monitoring or electrophysiologic study was performed in 56 patients. Three patients have required a pacemaker for junctional rhythm or sinus node dysfunction, and two have symptomatic or inducible supraventricular tachycardia. Three additional patients have junctional rhythm or sick sinus syndrome requiring no therapy at this time. There have been no late deaths owing to dysrhythmia in this series. Although early results in the Senning operation point to less dysrhythmia than in the Mustard series, it is likely that as Senning children experience longer follow-up time, the incidence of dysrhythmia will rise.

The most common need for reoperation in patients following the Mustard procedure is baffle obstruction or leakage. Although baffle complications are identified fairly frequently, most are mild and have no consequence. In 457 survivors of the Mustard procedure in Toronto, there were 101 baffle complications with 33 of these being significant. There were 24 reoperations for these complications with

10 operative deaths. Early in the experience of the Mustard procedure, the use of synthetic baffles lead to a higher incidence of baffle obstruction. The use of autologous pericardium constructed in the manner described previously appears to result in a very low incidence (<10%) of baffle obstruction or leaks and rarely requires reoperation. It is quite common for the junction between the superior vena cava and the neo-right atrium to be narrowed in both the Mustard and the Senning procedure. If the azygos vein is patent, this allows an additional conduit for systemic venous blood from the upper extremities and head to be routed into the inferior vena cava by the splanchnic connections of the azygos vein. Baffle obstruction appears to be less prominent in the Senning operation, perhaps owing to the use of atrial tissue for the repair rather than pericardium. In a group of 93 infants operated at Vanderbilt University Medical Center, mild obstruction of the superior vena cava was noted in four patients, and a baffle leak requiring reoperation occurred in one patient (Bender 1989).

INDICATIONS FOR ATRIAL SWITCH REPAIR

In the 1990s, it appears that most surgeons dealing with patients with TGA are performing the arterial switch operation in greater numbers than even 5 years ago. For that reason the primary indication for an atrial switch operation would have to be the inability to perform the arterial switch operation. Some reasons for this would be abnormalities of the pulmonic valve or outflow tract, such that it could not be formed into a neo-aortic valve. Some coronary artery distribution anomalies, such as the intramural left coronary pattern, could lead some surgeons into performing an atrial switch procedure. Also in the rare instance of an older child who presents with simple transposition, atrial switch operation is certainly as viable a procedure as pulmonary artery banding (to prepare the left ventricle for systemic pressure work) followed by an arterial switch procedure.

At Vanderbilt University Medical Center, we have been preferentially performing the arterial switch procedure since 1988. Careful follow-up has revealed progressive pulmonic stenosis, requiring reoperation in 8% of these patients similar to baffle obstruction following the Mustard procedure. Of more concern is the finding of an abnormality of ventricular function in patients subjected to methoxamine stress following arterial switch (Horne et al. 1989). These findings are similar to those found in past Senning patients and cause concern about long-term ventricular function.

It is generally believed that the Senning operation is superior to the Mustard procedure, especially in neonates, because atrial transport function is preserved, and the incidence of reoperation for baffle/flap obstruction or leakage is less (Marx et al. 1983). However, in children who combine transposition with anomalous systemic venous drainage, a Mustard operation is necessary to baffle adequately all systemic venous blood to the mitral valve.

REFERENCES

Albert HM. Surgical correction of transposition of the great vessels. Surg Forum 1955; 5:74.

Bender HW Jr, Graham TP Jr, Boucek RJ Jr, Walker WE, Buerth RG. Comparative operative results of the Senning and Mustard procedures for transposition of the great arteries. Circulation 1980; 62(suppl 1):197.

Bender HW Jr, Stewart JR, Merrill WH, Hammon JW, Graham TP Jr. Ten years' experience with the Senning operation for transposition of the great arteries: Physiological results and late follow-up. Ann Thorac Surg 1989; 47:218.

Benson JN, Bonet J, McLaughlin P, et al. Assessment of right ventricular function during supine bicycle exercise after Mustard's operation. Circulation 1982; 65:1052.

Byrne J, Clark D, Taylor JFN, et al. Treatment of patients with transposition of the great arteries and pulmonary vascular obstructive disease. Br Heart J 1978; 40:221.

Graham TP, Burger J, Bender HW, Hammon JW, Boucek RJ, Appleton S. Improved right ventricular function after intraatrial repair of transposition of the great arteries. Circulation 1985; 72(suppl 2):1145.

Horne BS, Graham TP Jr, Bender HW Jr, et al. Abnormal left ventricular functional reserve after arterial switch repair. Circulation 1989; 80(4):II.

Kirklin JW, Barratt-Boyes BG. Cardiac Surgery. New York: Wiley, 1986:p 1182.

Marx GR, Hougen TJ, Norwood WI, et al. Transposition of the great arteries with intact ventricular septum: Results of Mustard and Senning operations in 123 consecutive patients. J Am Coll Cardiol 1983; 2:476.

Pacifico AD, Stewart RW, Bargeron LM Jr. Repair of transposition of the great arteries with ventricular septal defect by an arterial switch operation. Circulation 1983; 68(suppl II):49.

Quaegebeur JM, Rohmer J, Brom AG, Tinkelenberg J. Revival of the Senning operation for treatment of transposition of the great arteries. Thorax 1977; 32:517.

Rashkind WJ, Miller WW. Transposition of the great arteries. Results of palliation by balloon atrioseptostomy in thirty-one infants. Circulation 1968; 38:453.

Trusler GA, Castaneda AR, Rosenthal A, et al., and the Congenital Heart Surgeons Society. Current results of management in transposition of the great arteries with special emphasis on patients with associated ventricular septal. J Am Coll Cardiol 1987a; 10:1061.

Trusler GA, Freedom RM. Transposition of the great arteries: I: The Mustard Procedure. In Sabiston DC Jr, Spencer FC, eds. Surgery of the chest, ed 5. Philadelphia: WB Saunders, 1990:p 1421.

Trusler GA, Williams WG, Duncan KF, et al. Results of the Mustard operation in simple transposition of the great arteries 1963–1985. Ann Surg 1987b; 206:251.

Turley K, Mavroudis C, Ebert PA. Repair of congenital cardiac lesions during the first week of life. Circulation 1982; 66:1.

Tynan M. Survival of infants with transposition of great arteries after balloon atrial septostomy. Lancet 1971; 1:621.

4

Surgical Options in Univentricular Atrioventricular Connection

Robert M. Sade

In hearts with univentricular atrioventricular connection (UVAVC), only one functional ventricle is present; this group of malformations includes tricuspid atresia, mitral atresia, double inlet ventricle, and hypoplastic left and right heart syndrome. Surgical cure for these lesions is not possible. Correction (more precisely, orthoterminal correction [Sade 1975]) can be achieved by the Fontan operation (Fontan and Baudet 1971), and several palliative procedures are available. Because of pulmonary arterial physiology, correction cannot be done in the very young, so palliation must be used in the newborn and small infant. Advances in surgical management have blurred the distinction between palliative and definitive surgery, but for purposes of this presentation, they are discussed separately.

PALLIATION

Palliative surgery is now virtually limited to the newborn and very young infant in our practice. Three clinical circumstances may require surgical intervention in patients with UVAVC: Inadequate pulmonary blood flow resulting in cyanosis, inadequate atrial communication resulting in symptoms of heart failure, and increased pulmonary blood flow resulting in congestive heart failure.

Palliation for Cyanosis

SYSTEMIC TO PULMONARY ARTERIAL ANASTOMOSIS

Many patients with UVAVC have restricted pulmonary blood flow, and palliation is usually required early in infancy. Newborns who become severely cyanotic can be resuscitated by infusion of prostaglandin E_1 to restore patency of the ductus arteriosus, thus maintaining pulmonary blood flow and allowing correction of metabolic derangements that may have occurred (Olley et al. 1976). Surgery may then be carried out electively in a stable patient.

Because of high pulmonary vascular resistance in the newborn, cavopulmonary anastomosis is not an option: A systemic to pulmonary artery shunt must be carried out. Direct anastomosis of the aorta to a branch pulmonary artery in the manner of Waterston or Potts is now rarely done because of the potentials for deformity of the pulmonary arteries and for producing excessive pulmonary blood flow and congestive heart failure.

Therefore, we use the modified Blalock-Taussig shunt in most cases, connecting a subclavian artery to the ipsilateral pulmonary artery with a 5-mm Gore-Tex (W.L. Gore and Associates, Flagstaff, AZ) graft (Ullom et al. 1987). If either the subclavian or the pulmonary artery is 3 mm or less in diameter, deformity or obstruction of the vessels is more likely with a larger graft, so in those cases a 4-mm graft is chosen. The modified Blalock-Taussig shunt has a major advantage over other aortopulmonary shunts: The lumen of the subclavian artery limits blood flow, so the interposition of a large graft rarely results in congestive heart failure, yet the systemic arterial oxygen saturation (SaO_2) is adequate.

A modified Blalock-Taussig shunt may not be possible for some reason, such as inaccessibility or hypoplasia of the subclavian artery. In such cases, a central shunt using a short tubular graft of 4-mm Gore-Tex can be used to connect the ascending aorta to the right pulmonary artery. The 4-mm aorta to pulmonary graft has proved to be quite satisfactory for palliation of newborns, permitting pulmonary blood flow adequate to produce a satisfactory SaO_2 but not enough to produce ventricular volume overload and consequent congestive heart failure.

Several adverse anatomic and physiologic sequelae of systemic to pulmonary artery shunt may increase the risk of a future Fontan operation (Mietus-Snyder et al. 1987). These complications include distortion of the pulmonary arteries, pulmonary artery hypertension with increased pulmonary vascular resistance, and ventricular systolic and diastolic dysfunction because of volume load consequent to the shunt. Pulmonary artery hypertension is fortunately uncommon after the shunts described here. Distortion of the pulmonary arteries due to a shunt may require reconstruction before or at the time of Fontan operation or may produce permanent hypoplasia of the pulmonary arteries, making orthoterminal correction impossible. Ventricular hypertrophy in patients with large shunt flow or ventricular outflow obstruction is a substantial risk factor for the Fontan operation (Kirklin et al. 1986; Freedom 1987).

One or more adverse anatomic or physiologic effects of aortopulmonary shunt are frequently seen in infants who undergo such shunts. For this reason, we now reserve systemic to pulmonary anastomosis for newborn and small infants up to 3 to 4 months of age. A Fontan operation, either staged or complete, is preferred for older infants and children.

CAVOPULMONARY ANASTOMOSIS

Anastomosis of the superior vena cava directly to the right pulmonary artery has been used clinically for over 30 years (Glenn 1958; Bakulev and Kolesnikov 1959). Its major advantage is that the superior vena caval return flows directly through the pulmonary capillary bed, so the left ventricle is not volume loaded, as it is after aortopulmonary shunt. In addition, pulmonary artery hypertension and endocarditis are rare after cavopulmonary anastomosis.

An important early postoperative complication is superior vena caval hypertension with consequent superior vena cava syndrome. This complication may occur with inadequate size of the pulmonary artery or anastomotic stenosis (Trusler and Williams 1980). Therefore, cavopulmonary anastomosis should not be done unless the right pulmonary artery is nearly the same diameter as the superior vena cava. Anastomotic stenosis due to technical errors is fortunately an uncommon problem. This anastomosis grows well with the child.

Late clinical deterioration after classic cavopulmonary anastomosis may have several causes (Sade and Fyfe 1990). Development of collateral veins from superior to inferior vena cava may steal blood from the pulmonary arteries, reducing pulmonary artery flow. Pulmonary arteriovenous fistulas may appear, allowing systemic venous blood to bypass the pulmonary capillary bed. Ventilation-perfusion imbalance may develop when bronchial arterial collaterals displace caval flow from the upper and middle lobes to the lower lobe of the right lung.

For these reasons, the cavopulmonary anastomosis has not enjoyed broad usage in the palliation of children with tricuspid atresia in recent years, even though cavopulmonary anastomosis is a safe operation and provides good palliation. Patients with a previous cavopulmonary anastomosis who undergo Fontan operation may have shorter hospital stays and a lower incidence of pericardial and pleural effusions than patients who have had previous aortopulmonary shunts (Pennington et al. 1981; DeLeon et al. 1983; Zellers et al. 1989).

Because of the demonstrable advantages of cavopulmonary anastomosis, a modification of the anastomosis has had advocates recently: The superior vena cava is divided and connected directly to the undivided right pulmonary artery, resulting in superior vena caval flow to both pulmonary capillary beds (Hopkins et al. 1985). This avoids two important problems of the classic shunt: Commitment of one third of the systemic venous return (superior vena cava) to 55% of the pulmonary capillary bed (right lung) and discontinuity of the pulmonary arteries. The bidirectional Glenn shunt sets the stage for a future Fontan operation that will result in return of all the systemic venous return to the entire pulmonary capillary bed. The principle of the bidirectional cavopulmonary anastomosis underlies the first stage of the recently advocated staged Fontan procedure (see later).

□ Palliation for Inadequate Atrial Communication

In tricuspid atresia, the entire systemic venous return must cross the atrial septum into the left atrium. The communication is a patent foramen ovale two thirds of the time and an atrial septal defect in the remainder. The pressure gradient across the communication can be measured by echocardiography or at cardiac catheterization (Fyfe et al. 1987).

There may be a physiologic advantage to a restrictive interatrial communication in tricuspid atresia. Chronic exposure of the systemic venous bed to higher than normal pressure may condition the vasculature and permit a smoother postoperative course after Fontan operation.

Current practice in our institution is balloon atrial septostomy (Rashkind and Miller 1966) at initial cardiac catheterization in the newborn period if the atrial communication is anatomically small or if there is a substantial pressure gradient across it, particularly in the form of UVAVC in which pulmonary venous return must traverse the atrial septum. Rarely, interatrial obstruction may develop in babies 1 to 4 months of age; then an atrial septal defect may be created by blade septostomy (Park et al. 1982) or surgically. For patients over the age of 4 months with severely obstructed septal communication, we now would do a staged Fontan (over age 4 months) or Fontan (over age 1 to 2 years) procedure.

□ Palliation for Increased Pulmonary Blood Flow

Some patients with UVAVC have increased pulmonary blood flow with congestive heart failure (Keith et al. 1978). Many of this small group of patients respond well to anticongestive medical management, so only a few eventually need palliative surgery.

Anatomically, UVAVC hearts tend to have an inverse relation between the size of the systemic and the pulmonary ventricular outlets. Hearts that permit unrestricted pulmonary blood flow often have a large pulmonary annulus and so are likely to have a narrow subaortic flow pathway (Ottenkamp et al. 1985). Even in patients without substantial subaortic obstruction, the outlet foramen diameter may decrease over time, leading to increasing subaortic obstruction (Rao 1983). Ventricular hypertension associated with subaortic obstruction and volume overload in these patients leads to ventricular hypertrophy. The consequent decrease in compliance and poor diastolic function of the left ventricle is well established as an important risk factor for orthoterminal correction (Freedom et al. 1986; Kirklin et al. 1986).

When congestive heart failure due to increased pulmonary blood flow is refractory to medical therapy, it can be effectively treated by banding the pulmonary artery. A constrictive band around the pulmonary artery increases resistance to flow, thus decreasing pulmonary blood flow, pulmonary artery pressure, and ventricular volume overload. In patients with UVAVC, the benefits of pulmonary artery band are improvement of symptoms of congestive heart failure, decrease in the potential for the development of pulmonary vascular disease, and reduction of the degree of left ventricular hypertrophy due to volume overload.

Pulmonary artery banding, however, may be associated with harmful effects. Distortion of the pulmonary arteries, particularly the origin of the right pulmonary artery, has been a risk factor for Fontan operation (Mayer et al. 1986), but technical improvements have rendered pulmonary artery distortion of this type less dangerous than it once was (Kirklin et al. 1986). The pulmonary artery band does not completely protect against the development of pulmonary vascular obstructive disease: Even in patients who have had a clinically successful banding with reduction of pulmonary artery pressure, increased pulmonary arteriolar smooth muscle and small organized thrombi have been found in the branch pulmonary vessels (Juaneda and Haworth 1984). These vascular changes mitigate against successful orthoterminal correction by increasing the pressure gradient across the pulmonary vascular bed postoperatively, leading to a higher right atrial pressure than would otherwise occur. Most importantly, pulmonary artery banding may accelerate the development of subaortic stenosis and left ventricular hypertrophy (Freed et al. 1973). If subaortic stenosis is associated with a pulmonary artery band, it may be bypassed (aortopulmonary window proximal to the band) (Penkoske et al. 1984) or resected at the time of Fontan operation or at a preliminary operation.

Because of these problems, alternatives to pulmonary artery band for young infants have been explored. The pulmonary artery can be divided and an aortopulmonary anastomosis created by anastomosing the distal end of the pulmonary artery to the side of the aorta or by connecting the distal pulmonary artery to the aorta by way of a 4-mm Gore-Tex graft. Alternative procedures like these have been reported in small numbers of patients (Jonas et al. 1985; Lin et al. 1986; Freedom 1987; Rychik et al. 1990), and the approach has seemed promising.

The introduction of the staged Fontan operation has obviated many problems consequent to pulmonary artery banding. This is discussed in greater detail later. For the few newborns with tricuspid atresia who require surgery for increased pulmonary blood flow, we now treat them with a pulmonary artery band, avoiding its late complications by planning a staged Fontan repair by 6 to 8 months of age.

ORTHOTERMINAL CORRECTION

□ Preoperative Evaluation and Indications for Surgery

Orthoterminal correction became possible when Fontan recognized that pulmonary vascular resistance in the normal lung is so low that only a small increase in pulmonary artery pressure is needed to move the systemic venous return across the pulmonary capillary bed to the left atrium. Fontan did the first such operation in 1968; he reported three cases and described the principle in 1971 (Fontan and Baudet 1971). The operation was first proposed for tricuspid atresia but was later used for virtually all forms of UVAVC.

The best method for achieving orthoterminal correction depends on each patient's specific preoperative anatomy and physiology. Several risk factors have been identified that affect the operability and choice of operation. Most contraindications to the Fontan procedure are now known to be relative rather than absolute.

Because of the absence of a pump for the pulmonary circuit after the Fontan operation, the pulmonary vascular resistance must be low. The operation should not be done if the pulmonary vascular resistance is more than 4 clinical units (Mair et al. 1985). Operation is safest when resistance is less than 2 clinical units (Mayer et al. 1986); in infants under 2 years of age, it should be less than 1 clinical unit for optimal safety.

The lower age limit for operation has been decreasing in recent years. Young age is an absolute contraindication to orthoterminal correction only in small infants, because of their relatively high pulmonary vascular resistance. In patients with ideal anatomy and physiology, the operation is probably safe above the age of 1 year. The recently introduced staged Fontan operation permits reasonably safe repair at ages considerably under 1 year. The lower age limit for safety of the first stage of the staged Fontan operation is not known but may be in the range of 4 to 6 months.

Small pulmonary arteries probably increase the risk of operation, insofar as small size contributes to total pulmonary arterial resistance. A precise lower limit of pulmonary artery size has not been found. The normal pulmonary artery area index is 330 mm^2/M^2; Nakata and co-workers found an index above 250 to be safe for a Fontan operation (Nakata et al. 1984). In the Mayo Clinic series (Girod et al. 1985), however, mortality risk was unrelated to pulmonary artery size down to the lowest pulmonary artery area index in the series, 188 mm^2/M^2. Fontan and co-workers have found that risk of mortality or need for takedown of corrective operation increases sharply when the McGoon ratio (sum of diameters of right and left pulmonary arteries immediately before branching divided by supradiaphragmatic aortic diameter) is below 1.8 (Fontan et al. 1989a).

Pulmonary artery stenosis proximal to branch bifurcation is not a major risk factor if it can be corrected with surgery, but correcting a stenosis at the site of previous aortopulmonary shunts may be quite difficult (Mietus-Snyder et al. 1987). The presence of only one pulmonary artery may not be a contraindication to a Fontan operation, particularly if the opposite lung is hypoplastic (Sade and Gillette 1989).

Pulmonary artery pressure ideally should be less than 15 mmHg, but much higher pressure may be acceptable if it is associated with high pulmonary blood flow and low resistance (Mair et al. 1985; Mayer et al. 1986). Unfortunately, resistance calculation requires knowledge not only of pulmonary artery pressure but also of pulmonary blood flow, and this estimation is often not available from cardiac catheterization. Therefore, acceptability of high pulmonary arterial pressure often rests on indirect evidence of increased pulmonary blood flow and qualitative estimates of resistance.

Good ventricular function is important to successful outcome of a Fontan operation. The ventricular end diastolic pressure ideally should be less than 12 mmHg, but all patients with univentricular atrioventricular connection who have not had previous cavopulmonary shunt have volume loading of the single ventricle. High ventricular end diastolic pressure, up to 25 mmHg, may be acceptable if associated with a large volume load of the ventricle, which is reduced to normal after orthoterminal correction (Mair et al. 1985).

Diastolic ventricular function has received much attention. It is now clear that severe ventricular hypertrophy and consequent poor diastolic compliance are associated with substantially increased risk of mortality after Fontan operation (Kirklin et al. 1986; Freedom 1987; Saliem et al. 1989). In fact, pre-existing severe ventricular hypertrophy may be the cause of most deaths after orthoterminal correction (Caspi et al. 1989). Ventricular hypertrophy is likely to occur in the context of subaortic obstruction, particularly when transposition of the great arteries is present, and may be associated with increasing age of the patient. Pulmonary artery banding may exacerbate potential or actual subaortic stenosis over time (Freed et al. 1973). Severe ventricular hypertrophy leads to need for high ventricular filling pressure, so the consequent elevated left atrial pressure after orthoterminal correction produces high pulmonary artery pressure, and death may result from complications caused by vena caval hypertension. Therefore, operations before Fontan repair have been suggested to remove subaortic obstruction or other causes of ventricular hypertrophy, to allow resolution of myocardial hypertrophy. We now treat patients who have correctable causes of ventricular hypertrophy with a staged Fontan operation, as described subsequently.

Abnormal rhythms do not contraindicate orthoterminal correction. Supraventricular arrhythmias, in fact, may be easier to control after operation than before, because of better myocardial oxygenation and resolution of ventricular hypertrophy (Alboliras et al. 1985). Heart block existing before operation or appearing after operation can be effectively treated with a permanently implanted pacemaker (Case et al. 1989). Although normal sinus rhythm is helpful in assisting ventricular function early postoperatively, many patients ultimately do not have sinus rhythm (as many as 25% at 5 years after operation), yet most continue to have a satisfactory clinical course (Porter et al. 1986).

Anomalous venous connections, both systemic and pulmonary, can usually be accommodated during corrective operation (Mair et al. 1985; Vargas et al. 1987).

SURGICAL TECHNIQUES

In general, it is of critical importance to the outcome of orthoterminal correction that all flow pathways through the reconstructed right side of the heart be widely patent and that the atrial pressures be as low as possible at the conclusion of the operation. Attention to technical details helps to achieve these goals.

Open flow pathways in the right side of the heart require reconstruction of any pulmonary artery stenoses. In general, this is easy to achieve if the stenoses are proximal to the branching of the pulmonary arteries but can be difficult when associated with pulmonary artery deformity related to a surgical shunt. The aortopulmonary anastomosis should be constructed to leave as large and circular an opening as possible; this usually requires the use of an anterior patch to augment the anastomosis.

The lowest possible left atrial pressure requires complete closure of all communications between the pulmonary and systemic circuits. All shunts must be completely ligated. Atrial septal defect closure should be done nearly always with a patch to ensure a tension-free suture line. Some surgeons believe that the coronary sinus should be left to drain on the left side of the patch to avoid impairment of ventricular function by high coronary vein pressure (Ilbawi et al. 1986).

Simple ligation of the main pulmonary artery, when this is required, is usually complete, but a ventricle to pulmonary artery residual shunt can be certainly avoided by division of the main pulmonary artery. In addition, repair or replacement of a mitral valve that is either insufficient or stenotic reduces left atrial pressure. Finally, meticulous attention to myocardial preservation throughout the procedure is of particular importance to optimize early postoperative ventricular performance.

□ Anterior Anastomosis

When the retrosternal space is adequate to accommodate an anterior conduit, anterior anastomosis can be achieved to either the pulmonary artery or the right ventricle in some cases of tricuspid atresia (Figure 4.1). In Fontan's experience, the mortality rate after orthoterminal correction for tricuspid atresia is lowest with a right atrium to right ventricle anastomosis (Fontan et al. 1989b). When a valve is included in that connection and the right ventricle is large enough, the potential exists for the ultimate growth of the right ventricle and the development of a four-chambered heart (Fontan et al. 1983; Bull et al. 1983; Laks et al. 1984; Gussenhoven et al. 1986) (Figure 4.2).

Achieving a four-chambered heart in patients with tricuspid atresia may be possible if the malformation is associated with normally related great arteries, normal or nearly normal sized pulmonary annulus and arteries, and a right ventricle that is at least one-third normal size (Ilbawi et al. 1989). Interposition of a valve-bearing conduit (usually a homograft) between the right atrium and right ventricle is required, so there must be adequate space between the heart and the sternum to accommodate such a graft. Sufficient retrosternal space is often not available, particularly in small children, in whom repair is being done increasingly frequently.

Few patients are likely to meet these criteria. When it can be done, however, the operation may result in growth of the right ventricle to accommodate the

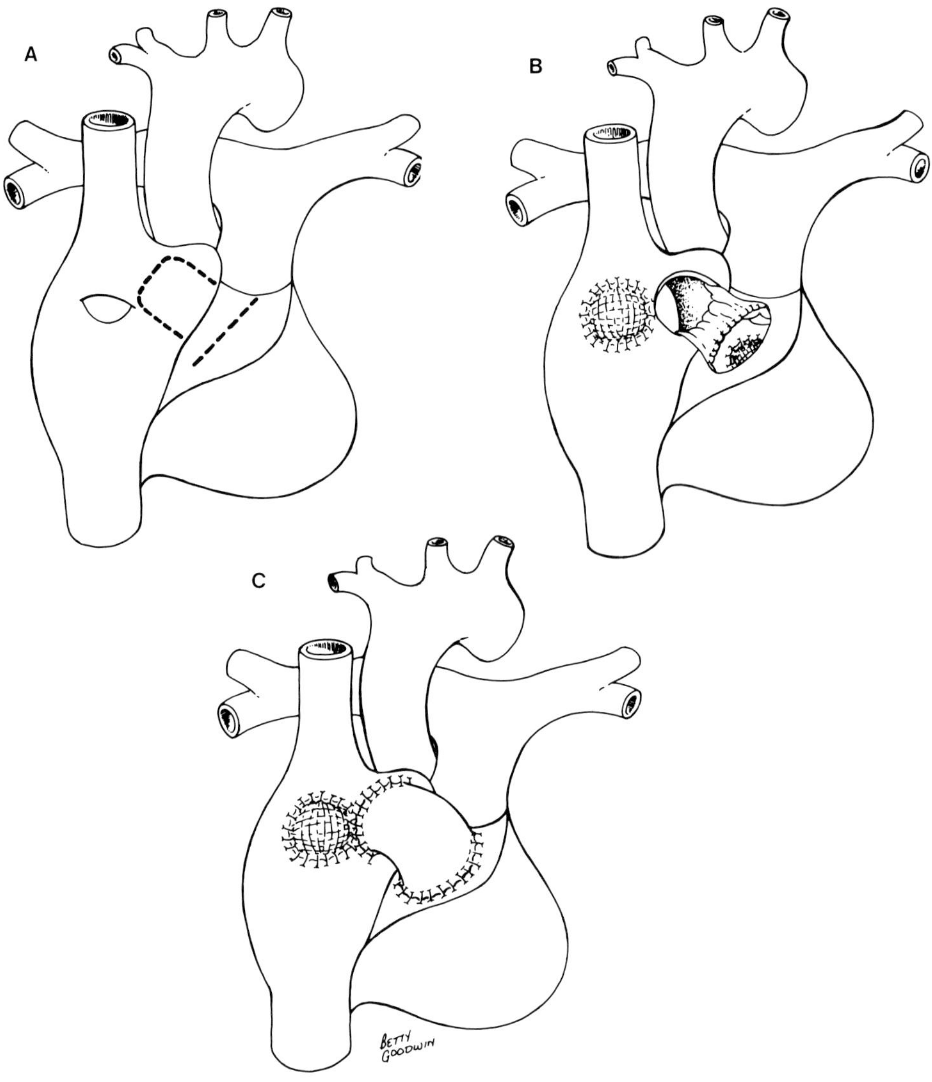

Figure 4.1. Anterior anastomosis to the right ventricle in a heart with tricuspid atresia. (A) A rectangular flap incision is made in the right atrial appendage to create a large opening, and a linear incision is made in the right ventricle. (B) The atrial septal defect is closed with a Gore-Tex patch secured with continuous 4–0 polypropylene suture. The ventricular septal defect is closed in a similar manner, and all obstructive muscle from sinus to pulmonary valve is excised. The free edge of the atrial flap is sewn to the right edge of the ventriculotomy with running 4–0 polydioxanone suture. (C) A large patch of pulmonary artery homograft or autogenous pericardium is sewn to the remaining opening of the right atrium and right ventricle and along the lateral edges of the atrial flap to complete a large conduit between right atrium and right ventricle.

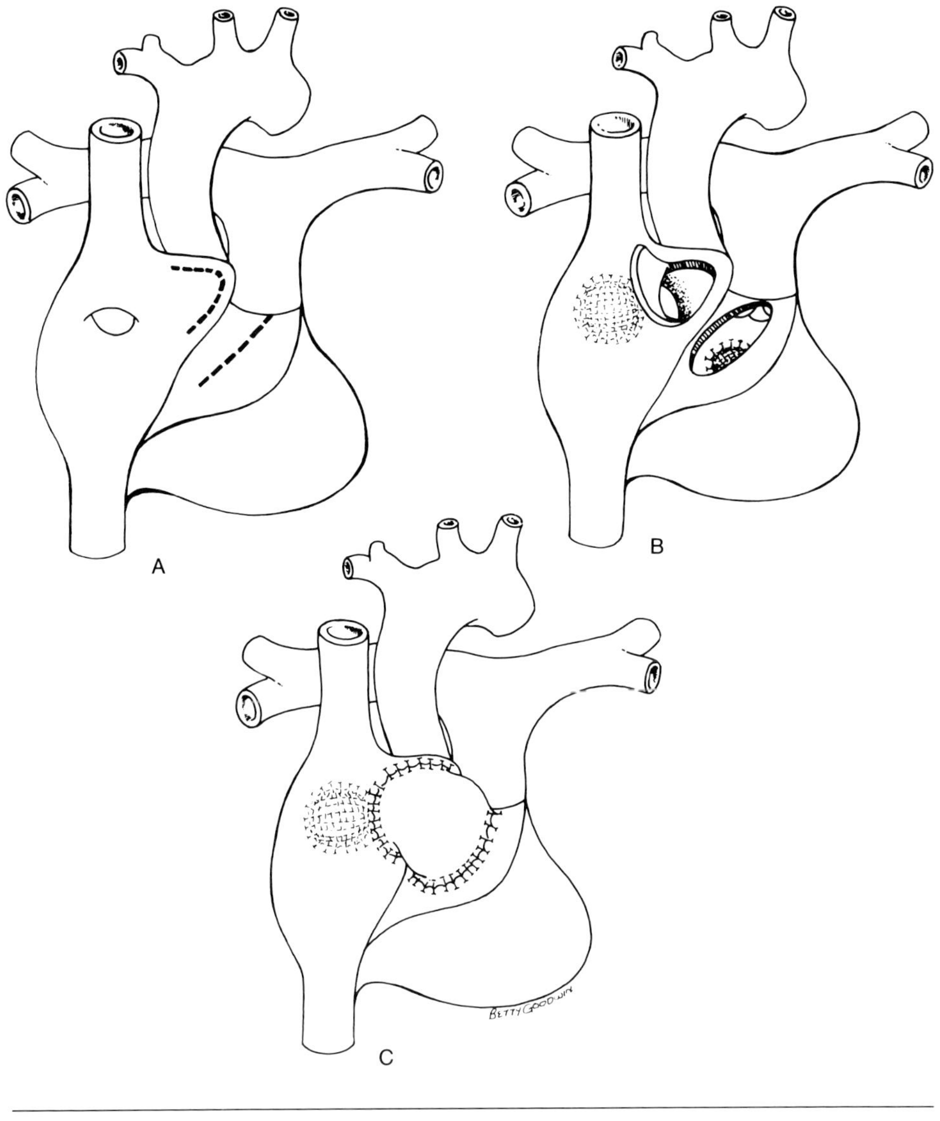

Figure 4.2. Homograft from right atrium to right ventricle in a heart with tricuspid atresia. (A) In this heart with moderate size right ventricle (greater than one-third normal) and normally related great arteries, a rectangular flap incision is made in the right atrial appendage to produce a large opening, and the right ventricle is opened. (B) The atrial septal defect is closed with a Gore-Tex patch secured with running 4–0 polypropylene suture. The ventricular septal defect is closed in a similar manner, and all trabeculations that may obstruct continuity from the ventricular sinus to the pulmonary valve are excised. The pulmonary valve is visible through the right ventriculotomy. (C) An appropriate size aortic or pulmonary homograft is inserted between the right atrium and right ventricle, being sutured in place with continuous 3–0 or 4–0 polypropylene suture. The atrial rectangular flap is used as a baffle to permit the valve annulus to lie in a vertical plane, avoiding distortion.

entire systemic venous return, a well-functioning four-chambered heart, and normally low systemic venous pressure (Fontan et al. 1983; Laks et al. 1984; Gussenhoven et al. 1986).

□ Posterior Anastomosis

In general, the most widely patent, nonobstructive atriopulmonary anastomosis is the posterior anastomosis, in which the right atrium and vena cavas are connected to the right or main and right pulmonary arteries (Kreutzer et al. 1982; Oelert and Borst 1984). This operation can be done for UVAVC hearts with either normally related or transposed great arteries. A large number of variations are possible, depending on local anatomic relations. The two variations depicted here (Figures 4.3 and 4.4) are the ones we use most commonly.

□ Total Cavopulmonary Anastomosis

In any type of UVAVC heart in which the tricuspid valve is functional, the preferred method of orthoterminal correction is total cavopulmonary anastomosis (Puga et al. 1987; de Leval et al. 1988; Jonas and Castaneda 1988). This operation is associated with fewer complications and a lower mortality rate than previous methods (Figure 4.5). The principle of this procedure is to accomplish atriopulmonary anastomosis by one of the methods described previously, then to baffle the inferior vena caval return directly into the atriopulmonary anastomosis. This avoids complications associated with baffling of the pulmonary venous return into the tricuspid valve (baffle obstruction is not uncommon) or, in cases of double inlet ventricle, dehiscence of the patch used to close the tricuspid valve.

A specific long-term complication may be associated with this procedure: The development of pulmonary arteriovenous malformations (Moore et al. 1989). Only a few such cases have been described, but they are worrisome, and vigilant follow-up of these patients is required.

□ Staged Fontan Operation

Many patients who require corrective operation are subjected to a relatively high risk because of need for complex reconstruction of the pulmonary arteries, small pulmonary artery size, ventricular hypertrophy, previous pulmonary artery band, young age, or moderately elevated pulmonary vascular resistance. Such patients may be treated with orthoterminal correction in two stages.

The first stage, the Hemi-Fontan operation (Douville et al., 1991), is in principle a bidirectional Glenn shunt, the superior vena cava being connected to both pulmonary arteries. The bidirectional Glenn shunt was first described experimentally by Haller et al. (1966) then applied clinically by several surgeons (Azzolina

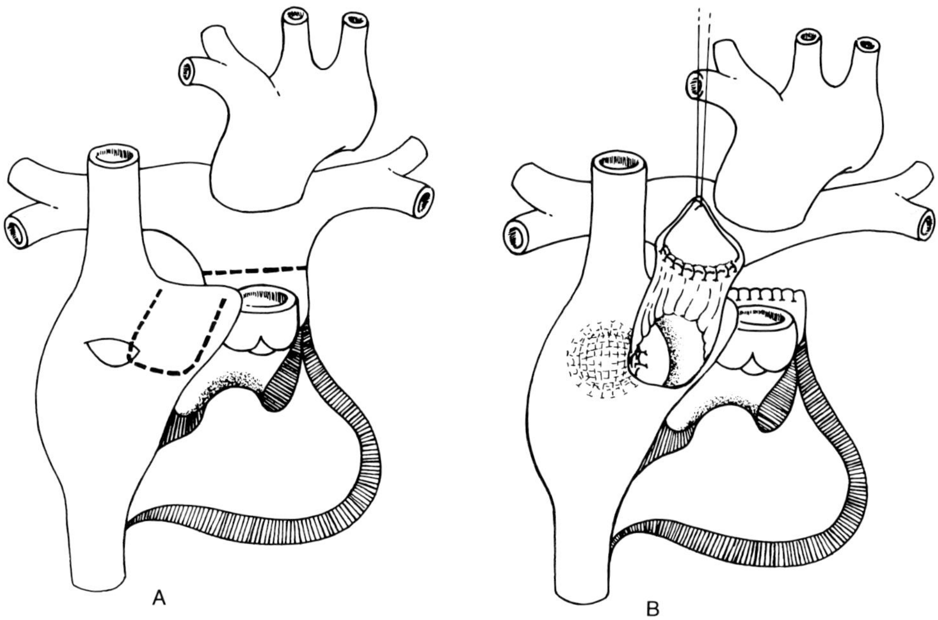

Figure 4.3.
Posterior flap anastomosis. This heart with tricuspid atresia also has transposition of the great arteries, but the operation can be done as well with normally related great arteries. The central portion of the ascending aorta has been removed to facilitate visualization of the atriopulmonary anastomosis. (A) A rectangular flap incision is made in the right atrial appendage, and the pulmonary artery is transected. (B) The atrial septal defect is closed with a Gore-Tex patch secured with a running suture of 4–0 polypropylene. The free edge of the rectangular flap is sewn to the posterior edge of the divided pulmonary artery. For a larger anastomosis, the pulmonary artery incision can be extended into the right pulmonary artery. The stump of the proximal pulmonary artery has been oversewn with a running suture of 4–0 polypropylene. (C) A large patch fashioned from homograft pulmonary artery or autogenous pericardium has been sewn to the remaining opening of the right atrium and pulmonary artery and along the lateral edges of the atrial flap, to complete a large conduit between the right atrium and pulmonary artery.

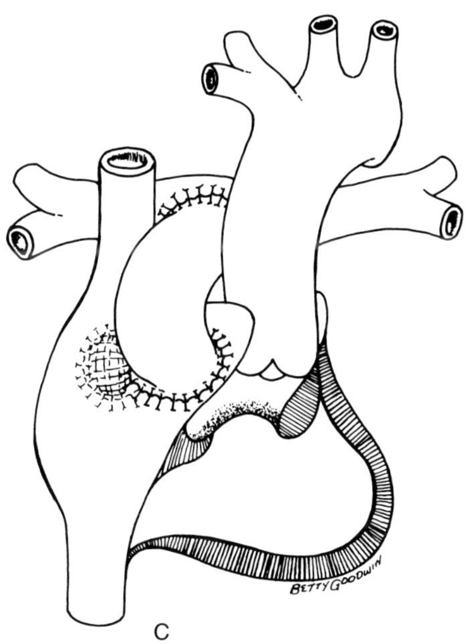

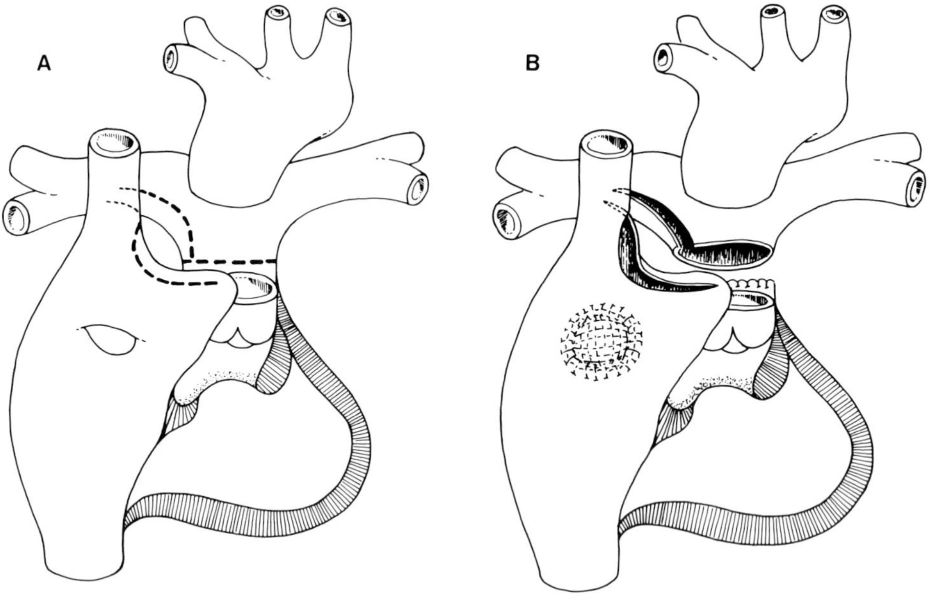

Figure 4.4. Posterior direct anastomosis. (A) The right atrium and superior vena cava are incised as depicted, the incision's upper end spiraling around the superior vena cava to end posteriorly adjacent to the anterior surface of the right pulmonary artery. The main pulmonary artery is divided, and the opening is extended into the right pulmonary artery to a point immediately opposite the corner of the pulmonary artery incision. (B) The atrial septal defect is closed with a Gore-Tex patch secured with a running suture of 4–0 polypropylene. The proximal stump of the main pulmonary artery is

et al. 1972; Laks et al. 1980; Hopkins et al. 1985; Kawashima et al. 1984; Mazzera et al. 1989; Drinkwater and Laks 1990). Norwood's modification has special advantages in preparing the patient for a Fontan procedure (Norwood 1990).

The operation is exactly the same as the Fontan technique appropriate for the specific anatomy except that the final step is not to separate the inferior caval return from the pulmonary venous return but to place a patch across the atriopulmonary anastomosis (Figure 4.6). This allows the superior vena cava to drain directly into both pulmonary arteries, while the inferior caval return goes to the ventricle by way of the atrioventricular valve. The ventricle pumps only the systemic venous return, which is composed of oxygenated blood from the superior vena cava and unoxygenated blood from the inferior vena cava. Unlike cardiovascular physiology after complete Fontan operation, cardiac output is not totally dependent on pulmonary blood flow.

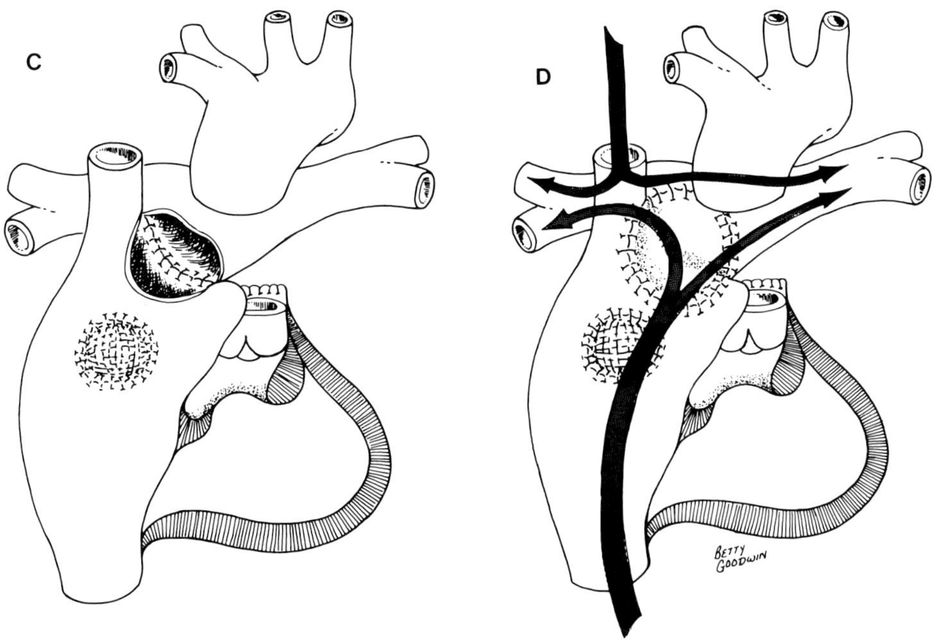

oversewn with a running suture of 4–0 polypropylene. (C) The posterior wall of the cavoatrial incision and inferior border of the pulmonary artery incision are anastomosed with a running suture of 4–0 or 5–0 polydioxanone. (D) The anterior portion of the anastomosis has been completed with a large patch of pulmonary artery homograft, with a running suture of 4–0 or 5–0 polypropylene. The arrows depict the flow of blood from both vena cavas into both pulmonary arteries.

Most patients do well after this procedure, with a very low incidence of prolonged pleural drainage, edema, or need for large intravascular volume infusion. In our early experience starting in late 1989, eight infants 6 to 15 months of age all survived hemi-Fontan operation. They had a median postoperative hospitalization of 6 days, none required pleural drainage for more than 3 days, and none had a pericardial effusion.

The second stage involves removal of the intraatrial patch to open the atriopulmonary anastomosis and closure of the interatrial communication by septal patch or inferior vena caval baffle, thus completing the Fontan repair. This procedure is simply done and may not be as physiologically challenging to the patient as a one-stage Fontan operation. We plan the final stage a few months after the first stage, because of uncertainty regarding the growth potential of pulmonary arteries that carry only the superior vena caval venous return.

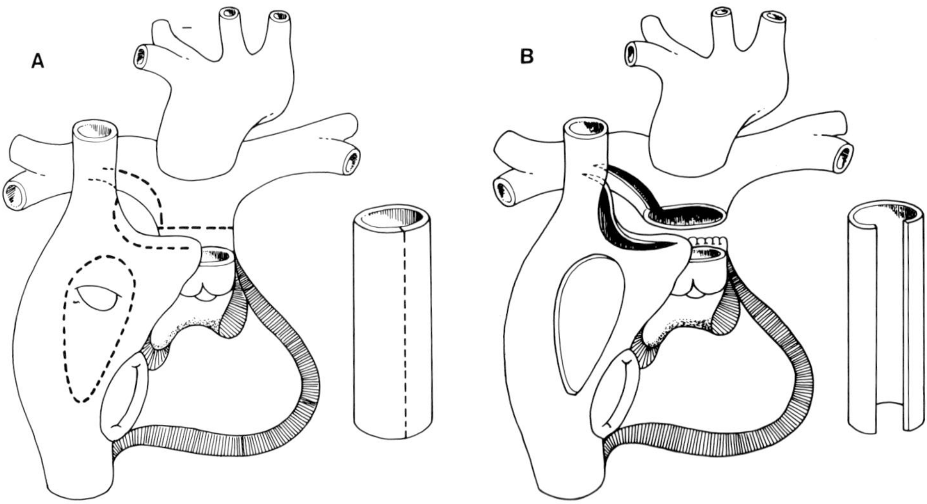

Figure 4.5. Total cavopulmonary anastomosis. This is the preferred operation whenever a functional tricuspid valve is present. The atriopulmonary connection can also be achieved by the posterior flap method (see Figure 4.3). The anteriorly transposed aorta has been cut away to permit visualization of the atriopulmonary anastomosis. (A) The atrial septum is excised (dotted line in atrium). The pulmonary artery is divided, and the opening is extended into the right pulmonary artery behind the superior vena cava. An incision is made along the superior border of the atrial appendage and extended into the superior vena cava, spiraling posteriorly to a point directly opposite the open pulmonary artery. A 10-mm Gore-Tex tube is cut to a length equal to the intercaval distance and incised on one side. The width of the graft can be reduced for small patients. (B) The proximal stump of the pulmonary artery is closed with a running suture of 4–0

Patients who have undergone a previous Glenn shunt are known to have a smoother postoperative course after orthoterminal correction than patients without a Glenn shunt (Pennington et al. 1981; DeLeon et al. 1983; Zellers et al. 1989; Bridges et al. 1989), and the expectation is that patients who undergo staged Fontan operation as described here will do as well because their physiology is that of a bidirectional Glenn shunt. Norwood's large early experience with this type of staged Fontan repair for hypoplastic left heart syndrome is described in Chapter 14.

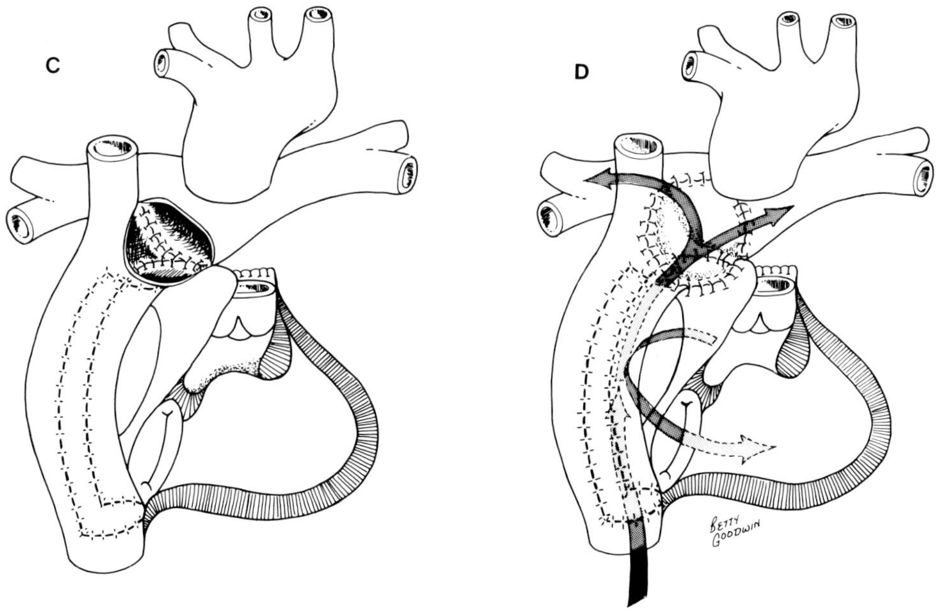

polypropylene. (C) The posterior edge of the cavoatriotomy is anastomosed to the posterior edge of the pulmonary arteriotomy with continuous 4–0 or 5–0 polydioxanone suture. Through a separate atriotomy (not shown here), the Gore-Tex graft is inserted between the vena cavas with a continuous suture of 4–0 polypropylene; the posterior suture line is carried along the rightward edge of the atrial septal communication, the inferior border around the vena caval orifice, the superior border around the atriopulmonary anastomosis, and the anterior border along the crista terminalis. (D) The reconstruction is completed by using a large patch (often needed to reconstruct stenotic pulmonary arteries or aid in closure of a large main pulmonary artery) of cryopreserved pulmonary artery homograft. The arrows demonstrate flow pathways of systemic venous return into the pulmonary arteries and pulmonary venous return through the tricuspid valve.

We now use this method of staging to treat patients with substantial risk factors for orthoterminal correction: For example, those with hypoplastic left heart syndrome, marginally small pulmonary arteries, severe ventricular hypertrophy due to outflow obstruction or large volume overload, marginally elevated pulmonary vascular resistance, and young age. Because the operation can be done in infancy, it permits avoidance of aortopulmonary shunts and their deleterious effects in all but the youngest (less than 3 to 4 months) patients. A possible long-term benefit of the earlier correction permitted by the staged Fontan operation may be better

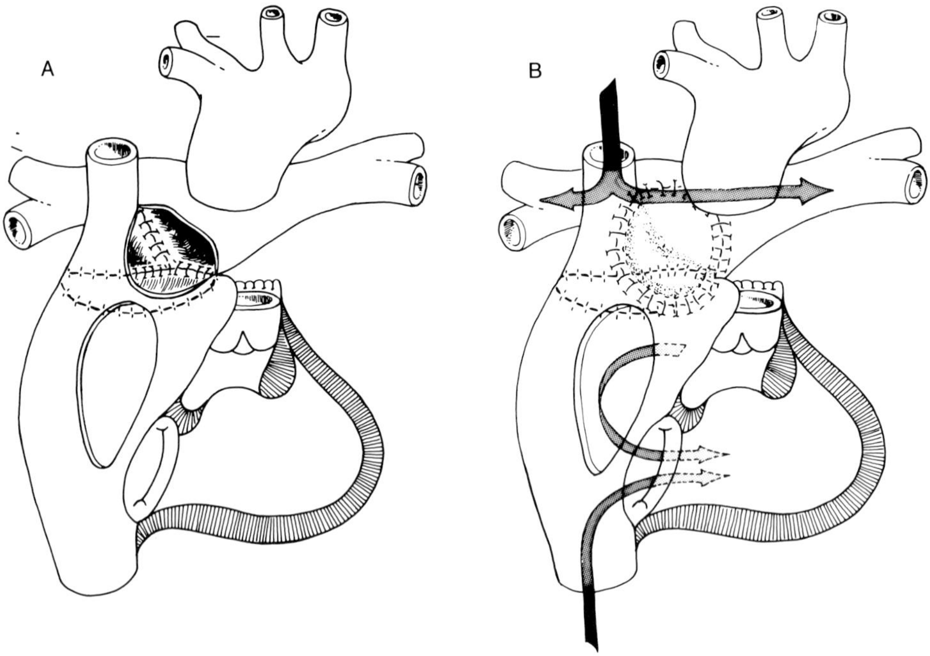

Figure 4.6. The staged Fontan operation: Hemi-Fontan procedure. (A) The Fontan operation is completed in an appropriate manner (shown here is a posterior anastomosis, as illustrated in Figure 5A,B). The inferior vena caval baffle, however, is not used; rather, a circular patch of Gore-Tex is placed within the atrium, across the atriopulmonary anastomosis, cutting off communication between the right atrium and the pulmonary arteries. (B) After reconstruction is completed with a homograft patch, the flow of blood, depicted by the arrows, is from the superior vena cava into pulmonary arteries and from inferior vena cava through the atrial septal defect into the ventricle.

long-term function of a ventricle that has not been subjected to volume and pressure overload for years, as is now the case for most orthoterminally corrected patients. Only very long-term follow-up will clarify this possibility.

A different approach to staging was first described by Laks (Laks et al. 1988; Laks and Billingsley 1989). The Fontan procedure is completed in the usual manner (see Figure 4.4), but an opening is left between the atria at the site of the intraatrial patch (Figure 4.7). At the second stage, the opening is closed by a tourniquet that is easily accessible subfascially (Laks and Billingsley 1989) or by a percutaneous transluminal device at cardiac catheterization (Bridges et al. 1990).

A major advantage of staging orthoterminal correction is the availability of interim cardiac catheterization to confirm the suitability of the patient's physiology

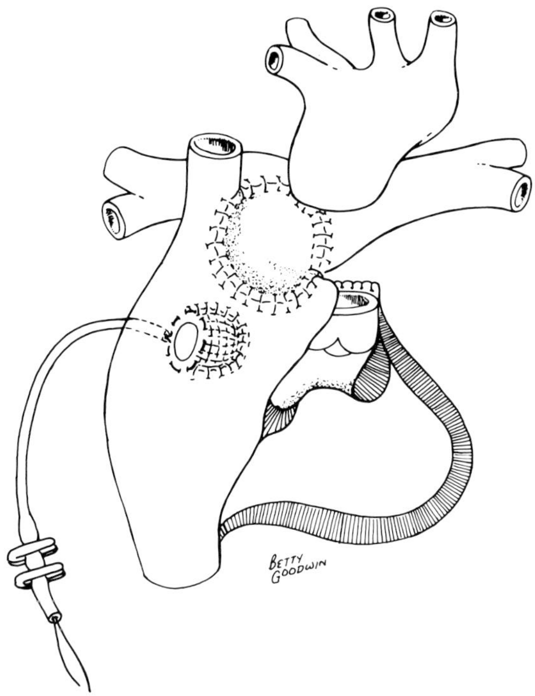

Figure 4.7. The staged Fontan operation: Controlled atrial septal communication. The operation is completed in a manner appropriate for the lesion (shown here is a posterior anastomosis for tricuspid atresia), but a 5- to 10-mm opening is left in or adjacent to the atrial septal patch. It is surrounded with a pursestring suture of 2–0 polypropylene, the ends of which are brought through the atrial wall at the interatrial groove and placed through a polyethylene tube. The end of the tube is placed immediately beneath the closure of the linea alba. The suture is secured with two metal clips. At a later time, depending on the condition of the patient, the inferior end of the incision is opened, the polyethylene tube retrieved below the fascia, the clips removed, and the atrial septal communication closed by tightening the snare and resecuring it with metal clips. Alternatively, the defect can be closed with a percutaneous transluminal device (see text).

for complete repair before the entire systemic venous return is committed to the pulmonary capillary bed.

Staging the Fontan operation has been introduced too recently to define precisely the advantages over ordinary Fontan repair. The logic of these procedures is impressive: Preparation of the heart for final correction by repairing risk factors (pulmonary artery deformities, subaortic stenosis, mitral valve abnormalities) and permitting resolution of myocardial hypertrophy. Staging has allowed application of the Fontan operation to infants. It remains to be seen how great an advantage these procedures bestow in the long term.

REFERENCES

Albaliris ET, Porter CJ, Danielson GK, et al. Results of the modified Fontan operation for congenital heart lesions in patients without preoperative sinus rhythm. J Am Coll Cardiol 1985; 6:228.

Azzolina G, Eufrate S, Pensa P. Tricuspid atresia. Experience in surgical management with a modified cavopulmonary anastomosis. Thorax 1972; 27:111.

Bakulev AN, Kolesnikov SA. Anastomosis of superior vena cava and pulmonary artery in the surgical treatment of certain congenital defects of the heart. J Thorac Surg 1959; 37:693.

Bridges ND, Locke JE, Castaneda AR. Fontan repair with baffle fenestration and subsequent transcatheter closure in high risk patients. J Am Coll Cardiol 1990; 15:203A.

Bridges ND, Jonas RA, Flanagan MF, Mayer JE, Castaneda AR. Bidirectional Glenn shunt for patients at high risk for Fontan repair: Early results. Circulation 1989; 80(suppl II):69.

Bull C, de Leval MR, Stark J, Taylor JFN, Macartney FJ. Use of a subpulmonary ventricular chamber in the Fontan circulation. J Thorac Cardiovasc Surg 1983; 85:21.

Case CL, Gillette PC, Ziegler V, Sade RM. Problems with permanent atrial pacing in the Fontan patient. PACE 1989; 12:92.

Caspi J, Coles JG, Rabinovitch M, et al. Morphological findings contributing to a failed fontan procedure in the current era. Circulation1989; 80(suppl II):365.

DeLeon Sy, Idriss FS, Ilbawi MN, et al. The role of the Glenn shunt in patients undergoing the Fontan operation. J Thorac Cardiovasc Surg 1983; 85:669.

de Leval MR, Kilner P, Gewillig M, Bull C. Total cavopulmonary connection: A logical alternative to atriopulmonary connection for complex Fontan operation. J Thorac Cardiovasc Surg 1988; 96:682.

Douville EC, Sade RM, Fyfe, DA. Hemi-Fontan operation for surgery in single ventricle: A preliminary report. Ann Thorac Surg 1991; 51:893.

Drinkwater DC Jr, Laks H. The use and modification of the Glenn shunt. J Am Coll Cardiol 1990; 15:204A.

Fontan F, Baudet E. Surgical repair of tricuspid atresia. Thorax 1971; 26:240.

Fontan F, Deville C, Quaegebeur J, et al. Repair of tricuspid atresia in 100 patients. J Thorac Cardiovasc Surg 1983; 85:647.

Fontan F, Fernandez G, Costa F, et al. The size of the pulmonary arteries and the results of the Fontan operation. J Thorac Cardiovasc Surg 1989a; 98:711-724.

Fontan F, Kirklin JW, Gernandez G, et al. Outcome after a perfect Fontan operation. Circulation 1989b; 80(suppl II):69.

Freed M, Rosenthal A, Plauth WH Jr, Nadas AS. Development of subaortic stenosis after pulmonary artery banding. Circulation 1973; 47(suppl 3):7.

Freedom RM. The dinosaur and banding of the main pulmonary trunk in the heart with functionally one ventricle and transpositon of the great arteries: a saga of evolution and caution. J Am Coll Cardiol 1987; 10:427.

Freedom RM, Lee NB, Smallhorn JF, et al. Subortic stenosis, the univentricular heart, and banding of the pulmonary artery. An analysis of the courses of 43 patients with univentricular heart palliated by pulmonary artery banding. Circulation 1986; 73:758.

Fyfe DA, Taylor AB, Gillette PC, Kline CH, Crawford FA Jr. Doppler echocardiographic confirmation of recurrent atrial septal defect stenosis in infants with mitral valve atresia. Am J Cardiol 1987; 60:410.

Girod DA, Rice MJ, Mair DD, et al. Relationship of pulmonary artery size to mortality in patients undergoing the Fontan operation. Circulation 1985; 72(suppl 2):93.

Glenn WWL. Circulatory bypass of the right side of the heart. IV. Shunt between superior vena cava and distal right pulmonary artery—report of a clinical application. N Engl J Med 1958; 259:117.

Gussenhoven WJ, The HK, Schippers L, et al. Growth and function of the right ventricular outflow tract after Fontan's procedure for tricuspid atresia: A two-dimensional echocardiographic study. J Thorac Cardiovasc Surg 1986; 34:236.

Haller JA, Adkins JC, Worthington J, et al. Experimental studies on permanent bypass of the right heart. Surgery 1966;59:1128.

Hopkins RA, Armstrong BE, Serwer GA, Peterson RJ, Oldham HN Jr. Physiological rationale for a bidirectional cavopulmonary shunt: A versatile complement to the Fontan principle. J Thorac Cardiovasc Surg 1985; 90:391.

Ilbawi MN, Idriss FS, DeLeon SY, et al. When should the hypoplastic right ventricle be used in a Fontan operation? An experimental and clinical correlation. Ann Thorac Surg 1989; 47:533.

Ilbawi MN, Idriss FS, Muster AJ, et al. Effects of elevated coronary sinus pressure on left ventricular function after the Fontan operation. An experimental and clinical correlation. J Thorac Cardiovasc Surg 1986; 92:231.

Jonas RA, Castaneda AR. Modified Fontan procedure: Atrial baffle and systemic venous to pulmonary artery anastomotic techniques. J Cardiol Surg 1988; 3:91.

Jonas RA, Castaneda AR, Lang P. Single ventricle (single- or double-inlet) complicated by subaortic stenosis: Surgical options in infancy. Ann Thorac Surg 1985; 39:361.

Juaneda E. Haworth SG. Pulmonary vascular structure in patients dying after a Fontan procedure. The lung as a risk factor. Br Heart J 1984; 52:575.

Kawashima Y, Kitamura S, Matsuda H, et al. Total cavopulmonary shunt operation in complex cardiac anomalies. J Thorac Cardiovasc Surg 1984; 87:74.

Keith JD, Rowe RD, Vlad P. Heart Disease in Infancy and Childhood. New York: MacMillan Company, 1978:3.

Kirklin JK, Blackstone EH, Kirklin JW, Pacifico AD, Bargeron LM Jr. The Fontan operation. Ventricular hypertrophy, age, and date of operation as risk factors. J Thorac Cardiovasc Surg 1986; 92:1049.

Kreutzer GO, Vargas FJ, Schlichter AJ, et al. Atriopulmonary anastomosis. J Thorac Cardiovasc Surg 1982; 83:427.

Laks H, Williams WG, Hellenbrand WE, et al. Results of right atrial to right ventriuclar and right atrial to pulmonary artery conduits for complex congenital heart disease. Ann Surg 1980; 192:382.

Laks H, Billingsley AM. Advances in the treatment of pulmonary atresia with intact ventricular septum: Palliative and definitive repair. Cardiol Clin North Am 1989; 7:387.

Laks H, Haas GC, Pearl JM, et al. The use of an adjustable intraatrial communication in patients undergoing the Fontan and definitive heart procedures. Circulation 1988; 78(suppl II):357.

Laks H, Milliken JC, Perloff JK, et al. Experience with the Fontan procedure. J Thorac Cardiovasc Surg 1984; 88:939.

Lin AE, Laks H, Barber G, Chin AJ, Williams RG. Subaortic obstruction in complex congenital heart disease: Management by proximal pulmonary artery to ascending aorta end to side anastomosis. J Am Coll Cardiol 1986; 7:617.

Mair DD, Rice MJ, Hagler DJ, et al. Outcome of the Fontan procedure in patients with tricuspid atresia. Circulation 1985; 72(suppl 2):88.

Mayer JE Jr., Helgason H, Jonas RA, et al. Extending the limits for modified Fontan procedures. J Thorac Cardiovasc Surg 1986; 92:1021.

Mazzera E, Corno A, Picardo S, et al. Bidirectional cavopulmonary shunts: Clinical applications as staged or definitive palliation. Ann Thorac Surg 1989; 47:415.

Mietus-Snyder M, Lang P, Mayer JE, et al. Childhood systemic-pulmonary shunts: Subsequent suitability for Fontan operation. Circulation 1987; 76(suppl 3 pt. 2):39.

Moore JW, Kirby WC, Madden WA, Gaither NS. Development of pulmonary arteriovenous malformations after modified Fontan operations. J Thorac Cardiovasc Surg 1989; 98:1045.

Nakata S, Imai Y, Takanashi Y, et al. A new method for the quantitative standardization of cross-sectional areas of the pulmonary arteries in congenital heart diseases with decreased pulmonary blood flow. J Thorac Cardiovasc Surg 1984; 88:610.

Norwood WI. Personal communication, 1990.

Oelert H, Borst HG. Modified Fontan procedure using a retroaortic atriopulmonary anastomosis. J Thorac Cardiovasc Surg 1984; 32:392.

Olley PM, Coreani F, Badoch E. E-type prostaglandins. A new emergency therapy for certain cyanotic congenital heart malformations. Circulation 1976; 53:728.

Ottenkamp J, Wenink ACG, Quaegebeur JM, et al. Tricuspid atresia. Morphology of the outlet chamber with special emphasis on surgical implications. J Thorac Cardiovasc Surg 1985; 89:597.

Park SC, Neches WH, Mullins CE, et al. Blade atrial septostomy: Collaborative study. Circulation 1982; 66:258.

Penkoske PA, Freedom RM, Williams WG, Trusler GA, Rowe RD. Surgical palliation of subaortic stenosis in the univentricular heart. J Thorac Cardiovasc Surg 1984; 87:767.

Pennington DG, Nouri S, Ho J, et al. Glenn shunt: Long-term results and current role in congenital heart operations. Ann Thorac Surg 1981; 31:532.

Porter CJ, Battiste CE, Humes RA, et al. Risk fctors for supraventricular tachyarrhythmias after Fontan procedure for tricuspid atresia. Am Heart J 1986; 112:645.

Puga FJ, Chiavarelli M, Hagler DJ. Modifications of the Fontan operation applicable to patients with left atrioventricular valve atresia or single atrioventricular valve. Circulation 1987; 76(suppl III):53.

Rao PS. Further observations on the spontaneous closure of physiologically advantageous ventricular septal defects in tricuspid atresia: Surgical implications. Ann Thorac Surg 1983; 35:121.

Rashkind WJ, Miller WW. Creation of an atrial septal defect without thoracotomy. A palliative approach to complete transposition of the great arteries. JAMA 1966; 196:991.

Rychik J, Murdison KA, Chin AJ, Norwood WI. Relief of aortic outflow obstruction in infancy: Use of the pulmonary artery to aortic anastomosis. J Am Coll Cardiol 1990; 15:204A.

Sade RM. Orthoterminal correction of congenital cardiovascular defects. Ann Thorac Surg 1975; 19:105.

Sade RM, Fyfe DA. Tricuspid Atresia. In: Sabiston DC, Spencer FC, eds. Gibbon's Surgery of the Chest. Philadelphia: WB Saunders, 1990:1461.

Sade RM, Gillette PC. Fontan operation in a case of single functional pulmonary artery. J Thorac Cardiovasc Surg 1989; 98:153.

Seliem M, Muster AJ, Paul MH, Benson DW. Relation between preoperative left ventricular muscle mass and outcome of the Fontan procedure in patients with tricuspid atresia. J Am Coll Cardiol 1989; 14:750.

Trusler GA, Williams WG. Long-term results of shunt procedures for tricuspid atresia. Ann Thorac Surg 1980; 29:312.

Ullom RL, Sade RM, Crawford FA Jr, Ross BA, Spinale F. The Blalock-Taussig shunt in infants: Standard versus modified. Ann Thorac Surg 1987; 44:539.

Vargas FJ, Mayer JE Jr, Jonas RA, Castaneda AR. Anomalous systemic and pulmonary venous connections in conjunction with atriopulmonary anastomosis (Fontan-Kreutzer). Technical considerations. J Thorac Cardiovasc Surg 1987; 93:523.

Zellers TM, Driscoll DJ, Hume RA, et al. Glenn shunt: Effect on pleural drainage after modified Fontan operation. J Thorac Cardiovasc Surg 1989; 98:725.

5

Risk Factors for Modified Fontan Operations

John E. Mayer, Jr.

☐

Patients with an increasing variety of complex congenital heart defects who have a *functionally* single ventricular chamber are now being "physiologically repaired" by operations in which systemic venous return is separated from pulmonary venous return and is then rerouted directly into the pulmonary arteries without augmentation by a ventricular pump. Since the initial report of successful application of this concept in a patient with tricuspid atresia by Fontan in 1971 (Fontan and Baudet 1971), these operations have thereafter been termed "*Fontan operations*," although the technical details of the operation have undergone significant modification since the initial description. Based on their initial experience, Choussat, Fontan, et al. (1977) suggested a number of criteria to aid in the selection of patients for these procedures, and we (Mayer et al. 1986) and others (Kirklin et al. 1986; Fontan et al. 1989a, 1989b; Bartmus et al. 1990) have attempted to define the physiologic and anatomic limits of these and other selection criteria. This chapter includes an updated analysis of our results with modified Fontan operations at the Children's Hospital, Boston, from 1973 to 1988 with 282 patients and contains some supplemental information from the experience of other institutions, particularly regarding criteria for which we have been unable to retrieve data from our own experience.

It should be understood at the outset that in a biologic system as complex as the patient with a single ventricle, the physiologic and anatomic data that can be obtained with current technology remain imprecise, and there may well be important information that we have not even considered. Therefore, analyses based on such data cannot provide "rules" on which to base decisions regarding the individual patient, but they yield information on the factors that have *previously* been associated with either an increase or a decrease in the risk of the operation to be undertaken. Continuing improvements in patient selection, operative management, and postoperative care may nullify factors that were thought to be important and may uncover others not previously considered. Therefore, a continuing critical analysis of one's experience is necessary, and retention of an open

Minimum age of 4 years
Sinus rhythm
Vena cavae-normal drainage
Right atrium of normal volume
Mean pulmonary artery pressure of <16 mmHg
Pulmonary resistance of <4 units·m^2
Pulmonary artery–aortic diameter ratio >0.75
Normal function of primitive ventricle (E.F. >60%)
No mitral incompetence
No impairing effects of previous shunt

Table 5.1 Original Selection Criteria (Fontan and Choussat)

and imaginative mind-set is necessary to continue to make advances in the care of this heterogeneous and challenging group of patients.

Choussat and Fontan (Choussat et al. 1977) listed 10 criteria in the form of a "checklist" when selecting patients for Fontan procedures, and these are detailed in Table 5.1. Since these original 10 criteria were described, no truly new selection criteria have been described, and the majority of efforts have been directed at testing and refining the validity of each of the criteria. Therefore, this discussion is organized around the original 10 criteria, addressing in particular the topics of age, rhythm, anomalies of venous return, pulmonary vascular hemodynamics, pulmonary artery anatomic factors, and function of the single ventricle.

AGE

The issue of age at which the Fontan operation should be performed has been a controversial one, and disagreement remains about its importance. Our own data with age considered in a *univariant* fashion are shown in Table 5.2. Based on these data alone, the conclusion may be reached that younger age at operation is

Age (yrs)	0–3.2	3.3–6.2	6.3–11.3	11.4–18	>18
Survived	44	53	60	39	23
Failed	27 (38%)	17 (24%)	12 (17%)	5 (11%)	2 (8%)

Table 5.2 Age and Outcome

associated with an increased risk. However, when a multivariant analysis of risk factors is carried out considering multiple preoperative variables, age does not appear as an independent risk factor. A similar result was noted in the analysis of the first 167 patients undergoing Fontan operations at our institution. The explanation for the disparity between the univariant and multivariant analysis results is that the patients undergoing Fontan operations in this younger age group frequently had associated risk factors that independently placed them in higher risk categories. For example, 32% of patients under 4 years of age had pulmonary vascular resistance measurements of more than 2 Wood units compared with 9% of the older patients. Over the 15 years covered by our review, the timing of Fontan operations has been primarily driven by patient status; until recently, there has been no systematic attempt to carry out Fontan operations at a particular age. In general, patients operated on at younger ages were referred for worsening cyanosis or other symptoms, and it is therefore not surprising that they may have had more unfavorable risk characteristics (for example, pulmonary vascular resistance, pulmonary artery distortion, depressed ventricular function) than the patients who were referred later in life on a more elective basis.

These results conflict with those reported by the Mayo Clinic group (Bartmus et al. 1990). In their multivariant analysis of 500 patients undergoing Fontan operations, age under 4 years was an independent risk factor for mortality. However, in the subgroup of patients with one or fewer risk factors, the survival of patients younger than 4 years of age was not different from that of older patients. Similarly, we found that the presence of additional risk factors seemed to have a greater effect in this younger age group. The Mayo Clinic group also noted that the patients presenting after 4 years of age were likely to be inherently different from patients who did not survive without intervention before this age. Similar results were reported by Kirklin et al. (1986), who found that younger age at operation was associated with an increased risk for Fontan operation. However, they also pointed out that this factor was reduced by a more recent date of operation and recommended that Fontan operations be undertaken routinely before the age of 4 years to avoid the potentially deleterious effects of continuation in the palliated state. Of note, an analysis of the combined experiences at the University of Bordeaux and the University of Alabama indicated that *older* age at operation had a negative effect on long-term outcome (Fontan et al. 1989b). Thus, we believe that young age per se does not contraindicate a Fontan operation.

If one were to conclude, however, that there is a higher risk for the Fontan operation in the younger patient, the question may be reasonably posed as to why the Fontan operation should be undertaken in this age group. One answer lies in considering the disadvantages of the surgical alternative of additional palliation. In a study from our institution, the construction of a second palliative shunt after the first year of life was associated with a significant number of patients becoming less favorable candidates for a Fontan operation because of distortion of the pulmonary arteries, deterioration of ventricular function, or elevation of pulmonary vascular resistance (Meitus-Snyder et al. 1987). The report by Graham et al. (1986) on patients with tricuspid atresia is also of interest because they found a growing incidence of ventricular dysfunction in palliated patients with increasing age and duration of the palliated state. Patients of similar age with Fontan repairs had less volume overload and less hypertrophy than the palliated patients, although abnormal contractile function persisted in a significant number of the Fontan patients. In a follow-up study, many of these contractility abnormalities in the Fontan patients had disappeared (Gewillig et al. 1990). Therefore, additional palliative shunting operations for potential Fontan candidates can be associated with the acquisition of other problems, which can adversely affect a subsequent Fontan operation.

The use of the bidirectional Glenn operation as a "halfway" Fontan in patients whom we have judged to be at higher risk for a usual Fontan operation has been associated with low risk in our initial experience. Also, from a technical standpoint, it seems to be relatively easy to convert these patients to a full Fontan circulation in the future. This procedure avoids the imposition of an additional volume load on the single ventricle, which would be associated with a systemic to pulmonary artery shunt, while providing increased effective pulmonary blood flow and systemic oxygenation. This procedure may be particularly appropriate for the young patient who has other risk factors for a Fontan approach.

RHYTHM

Normal sinus rhythm was a requirement for the Fontan operation in the original 10 criteria, and the vast majority of patients who present for Fontan procedures are in this rhythm. The issue of rhythm has not been addressed in prior analyses of risk, but in review of our experience, five of 282 patients undergoing Fontan operations had had pacemakers placed before their Fontan procedure. Interestingly, all survived the Fontan procedure, suggesting that sinus rhythm is not an absolute requirement for a a successful outcome. Alboliras et al. (1985) from the Mayo Clinic found a similar lack of impact of non–sinus rhythm on the outcome of 12 of their patients. However, we have certainly observed that the overall hemodynamics early after Fontan operations can be influenced by the cardiac rhythm and have noted that temporary atrial pacing can lead to an improved blood pressure and cardiac output, particularly when junctional rhythm is transiently present postoperatively. This improvement seems to occur primarily by lowering of the pulmonary venous atrial pressure with a consequent lowering of the systemic venous atrial pressure. Therefore, atrial and ventricular temporary pacing wires are routinely placed at the time of the Fontan operation to allow pacing in the early postoperative period. If sinus rhythm is not present preoperatively, permanent atrial and ventricular pacing wires are placed and connected to a dual-chambered pacemaker generator.

VENOUS ANOMALIES

The anatomy of the connections of the systemic and pulmonary veins with the heart is of obvious importance to the construction of a Fontan circulation, since these two circulations must be separated and connected without obstruction to the pulmonary arteries and to the systemic ventricle, respectively. Because the right atrium was believed to perform an essential "pumping" function in the pulmonary circulation, it was believed that all systemic venous return should be gathered into a right atrium of normal volume, which would then "pump" blood out to the pulmonary arteries. However, as the Fontan principle was applied to lesions other than tricuspid atresia, it became more difficult from a technical standpoint to collect the systemic venous return into a normal volume right atrial chamber. In particular, patients with heterotaxy syndromes (asplenia or polysplenia) with bilateral superior vena cavae connecting to the ipsilateral atrial walls or pulmonary veins connecting to systemic veins or to the ipsilateral walls of a common atrium present difficult anatomic situations if one attempts to collect all of the systemic veins together to make a single connection to the pulmonary arteries. The construction of complex intraatrial baffles to achieve this goal was associated with increased mortality risk in our initial experience because of obstruction within either the systemic or the pulmonary venous pathways.

A second anatomic variation of venous return that presented problems was that of a left-sided superior vena cava draining to the coronary sinus in association with stenosis or atresia of the left atrioventricular valve. In this situation, an intraatrial baffle to collect all systemic venous return within the right atrium must be placed between the coronary sinus orifice and the annulus of the right-sided atrioventricular valve. In this position the baffle tends to prolapse leftward because of the higher right atrial pressure and potentially obstruct the valve orifice with resulting pulmonary venous obstruction. Both of these types of problems with the separation of systemic from pulmonary venous return can be more easily managed by the creation of direct anastomoses between the superior vena cavae and the pulmonary arteries and then constructing geometrically simple tubular pathways from the inferior vena cava–right atrial junction to the superior vena cava–right atrial junction. The contralateral vena cava is also connected directly to the adjacent pulmonary artery. With the use of these techniques, anomalies of systemic or pulmonary venous return did not appear as independent risk factors in our Fontan experience (Mayer et al. 1986). The results considering anomalies of systemic or pulmonary venous return univariantly are shown in Table 5.3. The Mayo Clinic group, in contrast, has identified the presence of asplenia as a factor contributing to an increased risk of Fontan operation in their experience (Humes et al. 1988).

The experimental work of deLeval et al. (1988) suggests that there may well be a hydrodynamic advantage to the construction of this type of intraatrial tubular pathway by reducing turbulence and energy dissipation. In view of these consid-

	Present			Absent		
	Survived	Total	%	Survived	Total	%
ASVD	38	49	78	181	233	78
APVD	7	11	64	212	271	78

ASVD, anomalous systemic venous drainage
APVD, anomalous pulmonary venous drainage

Table 5.3 Anomalies of Venous Drainage

erations, we now routinely employ this technique of separation of systemic and pulmonary venous return in the majority of Fontan operations.

PULMONARY VASCULAR HEMODYNAMICS

It is intuitively obvious that if blood is to flow through the pulmonary vascular bed without the additional energy input provided by a ventricular contraction, the pulmonary vascular resistance must be low. The issues are to define the resistance and then to determine what are the upper acceptable limits for this resistance to blood flow. Pulmonary vascular resistance has been traditionally estimated in a fashion analogous to a direct current (nonpulsatile) electrical system. The mean pressure gradient across the pulmonary vascular bed is divided by the mean pulmonary blood flow indexed to body surface area to yield pulmonary vascular resistance in Wood units. This approach to the assessment of the pulmonary vascular resistance is at best an approximation of the energy dissipation in the pulmonary vascular bed and ignores the pulsatile nature of pulmonary blood flow. The measurement of pulmonary vascular *impedance*, which requires the measurement of instantaneous flow and pressure, theoretically provides a more correct assessment of the resistance to blood flow, but the technology to make this assessment in the catheterization laboratory is not generally available. Because the pulmonary blood flow after a Fontan operation is nonpulsatile, the direct current analogy of measuring resistance rather than impedance may be theoretically reasonable and is currently the only means technologically available.

Of interest, in our experience, the pulmonary vascular resistance measured after Fontan operations is almost always higher than that measured before the Fontan, suggesting that the pulsatile component may have a significant effect. In addition to these theoretical problems with the determination of pulmonary re-

PVR (Wood units·m²)	Survived	Total	%
<.7	49	57	86
>.7, <1.2	50	56	89
>1.2, <1.7	30	41	73
>1.7	30	50	60

PVR, pulmonary vascular resistance.

Table 5.4 Tip Pulmonary Vascular Resistance

sistance, difficulties may arise in a number of anatomic situations. If there are multiple sources of pulmonary blood flow that have different levels of oxygen content, the determination of the true mixed pulmonary artery saturation becomes virtually impossible, and therefore no calculation of pulmonary blood flow can be made. Similar problems may exist in the determination of pulmonary venous saturation. If there are stenoses in the pulmonary artery tree, the determination of mean pulmonary artery pressure is more difficult. All these factors must be considered in assessing the reliability of any individual pulmonary vascular resistance determination. Finally, it must be remembered that the resistance measured in the catheterization laboratory is also only a "snapshot" of the patient's hemodynamic status, which may be influenced by hypoventilation, pulmonary parenchymal disease, or subclinical airway obstruction.

With these limitations in mind, pulmonary vascular resistance remains among the most important of the risk factors influencing the outcome of Fontan operations. The outcome of Fontan operations as a function of pulmonary vascular resistance in our experience is shown in Table 5.4. In multiple logistic regression model, higher levels of pulmonary vascular resistance were associated with increasing risk with a P value of <0.01. Because of the problems with calculation of pulmonary vascular resistance as outlined in the previous paragraph, resistance data were available for only 204 of the 282 patients in this study. Interestingly, the lack of data for this variable was also a highly significant risk factor for poor outcome of a Fontan operation. These results are similar to those obtained in our analysis of the first 167 patients reported previously (Mayer et al. 1986) but are different than those reported by the Mayo Clinic group (Bartmus et al. 1990). However, in their analysis, consideration was given only to whether the resistance was more than 4 Wood units. Our data would suggest that this variable may be better considered as a continuous variable or at least with multiple categorical levels rather than simply above or below an arbitrary level.

Pulmonary artery pressure was among the original 10 variables to be considered, but we have previously found that this variable was less significant than the pulmonary vascular resistance. Clearly, these variables are closely linked since the pulmonary artery pressure is one of the major components of the resistance calculation. The results for pulmonary artery pressure considered univariantly are

PAP (mean)	Survived	Total	%
4–8	51	59	86
9–11	60	74	81
12–14	58	77	75
15–19	41	45	91
>19	3	15	20

PAP, pulmonary artery pressure.

Table 5.5 Pulmonary Artery Pressure

shown in Table 5.5. These results suggest that pulmonary artery pressure up to 19 mmHg are still consistent with good initial outcome from a Fontan operation. In our previous report (Mayer et al. 1986), we found that patients with pulmonary artery pressure greater than 15 mmHg but with resistance less than 2 Wood units remained in a relatively low risk group, whereas the combination of elevated pulmonary artery pressure and resistance raised the risk to very high levels. In our more recent analysis, pulmonary artery pressure did have statistical significance in the multiple logistic regression model at the 0.023 level. The Mayo Clinic group also found that pulmonary artery pressure greater than 15 mmHg and pulmonary resistance more than 4 Wood units together were a significant risk factor in their analysis of 500 patients (Bartmus et al. 1990).

Based on these data, we consider patients with pulmonary vascular resistance more than 2 Wood units and pulmonary artery pressures greater than 19 mmHg to be at increased risk for Fontan operations. These limits, like all others, are not absolute; we have encountered individual patients with values that exceed either one of these limits who have survived and done well following Fontan operations.

PULMONARY ARTERY ANATOMY

The size of the pulmonary arteries was among the original selection criteria suggested by Choussat and Fontan, but the lower limits of pulmonary artery size that are compatible with successful outcome remain in dispute. It has previously been pointed out that the greatest contribution to pulmonary vascular resistance in the normal pulmonary circulation occurs at the precapillary arteriole and postcapillary venule level. However, the relative contributions of the various aspects of the pulmonary vascular bed to total resistance have not been evaluated in the nonpulsatile post-Fontan circulation. In review of our experience with Fontan operations, we were unable to collect sufficient data on pulmonary artery size to

PA Distortion	Survived	Total	%
Absent	183	215	85
Present	36	67	54

PA, pulmonary artery.

Table 5.6 Pulmonary Artery Distortion

include it in the risk factor analysis. We were, however, able to make a qualitative judgment about whether there was significant pulmonary artery distortion present that would be likely to compromise the post-Fontan circulation. This qualitative assessment was highly predictive of risk in the initial review as well as our more recent update with a P value of <0.01 in the multivariant analysis. The results considering pulmonary artery distortion alone are shown in Table 5.6. Of greater significance than the presence of distortion was the presence of residual distortion following the Fontan operation in which all 11 patients with significant distortion that could not be relieved did not survive the operation.

A number of authors have carefully examined the issue of pulmonary artery size and the outcome of a Fontan operation, but we have been unable to consider this variable in our own review because many of the early patients in our experience had inadequate angiograms to allow reliable estimation of pulmonary artery size. Nakata et al. (1984) described a method for quantifying pulmonary artery size by relating the cross-sectional area of the pulmonary arteries at the hilum to the body surface area. Based on a small series of patients, they recommended that patients with an index of less than 250 mm^2/M^2 should not undergo Fontan procedures (normal index = 330 mm^2/M^2). More recently Fontan et al. (1989a) reported the combined experience of the University of Bordeaux and the University of Alabama. In their analysis, they used the McGoon ratio (sum of the diameters of the right and left pulmonary arteries divided by the diameter of the descending aorta) and found that the risk of failure of the operation increased sharply when the ratio was less than 1.8. When the ratio was less than 1.2, the risk of death or takedown within 30 days was 55% when an atriopulmonary anastomosis was made and 34% when the right atrium was connected to a "right ventricular chamber" (in tricuspid atresia).

These results contrast with those reported by Girod et al. (1985) from the Mayo Clinic and Bridges et al. (1989) from the Children's Hospital of Philadelphia, who did not find a relationship between pulmonary artery size and the outcome of a Fontan operation. However, the Mayo Clinic group measured pulmonary artery size intraoperatively *after* any pulmonary artery reconstruction had been carried out, and the Philadelphia group reported that 24 of the 29 patients in their series underwent pulmonary artery augmentation at the time of their Fontan operation. These results in combination with our own experience with pulmonary artery distortion suggest to us that the important variable is the *postoperative* size of the pulmonary arteries. If the pulmonary arteries are "small" in discrete, surgically accessible locations and these areas are enlarged, it is likely that preoperative pulmonary artery size will not be a significant factor in the outcome of a Fontan operation. However, if the pulmonary arteries cannot be repaired, anything more than a mild stenosis is likely to affect outcome adversely.

VENTRICULAR FUNCTION

There seems to be uniform agreement that candidates for a Fontan operation should have "good" ventricular function, but currently the techniques for the quantification of ventricular function in the clinical setting remain imprecise. Most measures of systolic function such as ejection fraction or shortening fraction are both preload and afterload dependent. This factor makes it difficult to carry out meaningful comparisons among patients with the varying degrees of volume overload or systemic afterload that are present in patients before Fontan operations. Load independent variables have been described that assess the velocity of circumferential shortening compared with end systolic wall stress, but the calculation of wall stress is dependent on the ventricular geometry, which may be quite abnormal in patients with complex single ventricle anatomy.

Assessment of diastolic function in the clinical setting is equally problematic. The importance of preoperative assessments of ventricular function or postoperative function is further complicated by the significant circulatory alterations imposed by the creation of the Fontan circulation. Preoperatively, the ventricle is volume loaded (since it pumps all of the output to both the systemic and the pulmonary circulations), and total afterload is probably relatively low because the pulmonary circuit is in parallel to the systemic circuit. Postoperatively, the ventricle pumps a reduced volume, but it must provide sufficient energy to force the blood through the systemic and pulmonary resistances *in series*. To the best of my knowledge, the effects of these particular changes in loading conditions on the mechanical work performed by the heart have not been investigated.

Perhaps related to these limitations in the assessment of ventricular function as well as to the general adherence to the ejection fraction criterion suggested by Choussat et al. (1977) (ejection fraction >0.60), few investigators have been able to relate preoperative ventricular function to outcome after Fontan operations. The Mayo Clinic group (Bartmus et al. 1990) has reported that ejection fraction less than 0.60 was associated with increased risk, and Fontan et al. (1989b) found a relationship between ejection fraction and long-term outcome. We have not addressed systolic function in our studies because of the difficulties in calculating cavity volumes in abnormally shaped ventricles.

Diastolic function has been addressed only by the measurement of ventricular end diastolic pressure, and the Mayo Clinic group (Bartmus et al. 1990) found no relationship between end diastolic pressure and outcome. In their series, patients with values as high as 20 mmHg survived Fontan operations if these elevated values were associated with a significant volume load on the ventricle (large pulmonary blood flow). We have also been unable to demonstrate any relationship between end diastolic pressure and outcome. More recently, the Mayo group (Mair et al. 1989) has suggested an index of ventricular compliance that takes into account both the pulmonary and the systemic outputs that the single ventricle is pumping pre-Fontan. This variable is calculated as left ventricular end diastolic pressure divided by the sum of pulmonary and systemic blood flows, and when added to the preoperatively measured pulmonary vascular resistance, was strongly correlated with the level of postoperative right atrial pressure. Ventricular hypertrophy, which is presumably associated with diastolic abnormalities, was associated with increased operative risk in the report of Kirklin et al. (1986). Seliem et al. (1989) from the Children's Memorial Hospital in Chicago found an association between preoperative ventricular mass and the outcome of Fontan operations in 22 patients with tricuspid atresia.

OTHER FACTORS

This discussion of risk factors for Fontan operations has been centered around the original criteria suggested by Choussat et al. (1977) but some additional risk factors have been suggested, particularly the issue of anatomic diagnosis. In many of the earlier reports, it appeared that diagnoses other than tricuspid atresia were associated with an increased risk of operation, and in our previous report, we found that the presence of a normal left-sided mitral valve (as is found in tricuspid atresia, pulmonary atresia with intact septum, and some forms of single ventricle) was associated with a lower risk of operation. This variable had greater statistical weight than the diagnosis of tricuspid atresia per se (Mayer et al. 1986). Only hypoplastic left-heart syndrome was significantly associated with increased mortality. The outcome by diagnosis in our experience through June 1988 is shown in Table 5.7.

With increasing experience, this factor of anatomic diagnosis is likely to continue to decline in importance. Technical modifications have contributed significantly to a decrease in risk for morphologic categories in which the systemic venous return enters the heart on the same side as the dominant atrioventricular valve. Specifically, by constructing relatively small diameter conduit-like pathways from the inferior to superior vena cavae, obstruction of pulmonary venous drainage by baffle displacement can be avoided. Pulmonary venous obstruction and pulmonary artery distortion were the two most common causes of death in the hypoplastic left-heart patients in the experience outlined in Table 5.7. Since these data were compiled, Fontan operations have been carried out in eight additional patients with hypoplastic left-heart syndrome with six operative survivors.

Diagnosis	Survived	Total	%
Tricuspid atresia	74	85	85
Single left ventricle	62	76	82
Pulmonary atresia (IVS)	9	11	82
Heterotaxy	13	20	65
Single right ventricle	21	31	68
RV hypoplasia with VSD	26	33	79
Single ventricle (? type)	7	7	100
Hypoplastic left-heart syndrome	5	10	50

Table 5.7 Anatomic Diagnosis

DISCUSSION

Given the dismal natural history of patients with tricuspid atresia and univentricular heart, the Fontan approach continues to provide symptomatic improvement and is likely to provide an improvement in longevity as well. Therefore, it seems reasonable to offer Fontan operations to patients with single ventricle physiology for whom there are no conventional surgical options and for whom the operation can be carried out with reasonable risk. The most important factors undoubtedly continue to be the physiologic factors related to pulmonary vascular resistance and the function of the single ventricle. Anatomic factors such as anomalies of systemic and pulmonary venous drainage and proximity of the systemic and pulmonary venous pathways have already yielded to surgical ingenuity. The impact of newer techniques such as skeletal muscle cardiomyoplasty may further extend the physiologic limits to the modified Fontan approach. Continuing assessment of both short-term and long-term outcome will provide important information on which to base further modifications in our approach to the patient with single ventricle.

REFERENCES

Alboliras ET, Porter CJ, Danielson GK, et al. Results of the modified Fontan operation for congenital heart lesions in patients without preoperative sinus rhythm. J Am Coll Cardiol 1985; 6:228.

Bartmus DA, Driscoll DJ, Offord KP, et al. The modified Fontan operation for children less than 4 years old. J Am Coll Cardiol 1990; 15:429.

Bridges ND, Farrell PE, Pigott JD, Norwood WI, Chin AJ. Pulmonary artery index: A nonpredictor of operative survival in patients undergoing modified Fontan repair. Circulation 1989; 80(suppl I):216.

Choussat A, Fontan F, Besse P, Vallot F, Chauve A, Bricaud, H. Selection criteria for Fontan's procedure. In: Pediatric Cardiology, 1st ed. Anderson RN, Shinebourne EA, eds. Edinburgh: Churchill Livingstone, 1977:559.

deLeval MR, Kilner P, Gewilling M, Bull C. Total cavopulmonary connection: A logical alternative to atriopulmonary connection for complex Fontan operations. J Thorac Cardiovasc Surg 1988; 96:682.

Fontan F, Baudet E. Surgical repair of tricuspid atresia. Thorax 1971; 26:240.

Fontan F, Fernandez G, Costa F, et al. The size of the pulmonary arteries and the results of the Fontan operation. J Thorac Cardiovasc Surg 1989a; 98:711.

Fontan F, Kirklin JW, Fernandez G, et al. Outcome after a perfect Fontan operation [abstract]. Circulation 1989b; 80(suppl II):69.

Gewillig M, Lundstrom UR, Deanfield JE, et al. Impact of Fontan operation on left ventricular size and contractibility in tricuspid atresia. Circulation 1990; 81:118.

Girod DA, Rice MJ, Mair DD, et al. Relationship of pulmonary artery size to mortality in patients undergoing the Fontan operation. Circulation 1985; 72(suppl II):93.

Graham TP, Franklin RCG, Wyse RKH, Gooch V, Deanfield JE. Left ventricular wall stress and contractile function in childhood: Normal values and comparison of Fontan repair versus palliation only in patients with tricuspid atresia. Circulation 1986; 74(suppl):61.

Humes RA, Feldt RH, Porter CJ, et al. The modified Fontan operation for asplenia and polysplenia syndromes. J Thorac Cardiovasc Surg 1988; 96:212.

Kirklin JK, Blackstone EH, Kirklin JW, Pacifico AD, Bargeron LW. The Fontan operation: Ventricular hypertrophy, age, and date of operation as risk factors. J Thorac Cardiovasc Surg 1986; 92:1049.

Mair DD, Hagler DJ, Puga FJ, et al. The Fontan operation in 176 patients with tricuspid atresia: Results and a proposed new index for patient selection. Circulation 1989; 80(suppl II):69.

Mayer JE, Helgason H, Jonas RA, et al. Extending the limits for modified Fontan procedures. J Thorac Cardiovasc Surg 1986; 92:1021.

Mietus-Snyder M, Lang P, Mayer JE, et al. Childhood systemic-pulmonary shunts: Subsequent suitability of Fontan operation. Circulation 1987; 76(suppl III):39.

Nakata S, Imai Y, Takanashi Y, et al. A new method for the quantitative standardization of cross-sectional areas of the pulmonary arteries in congenital heart diseases with decreased pulmonary blood flow. J Thorac Cardiovasc Surg 1984; 88:610.

Seliem M, Muster AJ, Paul MH, Benson DW. Relation between preoperative left ventricular muscle mass and outcome of the Fontan procedure in patients with tricuspid atresia. J Am Coll Cardiol 1989; 14:750.

6

Heart Transplantation in Children with Cardiomyopathies

Vaughn A. Starnes, Joan L. Miller, Patricia L. Gamberg, Daniel Bernstein, David Baum, and Norman E. Shumway

Heart transplantation has gained acceptance as therapy for end-stage heart disease due to either cardiomyopathies or structural defects (Starnes et al. 1987; Baum et al. 1981; Fricker et al. 1987). At most centers, initial heart transplantation experience in children was in those with cardiomyopathies. As more experience has been gained, younger children with more complex heart lesions have undergone heart transplantation. This trend is evident by reports from the early 1980s as compared with more recent reports (Pennington et al. 1985; Starnes et al. 1989). From the experience of transplanting children with cardiomyopathies and complex congenital heart disease has come evidence that children with congenital heart disease represent a higher risk group.

We report our experience since 1980 in children undergoing heart transplantation for cardiomyopathies and make comparisons to the group transplanted for congenital heart disease.

MATERIALS AND METHODS

Since 1980, 51 children from the newborn period to 18 years have undergone heart transplantation. Of these 51 children, 37 (74%) underwent heart transplantation for cardiomyopathies. There were 18 boys and 19 girls, with ages ranging from 3 months to 18 years. Average follow-up was 3.7 years, with a range of 6 months to 8.5 years.

Cardiomyopathies were idiopathic in 23 (62%), viral in eight (22%), familial in three (8%) , and due to doxorubicin (Adriamycin) toxicity in three (8%). The three children with Adriamycin toxicity are free from recurrent tumor (lymphoma) 8, 31, and 35 months following transplantation.

RECIPIENT AND DONOR SELECTION

Recipients consisted of children with intractable heart failure with a limited life expectancy (<1 year). In addition, recipients were without hepatic and renal dysfunction and any systemic illness that could be potentially aggravated by immunosuppression.

Pulmonary vasculature was assessed with pretransplantation cardiac catheterization. As noted in Table 6.1, pulmonary artery systolic pressure ranged from 24 to 50 mmHg, with a diastolic pressure ranging from 15 to 33 mmHg. The calculated pulmonary vascular resistance index (PVRI) ranged from 0.3 to 5.6 L/min/m². The average PVRI was 3.9 ± 2.7 L/min/m². In children with elevated PVRI (≥4.0), pulmonary vasoreactivity was assessed either with administered of FIO_2 or pulmonary vasodilation (sodium nitroprusside or prostaglandin E_1 [PGE_1]). Being a

Patient	Age at Transplant	PA Pressure (mmHg)	PVRI (L/min)/m²
1	14	42/32/36	3.5
2	14	49/29/33	2.3
3	12	38/23/28	0.3
4	9	50/33/35	5.6
5	2	30/20/24	1.9
6	11	50/25/35	—
7	7	35/15/22	4.0
8	12	50/28/38	3.8
9	5	—	2.5
10	3	45/28/36	5.5
11	3	38/26/32	5.2
12	3	24/16/18	3.3
		Mean ± SD	3.9 ± 2.7

*Hemodynamic data of recipients before transplantation.
Abbreviations: PA, pulmonary artery; PVRI, pulmonary vascular resistance index.

Table 6.1 Stanford Cardiac Transplantation: Pediatric Transplantation with Cardiomyopathies*

calculated index, the PVRI provided only estimations of the likelihood of right ventricular failure in the transplanted heart. Other parameters analyzed for the suitability of the potential recipient involved duration of illness, associated valvular disease, and nutritional status of the patient. Pulmonary resistance calculations were particularly treacherous in children with shunts, previous cardiac operations, valvular disease, and pulmonary artery stenosis due to structural or congenital abnormalities.

Donors were selected according to ABO blood group, size, and absence of cardiac dysfunction. Most infant donors were resuscitated victims of child abuse and sudden infant death syndrome. These infants were evaluated with ECG, need for inotropic support, and detailed echocardiograms. Cardiac resuscitation in the donor did not preclude successful transplantation if careful evaluation was performed. Donors were usually as large as the prospective recipients; however, large discrepancies in weight have been reported between donor and recipient, provided that cardiac size is determined in the donor and recipient to be similar (Mavroudis et al. 1988).

OPERATIVE TECHNIQUE AND POSTOPERATIVE MANAGEMENT

Cardiac transplantation was performed using hypothermic cardiopulmonary bypass (25° to 28°C). Profound hypothermia (15° to 18°C) with circulatory arrest was not needed owing to structurally normal great vessels and absence of anomalous venous drainage. Cardiopulmonary bypass was discontinued, with the transplanted heart supported on dopamine, 5 to 7 μg/kg/min, and isoproterenol, 25 to 75 ng/kg/min. Pulmonary catheter inserted through the right ventricle in small children (<10 kg) and transvenously in older children was used in the postoperative period. Pulmonary vasoreactivity was prevalent in children less than 1 year, often requiring either sodium nitroprusside or PGE_1, 25 to 100 ng/kg/min. Mean graft ischemia time was 187 minutes, with a range of 95 minutes to 495 minutes with all grafts functioning well at termination of cardiopulmonary bypass.

IMMUNOSUPPRESSION

A three-drug protocol of cyclosporine, azathioprine, and prednisone was used. Preoperatively, children received cyclosporine, 3 to 5 μg/kg by mouth 3 hours before transplantation, and azathioprine, 4 μg/kg intravenously. On discontinuation of cardiopulmonary bypass, 10 mg/kg of methylprednisolone was administered. Postoperatively, cyclosporine was given in divided daily doses of 150 to 250 ng/ml to maintain a serum level by radioimmunoassay; azathioprine, 1 to 3 mg/kg/day to maintain leukocyte tolerance (WBC >4000 cells/ml); and prednisone, 0.6 mg/kg/day in divided doses, with a taper to 0.2 mg/kg/day by 6 weeks. Secondary to poor growth, children were converted to alternate-day steroids by 6 months if tolerated, and attempts were made to discontinue steroids at 12 months.

The murine monoclonal antibody, OKT_3^R, was used during the first 2 weeks following transplantation. The dose was adjusted over time, and currently 0.1 to 0.2 mg/kg/day of OKT_3 is given to pediatric patients. Total lymphocyte count was monitored, and this level was maintained at 5% to 10%. OKT_3 was substituted for rabbit antithymocyte globulin (RATG) in our current protocol.

DIAGNOSIS AND TREATMENT OF REJECTION

Children over 1 year of age underwent routine cardiac biopsies. The Billingham criteria for determination of the presence and severity of rejection was employed (Caves et al. 1973). Cardiac rejection was treated if myocyte necrosis was present on biopsy.

Cardiac rejection in children was treated with methylprednisolone, 15 mg/kg intravenously, with a follow-up biopsy performed to document clearance of the rejection episode. If after two courses of methylprednisolone rejection persisted, retreatment with OKT_3 or treatment with RATG was used.

Infants and toddlers underwent biopsies only when clinically indicated. Noninvasive methods of echocardiography, voltage changes on the ECG, and clinical signs were used to assess cardiac rejection. Viral-like syndromes, however, often confused the issue of rejection or infection, and a biopsy was performed.

STATISTICAL ANALYSIS

Actuarial curves were computed by the method of Kaplan and Meier (1958) and compared by the method of Gehan (1965). Linearized rates were compared with the maximum likelihood ratio (Gross and Clark, 1975). Actuarial curves and linearized rates were expressed as the mean ±1 standard deviation.

RESULTS

□ Survival

Thirty-seven children have undergone heart transplantation for end-stage cardiomyopathy. Actuarial survival (Figure 6.1) was 84%, 80%, and 77% at 1, 2, and 5 years, respectively. In comparison, children with congenital heart disease undergoing transplantation had inferior survival. The congenital heart group undergoing transplantation had an actuarial survival of 69%, 61%, and 61% at 1, 2, and 5 years, respectively (Figure 6.2). This difference was related to the early mortality rate associated with pulmonary hypertension. Of the six deaths occurring in children who underwent transplantation for congenital heart disease, three (50%) resulted from right ventricular dysfunction in the donor graft secondary to pulmonary hypertension.

Eight deaths occurred in children with cardiomyopathies owing to infection (three), rejection (two), pulmonary hypertension (two), and late coronary atherosclerosis (one).

As noted, survival in children undergoing transplantation for cardiomyopathies was good. Deaths occurring in the cardiomyopathy group occurred generally in the first year.

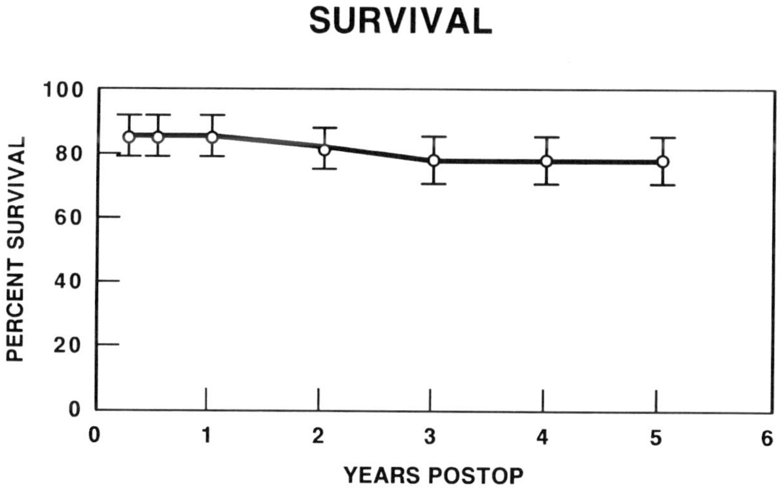

Figure 6.1 Actuarial survival of children undergoing heart transplantation for cardiomyopathies.

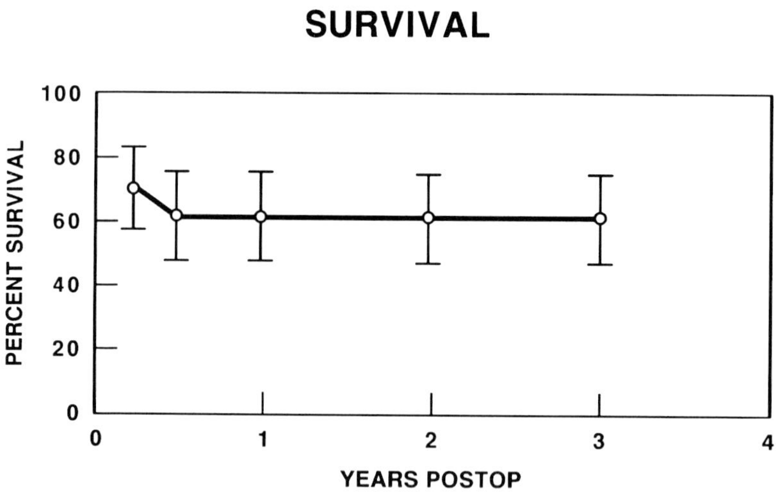

Figure 6.2 Actuarial survival of children undergoing heart transplantation for congenital heart disease.

□ Rejection

Allograft rejection was as frequent in children as in adults, with the possible exception of the children less than 1 year of age. The linearized rejection rate (events per 100 patient days) was 1.56 during the first 2 postoperative months, as compared with 2.31 and 1.52 in adults (P = N.S.). At the end of the third postoperative month, only 33% of children had never rejected. Again, a similar trend was noted in adults. With an average follow-up of 3.9 years, each child had an average of 2.7 ± 1.7 allograft rejection episodes. Two children successfully underwent total lymphoid irradiation for refractory allograft rejection. After irradiation, the first child was free of allograft rejection for 23 months before another episode occurred, and the last child has remained free from rejection for 15 months.

□ Hemodynamic Data and Coronary Anatomy

Annual cardiac catheterization has been part of the protocol since the recognition of accelerated coronary disease in the transplanted heart. Each child underwent annual catheterization with coronary angiograms. At cardiac catheterization, all children had normal hemodynamics. Mean pulmonary artery pressure and left ventricular end diastolic pressure were 10.0 ± 3.8 mmHg and 10.4 ± 3.1 mmHg, respectively. Mean cardiac index was 3.6 ± 1.4 L/min/m^2. Mild coronary disease was detected in four long-term survivors, and severe coronary disease was detected in one. Actuarial freedom from coronary disease was 97%, 89%, and 78% at 1, 3, and 5 years, respectively. All coronary disease occurred in children older than 10 years at transplantation. Four (80%) of the five children with coronary disease demonstrated only mild disease.

□ Rehabilitation

Twenty-nine children are currently alive. There are no physical limitations in any, and 100% are functioning in school and occupations.

DISCUSSION

Heart transplantation in children with cardiomyopathy has proved successful. Since 1981, 37 children have undergone transplantation at Stanford for cardiomyopathy. Actuarial survival at 1 and 5 years is 84% and 76%, respectively. At Stanford, survival in children has been equal to that of adults undergoing heart transplantation. Of note, the experience with heart transplantation for congenital heart disease has had somewhat inferior results with a 1- and 5-year survival of 69% and 61%, respectively. The estimation of pulmonary vascular resistance in children with shunts, altered pulmonary anatomy, and valvular disease represents the greatest uncertainty when evaluating a child with congenital heart disease. As further clinical experience has gained, survival with congenital heart disease will ultimately improve.

After periods of follow-up extending to 8 years, all the children have had normal hemodynamics with normal cardiac indices. The uncertainty arises with coronary artery disease. We have detected four children (20%) with mild coronary artery disease and one child with severe disease (5%) in need of retransplantation. Most coronary disease, however, has been mild (4/5, 80%) and has occurred in the older children. Etiologic factors have been proposed, with the most convincing data being the association of coronary artery disease occurrence and infection with cytomegaloviral disease (Grattan et al. 1989). Questions regarding optimal immunosuppression for prevention of graft rejection must also be posed for the prevention of coronary disease. Steroid-sparing protocols may predispose children to later graft atherosclerosis. The converse, inclusion of steroids, may also be true. At present, these questions remain unanswered and represent part of the challenge of caring for a child with a heart transplant. Although morbidities associated with heart transplantation are recognized, the overwhelming rehabilitation rate and quality of life of children with heart transplantations outweigh these morbid events.

REFERENCES

Baum D, Stinson EB, Shumway NE. The place for heart transplantation in children. In Godman MJ, ed. Pediatric Cardiology. New York: Churchill-Livingstone, 1981:741.

Caves PK, Stinson EB, Billingham ME, Shumway NE. Diagnosis of human cardiac allograft rejection by serial cardiac biopsy. J Thorac Cardiovasc Surg 1973; 66:461.

Fricker FJ, Griffith BP, Hardesty RL, et al. Experience with heart transplantation in children. Pediatrics 1987; 79:138.

Gehan EA. Generalized Wilcoxon test for comparing arbitrary singly-censored samples. Biometrics 1965; 52:203.

Grattan MT, Moreno-Cabral CE, Starnes VA, et al. Cytomegalovirus infection is associated with cardiac allograft rejection and atherosclerosis. JAMA 1989; 261(24):3561.

Gross AJ, Clark VA. Survival distribution: Reliability applications in the biomedical sciences. New York: Wiley, 1975:331.

Kaplan EL, Meier P. Nonparametric estimations from incomplete observation. J Am Stat Assoc 1958; 53:457.

Mavroudis C, Harrison H, Klein JB, et al. Infant orthotopic cardiac transplantation. J Thorac Cardiovasc Surg 1988; 96:912.

Pennington DG, Sarafrin J, Swartz M: Heart transplantation in children. J Heart Transplant 1985; 4:441.

Starnes VA, Bernstein D, Oyer PE, et al. Heart transplantation in children. J Heart Transplant 1989; 8(1):20.

Starnes VA, Stinson EB, Oyer PE, et al. Cardiac transplantation in children and adolescents. Circulation 1987; 76(suppl):43.

7

Reoperation after Initial Repair of Tetralogy of Fallot: Correction of Residual or Recurrent Defects

Carl L. Backer
Farouk S. Idriss

□

Since the first complete repair of tetralogy of Fallot was performed by Lillehei in 1954 (Lillehei et al. 1955), a tremendous volume of information has been accumulated with regard to the management of children with tetralogy of Fallot. Ongoing reevaluation of operative results with critical review has made possible precise intraoperative decision making based on accurate preoperative angiographic assessment (Blackstone et al. 1979). Improvements in the initial operative management of these patients has decreased the incidence of reoperation for residual or recurrent defects with respect to time (Table 7.1). Reoperation rates in reviews beginning prior to 1963 range from 4.8% to 13.3% (Fuster et al. 1980; Zhao et al. 1985; Lillehei et al. 1986). Reoperation rates in reviews beginning after 1963 range from 1.8% to 4.4% (Donahoo et al. 1974; Poirier et al. 1977; Katz et al. 1982). This improvement is certainly multifactorial in etiology, and the multiple different factors responsible are evaluated in detail. The total number of operative survivors in these six series was 1838 patients, with 96 reoperations for an overall reoperation rate of 5.2%. Mortality of reoperation is not insignificant and ranges from 12% to 26% (see Table 7.1). The average mortality in these six series was 17%. This makes avoidance of reoperation, if possible, of critical importance at the time of initial repair.

Indications for reoperation vary from institution to institution (see Table 7.2) (Castaneda et al. 1974; Uretzky et al. 1982; Backer and Idriss unpublished data). In a summation of seven different series, the most common indications for reoperation were residual ventricular septal defect (VSD), residual right ventricular outflow tract obstruction (RVOTO) or a combination of the two. Other common

Author	Period	Patients	Reoperation	Mortality
Lillehei et al. (1986)	1954–60	106	10 (9.4%)	2 (20%)
Fuster et al. (1980)	1955–64	396	19 (4.8%)	5 (26%)
Zhao et al. (1985)	1960–82	294	39 (13.3%)	5 (13%)
Donahoo et al. (1974)	1963–74	343	15 (4.4%)	2 (13%)
Poirier et al. (1977)	1964–70	285	5 (1.8%)	1 (20%)
Katz et al. (1982)	1967–77	414	8 (1.9%)	1 (12%)
Total		1883	96 (5.2%)	16 (17%)

Table 7.1 Incidence of Reoperation and Mortality after Intracardiac Repair of Tetralogy of Fallot

indications for reoperation were pulmonary insufficiency requiring pulmonary valve replacement, right ventricular outflow tract aneurysm, tricuspid insufficiency requiring tricuspid valve repair or replacement, atrial septal defect, and stenotic pulmonary arteries. Unusual indications for reoperation were collateral vessels requiring ligation, residual surgical shunts, heart block requiring pacemaker, and tachycardia intractable to medical management.

INDICATIONS FOR REOPERATION AND SURGICAL TECHNIQUES

□ Residual Ventricular Septal Defect

In seven large series of children with tetralogy of Fallot, reoperation for a residual or recurrent VSD was the most common indication for reoperation (Figure 7.1). A VSD was present in 91 of 256 reoperations (36% of reoperations). As techniques of myocardial protection have improved, more precise closure of the VSD has become possible, resulting in fewer recurrences. In Fuster's review of the Mayo Clinic experience from 1955 to 1964 (Fuster et al. 1980), 14 of 396 patients (3.5%) had residual VSDs. In Poirier's review of the Mayo Clinic experience from 1964 through 1970 (Poirier et al. 1977), only five of 285 patients (1.7%) had residual VSDs. In Katz's review of patients operated on from 1967 through 1977 at the University of Alabama (Katz et al. 1982), only 2 of 414 patients (0.5%) had a residual VSD.

A significant residual VSD was generally defined as one causing a pulmonary to systemic flow ratio (Qp/Qs) of 1.5 or greater. However, as Uretzky pointed out in his review of the Mayo Clinic experience (Uretzky et al. 1982), absolute criteria for reoperation are difficult to establish, and every patient should be evaluated

	Lillehei et al. (1986)	Uretzky et al. (1982)	Zhao et al. (1985)	Donahoo et al. (1974)	Katz et al. (1982)	Castaneda et al. (1974)	CMH (unpublished)	Total
VSD closure	2	33	12	9	2	9	3	70
PVR		8	11		1		37	57
RVOTO	3	11	12	4	1	7	8	46
VSD + RVOTO	2					19		21
RV aneurysm	1	5	6		3	5	1	21
TVR	1	6	5	2			1	15
ASD closure	1	3	3				1	8
PA reconstruction					1		4	5
Shunt closure		3	2					5
Collateral ligation			2				1	3
Pacemaker							3	3
Arrhythmia							2	2

Abbreviations: ASD, atrial septal defect; PA, pulmonary artery; PVR, pulmonary valve replacement; RV, right ventricle; RVOTO, right ventricular outflow tract obstruction; TVR, tricuspid valve replacement; VSD, ventricular septal defect.

Table 7.2 Procedures Performed at the Time of Reoperation for Residual or Recurrent Defects after Initial Repair of Tetralogy of Fallot

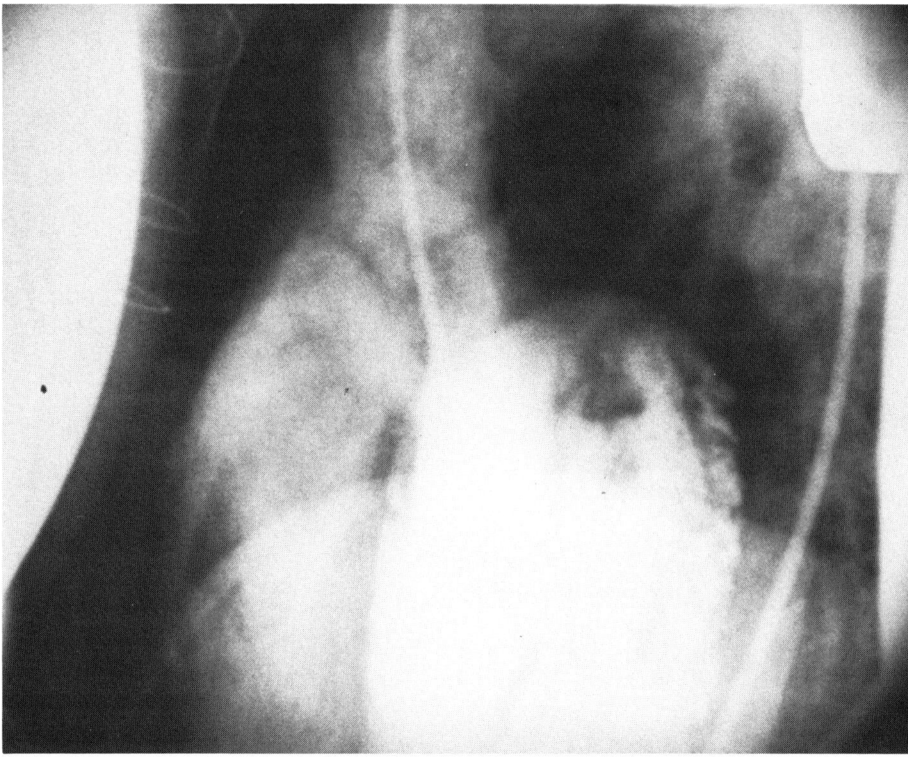

Figure 7.1 Left ventriculogram in a patient who underwent previous complete repair of tetralogy of Fallot. There is a significant shunt at the inferior portion of the VSD patch directed into the right ventricular outflow tract.

individually. In the Mayo experience, no clear correlation existed between symptomatic status and Qp/Qs. One patient with isolated residual VSD who was in functional class III had a Qp:Qs ratio of only 1.3 and became asymptomatic after reoperation. A small residual shunt may not be well tolerated after repair of tetralogy of Fallot, particularly if it is associated with other residual defects.

The importance of precise and accurate closure of the VSD at time of tetralogy repair was emphasized in the Stanford experience reported by Zhao (Zhao et al. 1985). Of 294 operative survivors of tetralogy of Fallot repair operated on between 1960 and 1982, 12 required reoperation for residual VSD, and this was identified as an incremental risk factor for late death.

The most common location for a residual VSD is in the posterior-inferior quadrant near the area of the conduction tissue. The next most common site of patch disruption is in the anterior-superior quadrant. This area is near the site of infundibular resection and may be related to loss of endocardium. The technique of closure of the VSD at the initial repair is of crucial importance. Pacifico (1989) has used a Dacron patch with continuous suture of 4–0 prolene. At the Children's Memorial Hospital in Chicago, we have used interrupted pledgeted sutures and a Dacron patch. The oxygen saturation of the right atrial blood should be compared with the oxygen saturation of the pulmonary artery blood. If there is more than a 10% step-up from the right atrium to pulmonary artery, a residual VSD should be suspected and repaired. If available, intraoperative echocardiography is useful to diagnose the residual VSD and identify its location.

Any patient with pulmonary dysfunction after repair of tetralogy of Fallot should be suspected of having a residual VSD. Patients discharged from the hospital who later have symptoms of exercise tolerance or congestive heart failure should also be suspected of having a residual VSD. Initial investigation for both groups should be with color Doppler echocardiography. This provides evidence confirming the presence or absence of a ventricular level shunt. If a VSD is demonstrated, left ventricular angiography with measurement of the pulmonary to systemic flow ratio is required.

The operative approach to a residual VSD is through a repeat median sternotomy. Using a chisel and hammer to open the sternum, the incidence of complications of repeat sternotomy at Children's Memorial Hospital have been less than 5% (DeLeon et al. 1986). Extracorporeal circulation is initiated using bicaval cannulation. The aorta is cross clamped and cold blood cardioplegia delivered in the aortic root to the coronary arteries. The left side of the heart is vented through the right superior pulmonary vein. The right atrium is opened, and the residual VSD is exposed with a quiet heart and bloodless field. Unless the defect is caused by obvious patch disruption, it should be closed with a separate Dacron patch, anchored in place with interrupted pledgeted sutures. The temptation for direct suture closure of residual defects should be avoided.

In Castaneda's review (Castaneda et al. 1974), 29 patients had repair of a residual VSD, all through a right atriotomy approach. The technique of closure was resuture of the original patch to the septal rim in 18 of the 29 patients (62%), insertion of a new patch in seven patients (24%), and total replacement of a completely disrupted patch in two patients (7%). In 19 of the 29 patients, disruption of the patch suture line was located at the posterior-inferior quadrant. Two of the 29 patients have a small residual VSD. Mortality in this series was two of 40 patients (5%).

□ Residual Right Ventricular Outflow Tract Obstruction

At most institutions, repair of residual RVOTO is the second most common indication for reoperation after initial repair of tetralogy of Fallot. In about one third of these patients, an associated VSD was also present. The obstruction can be at any of several levels: The infundibulum, the pulmonary annulus, the main pulmonary artery and bifurcation, or the branch pulmonary arteries. Diagnosis is suggested by Doppler echocardiography, but should be confirmed by cardiac catheterization. A peak systolic pressure gradient greater than 50 mmHg is considered significant and is generally considered an indication for reoperation, especially if the patient is symptomatic. In Uretzky's series from the Mayo Clinic (Uretzky et al. 1982), 11 of 41 patients undergoing reoperation after correction of tetralogy of Fallot had relief of a residual right ventricular outflow tract gradient. The right ventricular outflow tract gradient ranged from 51 to 88 mmHg before reoperation. The mean intraoperative $P_{RV/LV}$ after the initial repair was 0.72, and the mean $P_{RV/LV}$ at the time of catheterization was 0.89. In this series, there was no correlation between the severity of the right ventricular outflow tract gradient and the symptoms of the patient before reoperation.

In Castaneda's series of 40 patients undergoing reoperation for tetralogy of Fallot (Castaneda et al. 1974), 31 required opening of the right ventricular outflow tract. The site of residual obstruction was the infundibulum in 16 (51%), the valve annulus in eight (26%), and the pulmonary valve in seven (22%). At the time of the first operation, 21 patients had only infundibuloplasty, and 10 had an outflow patch. At the time of reoperation, 17 patients had an outflow patch, seven had valvotomy, and seven had extension of the outflow patch (five distal, two proximal).

In Zhao's series from Stanford (Zhao et al. 1985), of 39 reoperations, 18 were for residual RVOTO. Statistical analysis showed that extent of right ventricular outflow tract patch predicted likelihood of reoperation. If a right ventricular and/or a separate pulmonary arterial patch was used, the likelihood of reoperation at 10 years was 6%. If no right ventricular outflow tract patch was used, 11% of patients required reoperation by 10 years. If a transannular patch was used, 21% of patients required reoperation by 10 years.

Kirklin et al. have emphasized the importance of intraoperative measurement of the $P_{RV/LV}$ during the initial repair of tetralogy of Fallot (Kirklin and Blackstone 1980). They state that residual pulmonary stenosis of an amount resulting in a $P_{RV/LV}$ late postoperatively equal to or less than 0.65 to 0.70 is an acceptable post-repair $P_{RV/LV}$. Severe residual stenosis is a risk factor for reoperation, and to avoid this a transannular patch with its compromise of pulmonary incompetence is preferable.

At the Children's Memorial Hospital, we have liberally used a two-patch technique of patching the infundibulum and the pulmonary artery separately without crossing the valve annulus. Eight patients have required reoperation for residual RVOTO in the past 10 years (Backer and Idriss unpublished data).

The surgical techniques used depend on the level of obstruction. As with VSD closure, cardiopulmonary bypass with bicaval cannulation is employed. If there are residual intracardiac shunts, the heart should be electrically fibrillated or the aorta cross-clamped prior to opening the heart. The residual defects should then be closed and attention given to evacuating air from the heart prior to allowing the heart to beat. If the obstruction is at the infundibular level only, this can be managed by a longitudinal incision in the right ventricular outflow tract to just below the pulmonary valve annulus, provided that there is not anomalous origin of the anterior descending from the right coronary artery. The parietal and septal insertions of the infundibular septum are partially excised and the area patched with Dacron or Polytetrafluoroethylene (W. L. Gore & Associates, Inc., Elkton, MD). If an anomalous coronary artery is present, a conduit should be placed from the right ventricle to the pulmonary artery. If there is residual pulmonary valve stenosis, commissurotomy should be performed and the annulus size measured. If this dimension is smaller than 2 standard deviations from the mean normal value (Rowlatt et al. 1963), either a valve leaflet should be excised or the incision carried across the annulus. Distal pulmonary stenosis is best repaired with autologous pericardium, which can usually be harvested even at reoperation. Stenosis of the left pulmonary artery can be enlarged by extending the incision in the main pulmonary artery out to the left pulmonary artery. This can be carried to the branching of the left pulmonary artery if necessary. Reconstruction of the right pulmonary artery may require transection of the ascending aorta to facilitate exposure.

□ Pulmonary Insufficiency

Incompetence of the pulmonary valve is very common after intracardiac repair of tetralogy of Fallot (Figure 7.2). In particular, it is present in all patients who have had transannular patching as part of the repair and in those who have had excision

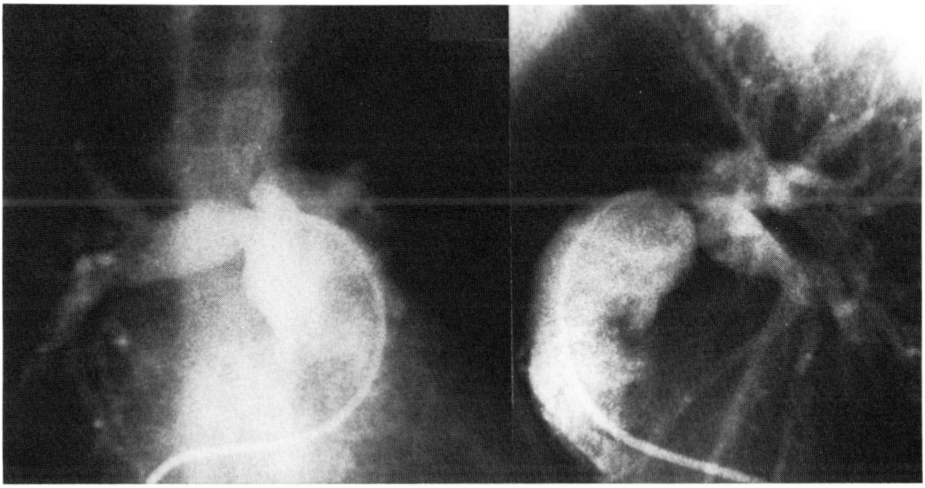

Figure 7.2 Pulmonary angiogram in a patient who underwent prior complete intracardiac repair of tetralogy of Fallot. There is four-plus regurgitation into the right ventricle, especially apparent on the lateral view. This patient required insertion of a pulmonary valve because of progressive cardiomegaly.

of a valve leaflet. Quantification of pulmonary insufficiency is difficult, but an assessment can be obtained by serial heart size on chest roentgenogram, color Doppler echocardiography, and, of course, cardiac catheterization. At Children's Memorial Hospital, we have employed serial exercise studies as a useful adjunct to the clinical and hemodynamic evaluation or tetralogy patients post-intracardiac repair (Wessel et al. 1980). Wessel et al. (1980) showed that exercise scores were significantly higher in 17 patients without angiographic evidence of pulmonary insufficiency than in 33 patients with definite pulmonary insufficiency by angiography.

The management of pulmonary insufficiency following initial repair of tetralogy of Fallot is controversial. Some surgeons believe that pulmonary valve replacement is almost never required and that pulmonary insufficiency is very well tolerated by the right ventricle for long periods of time. In the Mayo Clinic experience reported by Poirier et al. (1977), in 285 patients followed after repair of tetralogy of Fallot, no patient had a result classified as less than ideal because of pulmonary valvular insufficiency. There were no patients in their series who died or underwent reoperation because of this lesion. The experimental study of Ellison et al. (1970) showed that isolated pulmonary insufficiency in the dog is well tolerated unless it is associated with other defects such as a left to right shunt. The Mayo Clinic group recommended use of a valve only for patients with pulmonary insufficiency associated with impaired pulmonary artery runoff caused by peripheral stenosis, vascular obstructive disease, single pulmonary artery, or absent pulmonary valve with aneurysm of the central pulmonary artery.

At Children's Memorial Hospital, we have been somewhat more liberal than other institutions with regard to pulmonary valve insertion for pulmonary insufficiency. Ilbawi et al. (1986) reported 49 patients who underwent porcine valve insertion for pulmonary insufficiency between 1975 and 1985. The primary indications for valve implantation were progressive cardiomegaly and evidence of right ventricular dilatation or dysfunction. The previously mentioned experience with exercise testing reported by Wessel also influenced decisions to implant pulmonary valves for pulmonary insufficiency. There was one hospital death in this series (2%), and the functional actuarial life for the valves was 84% at 10 years.

Bove et al. (1983) also reported on the adverse effects of pulmonary insufficiency. They studied a group of 20 patients with pulmonary insufficiency with serial radionuclide angiography. They concluded that patients with clinically significant pulmonary insufficiency following repair of tetralogy of Fallot have impaired ventricular function late after operation. They recommended serial prospective assessment of right ventricular function in patients with pulmonary insufficiency following repair of tetralogy of Fallot to provide guidelines for future pulmonary valve replacement.

Misbach, Turley, and Ebert (1983) reported on 12 patients who had pulmonary valve replacement for pulmonary insufficiency following tetralogy of Fallot repair. All patients had progressive right ventricular failure not responsive to medical management. There was no mortality in their series, and they concluded that pulmonary valve replacement carries a low risk and prevents further deterioration of right ventricular function. Finck, Puga, and Danielson (1988) also concluded that pulmonary valve insertion should be considered during reoperation for tetralogy of Fallot when pulmonary insufficiency and right ventricular failure are present.

The technical details of pulmonary valve replacement at our institution were well detailed by Ilbawi et al. (1986). A median sternotomy approach was used in all patients. The procedure was performed using cardiopulmonary bypass, moderate hypothermia, and hemodilution. Bicaval cannulation was employed, the left side was vented, and coronary perfusion was not interrupted unless there was a residual intracardiac shunt, as described earlier. The right ventricular outflow tract was opened longitudinally to open all residual stenoses. A large patch of Dacron or Polytetrafluoroethylene was used enlarge the main pulmonary artery. The largest appropriate porcine valve was chosen and sutured posteriorly to the remnants of the pulmonary valve annulus using interrupted mattress sutures. A second path was used to enlarge the ventricular side of the incision. Closure was completed by suturing the free ends of the pulmonary and ventricular patches to the anterior aspect of the valve. Ilbawi noted that the incidence of bioprosthesis failure is much higher when the annulus diameter is less than 25 mm and becomes negligible with diameters of 27 mm or more.

□ Right Ventricular Aneurysm

A significant mediastinal mass can be formed by an aneurysm of the right ventricular infundibular patch following repair of tetralogy of Fallot (Figure 7.3). This occurs in somewhat fewer than 1% of patients following tetralogy repair. It can either be a false aneurysm as described by Rosenthal et al. (1972) or a true aneurysm of the right ventricular patch, particularly if pericardium is used, as noted by Seybold-Epting et al. (1977). In Rosenthal's series, of 135 patients in whom the right ventricular outflow tract was reconstructed with the use of autogenous pericardial tissue, eight (6%) developed an aneurysm of the patch. Six of the lesions were true aneurysms, and two were false. Pseudoaneurysms tend to increase rapidly in size and usually require operation soon after diagnosis. The development of right ventricular aneurysms seems more related to persistent right ventricular hypertension following repair than to the type of material used for the patch. In Castaneda's series (Castaneda et al. 1974), five of 40 patients having reoperation after repair of tetralogy of Fallot had a right ventricular aneurysm. Three had a true aneurysm, and two had false aneurysms. The residual right ventricular outflow tract gradient in these five patients was 60, 70, 80, and 100 mmHg. Similarly, Uretzky's group of 41 patients having reoperation after tetralogy of Fallot repair had five patients with a right ventricular aneurysm. The mean $P_{RV/LV}$ was 0.97. In three of their patients, the right ventricle had been closed primarily (Uretzky et al. 1982).

sudden death in seven of 243 patients followed for an average of 12 years after repair of tetralogy of Fallot. In his review, 30% of patients with right bundle branch block *and* premature ventricular contractions experienced sudden death. Likewise, 30% of patients with trifascicular block died suddenly. As Miller noted in the discussion of the Stanford experience (Zhao et al. 1985), aggressive electrophysiologic investigation of any patient with simple or complex arrhythmias is recommended regardless of symptoms.

Harken et al. (1980) reported the case histories of two patients with multiple episodes of ventricular tachycardia following complete repair of tetralogy of Fallot. Neither pharmacologic nor pacing regimens prevented the tachycardia. The source of the tachycardia was localized to the right ventricular scar by transvenous electrophysiologic mapping. Under extracorporeal circulation, epicardial mapping was performed to confirm sites of earliest electrical activity in the right ventricular outflow tract. In both patients, the former ventricular incision was widely excised and replaced with a pericardial patch. Ventricular tachycardia was not inducible following operation and has not clinically recurred. At Children's Memorial Hospital (Backer and Idriss unpublished data), we have performed similar operations in two patients. One did extremely well and was not inducible after surgery. The second patient had severe preoperative right ventricular dysfunction and died postoperatively of low cardiac output despite circulatory support with ECMO. If medical therapy fails, operation combined with extensive preoperative and intraoperative electrophysiologic studies may be a realistic option in the treatment of selected patients with ventricular tachycardia following complete repair of tetralogy of Fallot.

DISCUSSION

Tremendous advances have been achieved in the surgical management of patients with tetralogy of Fallot. In the current era, the incidence of reoperation for residual or recurrent defects following initial intracardiac repair is approximately 5%. The mortality rate of reoperation is approximately 15%.

Relatively common indications for reoperation include residual VSD with symptoms or a shunt greater than 1.5:1, residual right ventricular outflow tract gradient of more than 50 mmHg, pulmonary insufficiency with progressive right ventricular dysfunction, and right ventricular aneurysm. Less common indications for reoperation are tricuspid insufficiency, residual atrial septal defect, peripheral pulmonary artery stenosis, residual surgical shunts, collaterals, heart block, and ventricular arrhythmias.

Attention to surgical details at the initial operation can greatly decrease the need for reoperation in patients with tetralogy of Fallot.

REFERENCES

Backer CL, Idriss FS. Reoperation after repair of tetralogy of Fallot 1980–1990 at the Children's Memorial Hospital. Unpublished data.

Blackstone EH, Kirklin JW, Bertranou EG, et al. Preoperative prediction from cineangiograms of post repair right ventricular pressure in tetralogy of Fallot. J Thorac Cardiovasc Surg 1979; 78:542.

Bove EL, Byrum CJ, Thomas FC, et al. The influence of pulmonary insufficiency on ventricular function following repair of tetralogy of Fallot. Evaluation using radionuclide ventriculography. J Thorac Cardiovasc Surg 1983; 85:691.

Castaneda AR, Sade RM, Lamberti J, Nicoloff DM. Reoperation for residual defects after repair of tetralogy of Fallot. Surgery 1974; 76:1010.

DeLeon SY, LoCicero J III, Ilbawi MN, Idriss FS. Repeat median sternotomy in pediatrics. Experience in 164 consecutive cases. Ann Thorac Surg 1986; 41:184.

Donahoo JS, Brawley RK, Gott VL, Haller JA. Reoperation after total correction of tetralogy of Fallot. J Thorac Cardiovasc Surg 1974; 68:466.

Ellison RG, Brown WJ Jr, Yeh TJ, Hamilton WF. Surgical significance of acute and chronic pulmonary valvular insufficiency. J Thorac Cardiovasc Surg 1970; 60:549.

Finck SJ, Puga FJ, Danielson GK. Pulmonary valve insertion durıng reoperation for tetralogy of Fallot. Ann Thorac Surg 1988; 45:610.

Fuster V, McGoon DC, Kennedy MA, Ritter DC, Kirklin JW. Long-term evaluation (12 to 22 years) of open heart surgery for tetralogy of Fallot. Am J Cardiol 1980; 46:635.

Harken AH, Horowitz LN, Josephson ME. Surgical correction of recurrent sustained ventricular tachycardia following complete repair of tetralogy of Fallot. J Thorac Cardiovasc Surg 1980; 80:779.

Ilbawi MN, Idriss FS, DeLeon SY, et al. Long term results of porcine valve insertion for pulmonary regurgitation following repair of tetralogy of Fallot. Ann Thorac Surg 1986; 41:478.

James FW, Kaplan S. Sudden unexpected cardiac arrest in patients after surgical correction for tetralogy of Fallot. Am J Cardiol 1975; 35:146.

Katz NM, Blackstone EH, Kirklin JW, Pacifico AD, Bargeron LM Jr. Late survival and symptoms after repair of tetralogy of Fallot. Circulation 1982; 65:403.

Kirklin JW, Barratt-Boyes BG. Cardiac Surgery. Toronto: Wiley, 1986:767.

Kirklin JW, Blackstone EH. Editorial on papers by Naito, Wessel, and their colleagues. J Thorac Cardiovasc Surg 1980; 80:594.

Lillehei CW, Cohen M, Warden HE, et al. Direct vision intracardiac surgical correction of the tetralogy of Fallot, pentalogy of Fallot, and pulmonary atresia defects. Report of first ten cases. Ann Surg 1955; 142:418.

Lillehei CW, Varco RL, Cohen M, et al. The first open heart corrections of tetralogy of Fallot. A 26–31 year follow-up of 106 patients. Ann Surg 1986; 204:490.

Misbach GA, Turley K, Ebert PA. Pulmonary valve replacement for regurgitation after repair of tetralogy of Fallot. Ann Thorac Surg 1983; 36:684.

Pacifico AD. Reoperations after repair of tetralogy of Fallot. In Stark J, Pacifico AD, eds. Reoperations in Cardiac Surgery. London: Springer-Verlag, 1989:171.

Poirier RA, McGoon DC, Danielson GK, et al. Late results after repair of tetralogy of Fallot. J Thorac Cardiovasc Surg 1977; 73:900.

Quattlebaum TG, Varghese PJ, Neill CA, Donahoo JS. Sudden death among postoperative patients with tetralogy of Fallot. A follow up study of 251 patients for an average of twelve years. Am J Cardiol 1975; 35:164.

Rosenthal A, Gross RE, Pasternac A. Aneurysms of right ventricular outflow patches. J Thorac Cardiovasc Surg 1972; 63:735.

Rowlatt UF, Rimoldi HJA, Lev M. The quantitative anatomy of the normal child's heart. Pediatr Clin North Am 1963; 10:499.

Seybold-Epting W, Chiaviell L, Hallman GL, Cooley DA. Aneurysm of pericardial right ventricular outflow patches. Ann Thorac Surg 1977; 24:237.

Uretzky G, Puga FJ, Danielson GK, Hagler DJ, McGoon DC. Reoperation after correction of tetralogy of Fallot. Circulation 1982; 66(suppl I):202.

Wessel HU, Cunningham WJ, Paul MH, et al. Exercise performance in tetralogy of Fallot after intracardiac repair. J Thorac Cardiovasc Surg 1980; 80:582.

Zhao H, Miller DC, Reitz BA, Shumway NE. Surgical repair of tetralogy of Fallot. Long-term follow-up with particular emphasis on late death and reoperation. J Thorac Cardiovasc Surg 1985; 89:204.

8

Surgical Treatment of Critical Valvar Aortic Stenosis in the Neonate

Frank M. Midgley

□

The neonate with critical aortic valve stenosis usually presents with intractable congestive heart failure and associated low cardiac output due to severe left ventricular dysfunction. This clinical picture is frequently complicated by endocardial fibroelastosis, primary and secondary abnormalities of the mitral valve, and the associated defects of patent ductus arteriosus and coarctation of the aorta. Although aortic valve stenosis is uncommon, it is a major life-threatening malformation presenting in the neonatal period and demands aggressive interventional therapy for survival.

Intensive medical therapy directed at metabolic, respiratory, cardiac, and renal systems is essential to stabilize the patient during the evaluation period and to prepare the patient for mechanical intervention. Critical aortic valve stenosis in the neonate has been managed by many different strategies since first approached surgically. The evolution and evaluation of surgical modalities is the subject of this chapter.

ANATOMY

Malformation due to lack of maturation of aortic valve substance has variable forms, severities, and clinical consequences depending on the degree of abnormality. Those patients with the most severe forms of aortic valve stenosis realistically should be considered in the category of hypoplastic left-heart syndrome owing to associated hypoplasia of the aortic annulus, diminutive left ventricular volume, and associated hypoplasia of the mitral valve ring. Suggested lower limits have been proposed for the diameter of the aortic annulus of 6 mm (Edmunds et al. 1980), left ventricular volume of 25 ml/m^2 (Hammon et al. 1988), and mitral annulus of 11 mm diameter (Graham et al. 1971). At the other end of the pathologic and clinical spectrum, slight abnormalities of valve maturation as regards the number of leaflets, degree of commissural fusion, and thickness of the leaflets are of less clinical significance and often do not present until later in life. The valve abnormalities presenting in the first month of life are always severe and are due both to abnormalities of cusp division and to thickness of the leaflet tissues. These patients have varying degrees of associated hypoplasia of the aortic annulus, which limit the surgical expectations. Residual left ventricular outflow tract obstruction due to annular hypoplasia frequently persists despite the total relief of the valvar component. The valves, however, typically have poorly differentiated commissural landmarks and bulky thickening of the leaflet substance with resultant rigidity of the cusps. These less mature valves differ considerably from the more defined valves seen later in infancy and adolescence. It is probably this primitive anatomic substrate that is responsible for the high mortality reported in most clinical series in which different surgical therapies have been employed as well as for a significant reoperation rate.

DIAGNOSIS

The diagnosis of critical aortic valve stenosis is readily made on clinical grounds in the noncyanotic newborn who presents with a life-threatening illness characterized by severe dyspnea, intractable congestive heart failure, and progressive acidosis. In the earlier years, cardiac catheterization was usually performed for confirmation of diagnosis and measurement of gradient. The patient usually presents with such low cardiac output that any realistic measurement of gradient and its relation to severity of disease is impractical. Currently, echocardiographic studies are sufficient for these purposes. Echocardiography variably demonstrates a narrow aortic root, dysplastic or doming valve elements, and diminished left ventricular volume and muscle mass. Additionally, associated abnormalities of the mitral valve, ductus arteriosus, and thoracic aorta can be defined.

PREPROCEDURE MANAGEMENT

Neonates with a presumptive diagnosis of critical valvar aortic stenosis are admitted to an intensive care environment, where stabilization of clinical status and confirmation of diagnosis are carried out concurrently. Therapy involves appropriate utilization of cardiotonic and respiratory support with aggressive normalization of metabolic status. Full monitoring is instituted.

There have been many different interventional therapies and techniques used for the treatment of valvar aortic stenosis in the neonate. Basically they can be differentiated into two distinct strategies: Those in which relief of valvar stenosis is performed under direct vision and those accomplished using closed (blind) techniques.

OPEN TECHNIQUES

□ Inflow Occlusion

Swann in 1956 reported the first successful use of inflow occlusion (Swann and Korz 1956) to approach aortic valve stenosis under direct vision in a 5-year-old patient. Subsequent extensive use of this technique in neonates in many centers has established inflow occlusion as a standard approach (Keane et al. 1975; Sade et al. 1982; Sink et al. 1984; Pelech et al. 1987).

Through a median sternotomy at normothermia, the ascending aorta is controlled and tourniquets are placed around each cava. After a period of hyperventilation, the tourniquets are snared and the heart allowed to empty. After several beats, a clamp is placed on the ascending aorta. An oblique aortotomy is then made at the aortic root and the valve substance visualized and assessed. Discrete commissurotomy and valvuloplasty are then expeditiously accomplished. The tourniquets are released to evacuate air from the aortotomy just before closure by the last sutures. Resuscitation of the stressed myocardium may be necessary with blood transfusion, bicarbonate, and defibrillation. Inflow occlusion times can generally be kept to less than 3 minutes.

□ Cardiopulmonary Bypass

Lillehei in 1956 first approached the aortic valve using cardiopulmonary bypass to achieve a less hurried and more discrete commissurotomy (Lillehei et al. 1956). Increasingly sophisticated perfusion techniques with hypothermia, low flow, circulatory arrest, and cardioplegia have advanced this approach to the forefront as the method of support of choice used in most centers.

All procedures are done through a median sternotomy. After heparinization and aortic and atrial cannulation, cardiopulmonary bypass is instituted and some degree of hypothermia attained. Techniques using cardioplegia and low flow, profound hypothermia with circulatory arrest, and cold blood prime have been employed successfully in different centers. Ultimately the aortic root is opened, allowing for a direct vision procedure on the valve substance. This might be a direct, discrete commissurotomy when well-defined valve elements are encountered or dilatation

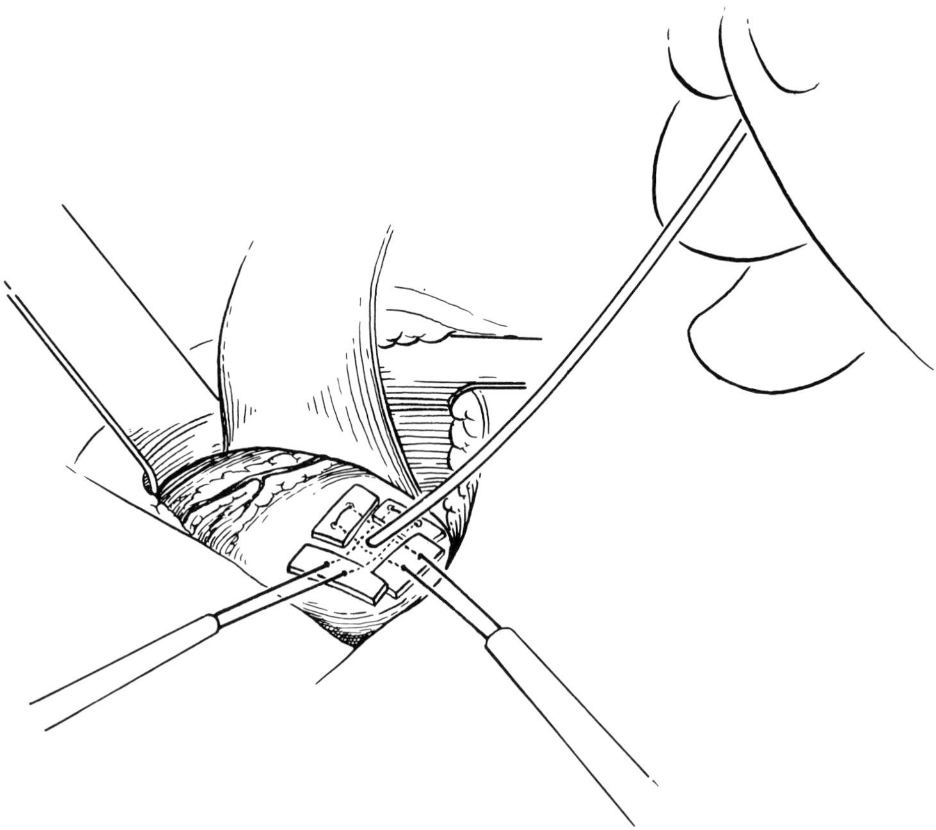

Figure 8.3 Large interlocking pledgeted sutures are shown in place on left ventricular apex. A dilator has been passed into the left ventricle.

of the left ventricle and aortic annulus. There is typically a popping sensation appreciated digitally with a correspondingly improved upstroke on the arterial pressure monitor. When the patient has stabilized, the residual gradient is assessed and the pledgeted sutures tied. Additional procedures, when indicated, can be undertaken for patent ductus ligation or repair of coarctation.

A variation on this theme was introduced by Brown, in which instead of graded dilators a Grüntzig balloon catheter was passed in antegrade fashion out the left ventricular outflow tract from a left ventricular approach (Brown et al. 1985). One infant that did not survive was shown at postmortem examination to have had the commissures of the dysmorphic aortic leaflets split appropriately to the diameter of the preselected 6-mm Grüntzig catheter.

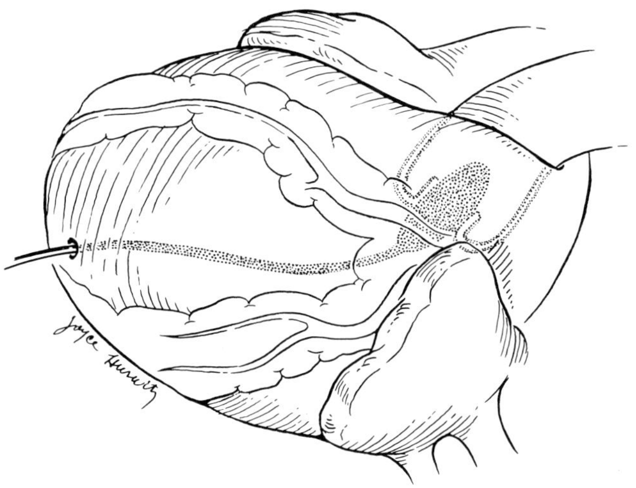

Figure 8.4
A dilator is shown silhouetted in the aortic valve orifice.

DISCUSSION

Proponents of repair of neonatal valvar aortic stenosis by the open approach argue that a more defined commissurotomy can be performed with care being taken to do a limited commissurotomy, not extending the lesion back entirely to the vessel wall. This acceptance of residual stenosis in preference to inducing aortic insufficiency is a basic tenet of aortic valve procedures in small infants.

Realistically, although the aortic root may be open and the valve substance directly visualized, the morphology of the valve as it presents in the neonate is often quite primitive in appearance with indistinct commissures and raphés, thickened, poorly compliant cusp tissues, and often with an underlying hypoplastic annulus. Procedures on such a valve lesion cannot be considered to be of optimum precision. As noted by various authors (Sade et al. 1982; Brown et al. 1988), dilatation with a hemostat under direct vision is often necessary. Valvotomy does not correct the thickened valve substance or annular hypoplasia.

Keane postulated that a maturation of the embryonic valve structure may occur in infants (Keane et al. 1975). This concept is given considerable support by the observation that those patients in their series undergoing reoperation 1 to 10 years later had flexible, noncalcified valves with more definition than when seen as neonates. Proponents of the closed approach use this postulate in support of the argument for blind intervention.

The experience with inflow occlusion at several centers has resulted in reports of mortality ranging from 12% to 50%. Follow-up results have been variable, but the combined experience from four centers indicted one late death and 10 reoperations during long-term follow-up of 38 patients who survived the initial operative procedure as a neonate (Keane et al. 1975; Sade et al. 1982; Swink et al. 1984; Pelech et al. 1987).

Most centers have reported disappointingly high mortalities for operations for neonatal aortic stenosis using various cardiopulmonary bypass techniques. One center did report more favorable results using a cold blood prime (4°C) and short perfusion (21 minutes) and cross clamp (7 minutes) times (Messina et al. 1984). Most centers have generally reported a low number of reoperations. In a combined group of 63 survivors of the primary operative procedure from six centers, followed up to 17 years, there were seven late deaths and 11 reoperations (Edmunds et al. 1980; Sandor et al. 1980; Messina et al. 1984; Grundy and Behrendt 1986; Treter et al. 1988; Wheeler et al. 1988).

Experience with closed transventricular valvotomy at Children's National Medical Center includes 10 neonatal patients operated on between 1973 and 1989 (Midgley et al. 1985). Since 1985 approximately six other neonates have been managed by balloon valvotomy in the cardiac catheterization laboratory. Patient selection for a specific therapeutic modality has been at the discretion of the cardiologist. There were two operative deaths early in the series, both patients having severely diminished left ventricular volumes and aortic annular hypoplasia. These patients would currently undergo other procedures for hypoplastic left-heart syndrome. Eight patients currently are surviving for periods of 2 months to 16 years postvalvotomy. None have required operative reintervention. Four patients have had follow-up catheterization 3 months to 10 years following closed valvotomy. Excellent left ventricular function was demonstrated in all patients with transvalvar gradients of less than 30 mmHg. No patient showed evidence of aortic insufficiency angiographically. These eight patients have remained free of symptoms with no clinical evidence of restenosis or insufficiency. Other centers (Duncan et al. 1987; Brown et al. 1988) have reported operative mortalities of 30% and 60% with reoperation in four of 14 survivors from both series.

Closed transventricular valvotomy is quick and easy and does not require utilization of techniques of cardiopulmonary bypass, inflow occlusion, hypothermia, or circulatory arrest. It allows easy repair of the often associated coarctation of the aorta. It preserves the median sternotomy for possible future surgery. There are no periods of left ventricular ischemia, and aortic insufficiency has historically not been a problem on follow-up of up to 16 years.

Inflow occlusion and techniques using cardiopulmonary bypass are equally effective in treating critical aortic valve stenosis in the neonate. Additionally, closed transventricular valvotomy has afforded equally good survival statistics and in some centers a lower or absent reoperation rate. Selection of technique would seem to be based on personal prejudice and recent experience. True comparison between techniques is not possible because of the small patient numbers and the years of study during which time so many factors have come into play to improve the results evidenced by all techniques. Earlier recognition, transport, and diagnosis; avoidance of catheterization; and better preoperative, intraoperative, and postoperative stabilization have clearly played a major role in the increased survival rates achieved by several approaches.

REFERENCES

Brown JW, Robinson RG, Waller BF. Transventricular balloon catheter aortic valvotomy in neonates. Ann Thorac Surg 1985; 39:376.

Brown JW, Stevens LS, Holly S, et al. Surgical spectrum of aortic stenosis in children: a thirty-year experience with 257 children. Ann Thorac Surg 1988; 45:393.

Duncan K, Sullivan I, Robinson P, et al. Transventricular aortic valvotomy for critical aortic stenosis in infants. J Thorac Cardiovasc Surg 1987; 95:546.

Edmunds LH, Wagner HR, Heymann MA. Aortic valvotomy in neonates. Circulation 1980; 61:421.

Graham TP, Jarmakani JM, Canent RV, Morrow MN. Left heart volume estimation in infancy and childhood. Circulation 1971; 43:895.

Grundy SR, Behrendt MD. Prognostic factors in valvotomy for critical aortic stenosis in infancy. J Thorac Cardiovasc Surg 1986; 92:747.

Hammon JW, Lupinetti FM, Maples MD, et al. Predictors of operative mortality in critical valvar aortic stenosis presenting in infancy. Ann Thorac Surg 1988; 45:537.

Keane JF, Bernard WF, Nadas AS. Aortic stenosis surgery in infancy. Circulation 1975; 52:1138.

Lillehei CW, Gott VL, Varco RL. Direct vision correction of calcific aortic stenosis by means of pump-oxygenator and retrograde coronary sinus perfection. Dis Chest 1956; 30:123.

Messina LM, Turley K, Stanger P, Hoffman JIE, Ebert PA. Successful aortic valvotomy for severe congenital valvular aortic stenosis in the newborn infant. J Thorac Cardiovasc Surg 1984; 88:92.

Margues RM, Logan R. Congenital aortic stenosis and its surgical treatment. Br Heart J 1955; 17:373.

Midgley FM, Perry LW, Shapiro SR, et al. Closed transventricular valvotomy for critical aortic stenosis in the neonate. In Doyle EF, ed. Proceedings of the Second World Congress of the Pediatric Cardiology. New York: Springer-Verlag, 1985:540.

Pelech AN, Dyck JD, Trusler GA, et al. Critical aortic stenosis: Survival and management. J Thorac Cardiovasc Surg 1987; 94:510.

Sade RM, Crawford FA, Hohn AR. Inflow occlusion for semilunar valve stenosis. Ann Thorac Surg 1982; 33:570.

Sandor GGS, Olley PM, Trusler GA, et al. Long-term follow-up of patients after valvotomy for congenital valvular aortic stenosis in children. J Thorac Cardiovasc Surg 1980; 80:171.

Sink JD, Smallhorn JF, Macartney FJ, et al. Management of critical aortic stenosis in infancy. J Thorac Cardiovasc Surg 1984; 87:82.

Swan H, Korz A. Direct vision trans-aortic approach to the aortic valve during hypothermia: Experimental observations and report of a successful clinical case. Ann Surg 1956; 144:205.

Treter KJ, Einzig S, Ring WS, Foker JE. Critical aortic stenosis in the newborn: early risk factors and later prognosis (abstract). J Am Coll Cardiol 1988; 11:70A.
Trinkle JK, Norton JB, Richardson JD, Grover FL, Noonan JA. Closed aortic valvotomy and simultaneous correction of associated anomalies in infants. J Thorac Cardiovasc Surg 1975; 69:758.
Wheeler JJ, Hosier DM, Teske DW, Craenen JM, Kilman JW. Results of operation for aortic valve stenosis in infants, children, and adolescents. J Thorac Cardiovasc Surg 1988; 96:474.

9

Invasive Catheter Techniques in the Management of Critical Aortic Stenosis in Infants

Benjamin Zeevi, John F. Keane, Stanton B. Perry, and James E. Lock

Neonates (less than 1 month) and occasionally infants (1 to 2 months) with critical valvar aortic stenosis present with severe congestive heart failure (Lakier et al. 1974; Mocellin et al. 1983). The symptomatic infant is irritable, pale, and hypotensive and has small pulse volume; pulmonary congestion is manifested by tachypnea and cyanosis. The systolic murmur is often unimpressive and very soft secondary to low cardiac output.

The seriously ill neonate with critical valvar aortic stenosis must be considered to be a medical emergency. In the neonatal period, in addition to inotropic and ventilatory support, infusion of prostaglandin E_1 maintains the ductus communication with a right to left shunt. This frequently improves systemic circulation and may relieve metabolic acidosis, thereby improving the patient's tolerance to further intervention, which is undertaken as soon as possible (Jonas et al. 1985; Messina et al. 1985). Death ensues in most patients with medical treatment alone. Survival past the neonatal period does not preclude subsequent difficulties, and deterioration may occur later with the onset of anemia or secondary to ongoing significant ischemia. In infants severe congenital valvar aortic stenosis is an indication for urgent but usually not emergent intervention.

Operative mortality for neonatal critical valvar aortic stenosis is high when the patient is less than 7 days old regardless of the surgical approach and ranges between 9% to 86% (Kugler et al. 1979; Edmunds et al. 1980; Pelech et al. 1982; Messina et al. 1984; Sink et al. 1984; Gundry and Behrendt 1986; Hammon et al. 1988). Contributing to the high mortality of neonatal critical valvar aortic stenosis are the poor clinical condition of the patients and the association of other anatomic abnormalities (40% of the neonates) (Bernhard et al. 1973). Factors such as left ventricular cavity hypoplasia, hypoplastic aortic annulus with valvar dysplasia, and poor myocardial performance resulting from subendocardial ischemia with or without endocardial fibroelastosis increase mortality. Other associated lesions are congenital mitral stenosis and insufficiency, patent ductus arteriosus, severe coarctation, and subaortic stenosis. Although surgical valvotomy can be an effective treatment, it must be considered palliative since restenosis and aortic regurgitation are not uncommon (Sandor et al. 1980; Dobell et al. 1981; Presbitero et al. 1982; Fulton et al. 1983).

Since the initial description of balloon aortic valvotomy by Lababidi (1983), several studies have demonstrated that the severity of childhood congenital valvar aortic stenosis can be reduced with minimal mortality and acceptable morbidity (Choy et al. 1987; Helgason et al. 1987; Sholler et al. 1988). Based on our experience in older children, we have, for the last 4 years, attempted balloon dilation in all neonates and infants with critical valvar aortic stenosis who were admitted to The Children's Hospital, Boston. The primary objective of the procedure is to improve the immediate condition of the patient, which may allow for later valve maturation and redilation if necessary (Fulton et al. 1983; Zeevi et al. 1989).

BALLOON DILATION TECHNIQUE

The methodology, outlined here, is our current approach and has been modified in response to our initial experience.

Patients are premedicated, usually with morphine sulfate (0.1 mg/kg body weight) and receive local anesthesia with 1% xylocaine if the femoral vessels are to be used. Critically ill neonates are intubated and commonly paralyzed. In neonates less than 72 hours of age, we attempt to use the umbilical artery. If the aortic valve cannot be crossed within 20 minutes using umbilical artery access, percutaneous femoral artery access is used. The arteries are cannulated with a 3.2 or 4.5 Fr pigtail catheter. Heparin is administered intravenously (100 units/kg body weight). Complete right-sided and left-sided heart catheterization includes measurements of peak systolic ejection gradient across the aortic valve using simultaneous measurement of left ventricular (antegrade) and ascending aorta (retrograde) pressures. Biplane cine angiograms of the left ventricle and the ascending aorta allow measurement of left ventricular size and function and the aortic annulus size as well as evaluation of associated lesions and the degree of aortic regurgitation (AR).

In almost all cases, the valves are unicommissural or bicommissural, and the open commissure is almost always between the left and noncoronary cusps (Van Praagh et al. 1986; Gittenberger-deGroot and Sauer 1987). Using a partially cut off 3.2 or 4 Fr pigtail catheter to direct the guidewire posteriorly and to the left toward the open commissure, the aortic valve is crossed retrograde using a soft 0.015- to 0.018-inch guidewire. The catheter is advanced over the wire and positioned in the left ventricle. The small wire is exchanged for a 0.021 to 0.028-inch guidewire with a preformed curve, which is curled in the apex of the left ventricle. Biplane fluoroscopy is used to avoid passing the wire through the tensor apparatus of the mitral valve. The neonatal aortic valves are soft and dysplastic and can easily be perforated with the guidewire. Thus accurate assessment of the location of the valve orifice using 2D-echocardiography and angiography and the use of very soft wires to cross the valves are important. Valve perforation with the wire and catheter should be suspected whenever the wire crosses the valve anteriorly, which may be identified angiographically or by using 2D-echocardiography. Valve perforation with the wire alone causes minimal AR; dilation of a valve through a perforated cusp causes severe AR.

The pigtail catheter is exchanged for a balloon dilation catheter (Cook Inc., Bloomington, IN; or Mansfield Scientific, Watertown, MA), which is positioned across the aortic valve and inflated by hand to 3 to 8 atmospheres or until the waist in the balloon produced by the valve disappears. The actual diameter of the inflated balloon varies with inflation pressure; small (less than 1 mm) increases in balloon diameter can be achieved by increasing pressure rather than changing to a larger balloon. Because a waist is commonly absent in neonates with aortic stenosis, two to four inflations are performed to ensure that the balloon was properly positioned. After each inflation, the balloon is deflated rapidly and withdrawn to the descending aorta. Inflation-deflation cycles last at most 15 seconds. In neonates we initially use a balloon that is 85% to 90% of the valve annulus diameter, modifying inflation pressure to adjust the actual balloon diameter and allow improved gradient reduction. A balloon to annulus ratio greater than 100% may adversely affect outcome and has been associated with increased AR (Waller et al. 1986; Phillips et al. 1987; Helgason et al. 1987; Sholler et al. 1988). Following balloon dilation, the transvalvar gradient and left ventricular end diastolic pressures are measured, and an aortogram is performed to evaluate the severity of AR. Neonates are observed, at least overnight, in the cardiovascular intensive care unit.

Assessing the immediate results of balloon dilation in the catheterization laboratory can be difficult. In many neonates, no definite waist is seen. The peak to peak systolic ejection gradient in these neonates may not accurately reflect the severity of the obstruction as a result of low cardiac output, left to right atrial shunts, and right to left ductal shunts. Results are therefore subjective in many cases. We currently consider the procedure successful when there is significant reduction in the transvalvar gradient, left ventricular end diastolic and left atrial pressures, no more than mild AR, and clinical improvement. An unquestionable relief in the stenosis occurs when the contractility of the left ventricle improves or when the right to left ductal shunting changes to left to right shunting.

NEONATES

Since January 1985, all 25 neonates admitted to The Children's Hospital with the diagnosis of critical valvar aortic stenosis have undergone attempted balloon dilation. No neonates were excluded on the basis of clinical condition, aortic valve morphology, left ventricular size or function, or degree of mitral regurgitation. The neonates ranged in age from 1 to 30 days (mean 10.5 ± 10.3 days) and in weight from 2.2 to 5 kg (mean 3.5 ± 0.8 kg). Associated lesions were present in 20 patients, including patent ductus arteriosus in 13, coarctation of the aorta in three, mitral regurgitation in 11 (moderate to severe in seven and mild in four), and a small left ventricle in 10. The anatomy of the aortic valves, as determined by inspection at surgery, autopsy, or by echocardiography were unicommissural in 15 and bicommissural in 10.

Emergency balloon dilation was performed in one neonate without hemodynamic measurements before the procedure. Thus predilation hemodynamic data are available in 24 neonates. The peak systolic ejection gradients ranged from 10 to 139 mmHg (mean 56.3 ± 28.5 mmHg) and the left ventricular end diastolic pressures from 10 to 33 mmHg (mean 19.9 ± 65 mmHg). The left ventricle was small (60% to 80% of predicted normal) in six, and hypoplastic (less than 60% of predicted normal) in four.

The diameter of the aortic annulus ranged from 4.5 to 8 mm (mean 6.0 + 0.9 mm) and the diameter of the balloon from 4 to 6 mm, resulting in a balloon to annulus diameter ratio of 67%:120% (mean 92% ± 15%). The immediate postdilation peak systolic ejection gradients ranged from 1 to 100 mmHg (mean 26.8 ± 20 mmHg), representing 0 to 95% (mean 57% ± 22%) reduction in the gradient. The immediate postdilation left ventricular end diastolic pressure ranged from 6 to 25 mmHG (mean 14.1 ± 5.5 mmHg) ($P<0.02$ compared with predilation). New AR developed in 10 neonates, being mild in seven and severe in three who died. Loss of pulse occurred in 12 neonates but returned to normal in eight following anticoagulation therapy, thrombolytic therapy, or both.

In the first 30 days following the initial balloon dilation, there were five deaths. In addition to these early deaths, two patients underwent stage I palliation for hypoplastic left-heart syndrome and were excluded from further follow-up.

Of the five early deaths, three occurred early in our experience and were probably related to procedural and technical errors. One neonate died from *Staphylococcus aureus* sepsis 2 days after a prolonged, unsuccessful dilation attempt performed through an umbilical artery and subsequent surgical aortic valvotomy. Autopsy showed numerous small infected vegetations on all four heart valves and in the great arteries. A second neonate developed severe AR after dilation with a balloon to annulus ratio of 120% and at surgery was found to have avulsion of the right and noncoronary cusps from the annulus. Although the left ventricular volume was initially normal, repeat catheterization showed a hypoplastic left ventricle, and the patient died 2 weeks following dilation during an attempt to perform stage I palliation for hypoplastic left-heart syndrome. The third neonate, a patient with uncorrectable acidosis, a unicommissural valve, and a small left ventricle (66% of predictable normal) developed severe AR following passage of a 0.025-inch guidewire through the valve tissue and dilation of a cusp rather than the valve orifice. He died 3 hours later from low cardiac output.

There were three late deaths, all following late repair of coarctation of the aorta. All three had small left ventricles and died secondary to low cardiac output.

Thus excluding the seven early failures and three late deaths, there were 15 patients available for follow-up. The systolic ejection gradient (peak to peak in six by cardiac catheterization, maximal instantaneous in nine by Doppler echocardiography) was 51 ± 17 mmHg, 7.6 ± 7.8 months after dilation. None of these patients had significant AR, and two had moderate mitral regurgitation.

Of the 25 patients undergoing balloon dilation, a total of eight died (32%), a total of six required a second procedure: three balloon dilations (one died), one surgical valvotomy (died), and two stage I palliations for hypoplastic left-heart syndrome (one died). Of 10 failures (eight deaths and two stage I palliation for hypoplastic left-heart syndrome), eight occurred in the 10 patients with small or hypoplastic left ventricles and only two in the 15 patients with normal or large left ventricles.

INFANTS

We have performed balloon aortic valvotomy in 22 infants with a mean age of 4 ± 2.7 months (range 1 to 10 months). The transvalvar gradient decreased from 78.8 ± 19.5 mmHg to 35.9 ± 23.2 mmHg. This represents a 53% ± 27% reduction in gradient, which is similar to published results for older children. The balloon to annulus ratio used was 0.98 ± 0.14 (range 0.75 to 1.25). None of the patients had AR before dilation. Following dilation, the regurgitation increased in eight but was at most mild. There were no deaths in this group. The only significant complications involved the femoral arteries. Nine patients had transient and two permanent loss of femoral artery pulse. One infant underwent surgery to repair a ruptured iliac artery.

DISCUSSION

Our results using balloon aortic valvotomy in 47 neonates and infants with valvar aortic stenosis support at least two conclusions. First, with proper evaluation of anatomy and proper technique, essentially all patients can be dilated. Second, the neonates with normal or dilated left ventricles and ill infants can be dilated effectively with low mortality and morbidity. Because very few previous reports in the literature of surgical or balloon valvotomy have clearly defined selection criteria or patient age, comparison of results is not possible. In an attempt to overcome these problems, we compared the last 16 consecutive neonates to undergo surgical valvotomy with the first 16 consecutive neonates to undergo balloon valvotomy in our institution (Zeevi et al. 1989).

This was a retrospective study comparing nonrandomized patients managed over different time periods for the groups, and therefore preintervention and postintervention care may differ. It should be emphasized that the balloon valvotomy group represented the first 16 neonates undergoing balloon dilation at our institution and that surgical results are from an era when myocardial protection may have been suboptimal. Despite these problems, both groups were comparable in terms of age, weight, hemodynamic data, left ventricular size, and associated lesions.

Early mortality was 38% following surgery with one late death compared with an early mortality of 20% and two late deaths after balloon valvotomy. Five out of six neonates requiring a second operation died. Left ventricular size had significant influence on survival. In the surgical group three of three with smaller hypoplastic left ventricles and three of 10 with normal sized left ventricles died. Following balloon valvotomy four of six with small hypoplastic left ventricles and two of nine with normal sized left ventricles died. At late follow-up (although shorter in the balloon valvotomy group), the degrees of aortic stenosis and AR were similar in each group. This is the only study to date comparing balloon valvotomy and surgical valvotomy in neonates. Our results suggest that percutaneous balloon valvotomy is as effective as surgical valvotomy in these neonates.

Previous reports of balloon aortic valvotomy in small series of neonates and infants have not compared the results directly with surgical results. Kasten-Sportes et al. (1989) reported an attempted balloon dilation in 10 neonates with critical valvar aortic stenosis, with results that are similar to our own experience. In one infant, the aortic valve could not be crossed, and in another infant, a technical error resulted in severe aortic insufficiency and death. Among the eight patients who had effective dilation, the stenosis was relieved in seven. None of the three newborns with a very small left ventricle recovered (two died and one underwent cardiac transplantation). Among the seven neonates with a left ventricle of acceptable size, three underwent subsequent aortic valvotomy; one of these died and two had good results. The mortality rate in the entire series was 30%. In a series of 13 patients less than 1 year of age published by Wren et al. (1987), mortality was 54%, with four out of six infants less than 1 month of age dying, and in two of the seven patients who died, they were unable to pass a catheter across the valve. The other reports on balloon dilation of the aortic valve in infants and neonates, some intraoperative, did not discuss the anatomic features or technical details (Sanchez et al. 1985; Rupprath and Neuhaus 1985; Brown et al. 1985; Lababidi and Weinhaus 1986; Waller et al. 1986; Phillips et al. 1987).

A small hypoplastic left ventricle has previously been reported to be a high risk factor in this group of patients (Pelech et al. 1982; Mocellin et al. 1983; Brown et al. 1988; Hammon et al. 1988), but caution is required in assessing operability based on left ventricular volume alone. In our group, there was a survivor with a left ventricular volume of 41% of the predicted normal. Obviously survival after valvotomy is multifactorial, and analysis of anatomic variables other than the gradient may be needed to improve the assessment of the adequacy of the left ventricle to maintain an adequate cardiac output. The development of these criteria will help us to select patients for either balloon dilation or palliation similar to the approach for hypoplastic left-heart syndrome.

Our data suggest that percutaneous balloon valvotomy may be as effective as surgical valvotomy in infants and neonates. Infants who are older than 1 month do very well and are more appropriately grouped with children and adults in terms of results, complications, and prognosis. Long-term evaluation of balloon dilation in these patients is necessary to provide a better basis for comparison with the surgical alternative.

REFERENCES

Bernhard WF, Keane JF, Fellows KE, Litwin SB, Gross RE: Progress and problems in the surgical management of congenital aortic stenosis. J Thorac Cardiovasc Surg 1973; 66:404.

Brown JW, Robison RJ, Waller BF. Transventricular balloon catheter aortic valvotomy in neonates. Ann Thorac Surg 1985; 39:376.

Brown JW, Stevens LS, Holly S, et al. Surgical spectrum of aortic stenosis in children: A thirty year experience with 257 children. Ann Thorac Surg 1988; 45:393.

Choy M, Beekman RH, Rocchini AP, et al. Percutaneous balloon valvuloplasty for valvar aortic stenosis in infants and children. Am J Cardiol 1987; 59:1010.

Dobell ARC, Bloss RS, Gibbons JE, Collins GF. Congenital valvular aortic stenosis, surgical management and long term results. J Thorac Cardiovasc Surg 1981; 81:916.

Edmunds LH, Wagner HR, Heymann MA. Aortic valvotomy in neonates. Circulation 1980; 61:421.

Fulton DR, Hougen TJ, Keane JE, et al. Repeat aortic valvotomy in children. Am Heart J 1983; 106:60.

Gittenberger-deGroot AC, Sauer U. The aortic valve in critical valvular aortic stenosis: A morphological approach [abstr.]. Pediatr Cardiol 1987; 8:229.

Gundry SR, Behrendt DM. Prognostic factors in valvotomy for critical aortic stenosis in infancy. J Thorac Cardiovasc Surg 1986; 92:747.

Hammon JW, Lupinetti FM, Maples MD, et al. Predictors of operative mortality in critical valvular aortic stenosis presenting in infancy. Ann Thorac Surg 1988; 45:537.

Helgason H, Keane JF, Fellows KE, Kulik TJ, Lock JE. Balloon dilation of the aortic valve. Studies in normal lambs and in children with aortic stenosis. J Am Coll Cardiol 1987; 9:816.

Jonas RA, Lang P, Mayer JE, Castaneda AR. The importance of prostaglandin E1 in resuscitation of the neonate with critical aortic stenosis [letter]. J Thorac Cardiovasc Surg 1985; 39:314.

Kasten-Sportes CH, Piechaud JF, Sidi D, Kachaner J. Percutaneous balloon valvuloplasty in neonates with critical aortic stenosis. J Am Coll Cardiol 1989; 13:1101.

Kugler JD, Campbell E, Vargo TA, et al. Results of aortic valvotomy in infants with isolated aortic valve stenosis. J Thorac Cardiovasc Surg 1979; 78:553.

Lababidi Z. Aortic balloon valvuloplasty. Am Heart J 1983; 106:751.

Lababidi Z, Weinhaus L. Successful balloon valvuloplasty for neonatal critical aortic stenosis. Am Heart J 1986; 112:913.

Lakier JB, Lewis AB, Heymann MA, et al. Isolated aortic stenosis in neonates: Natural history and hemodynamic considerations. Circulation 1974; 50:801.

Messina LM, Turley K, Stanger P, Hoffman JIE, Ebert PA. The importance of prostaglandins E1 in resuscitation of the neonate with critical aortic stenosis [reply]. J Thorac Cardiovasc Surg 1985; 89:315.

Messina LM, Turley K. Stanger P, Hoffman JIE, Ebert PA. The importance of prostaglandins E1 in resuscitation of the neonate with critical aortic stenosis [reply]. J Thorac Cardiovasc Surg 1985; 89:315.

Mocellin R, Sauer U, Simon B, et al. Reduced left ventricular size and endocardial fibroelastosis as correlates of mortality in newborns and young infants with severe aortic stenosis. Pediatr Cardiol 1983; 4:265.

Pelech AN, Dyck JD, Trusler GA, et al. Critical aortic stenosis: Survival and management. J Thorac Cardiovasc Surg 1982; 44:510.

Phillips RR, Gerlis LM, Wilson N, Waller DR. Aortic valve damage caused by operative balloon dilation of critical aortic valve stenosis. Br Heart J 1987; 97:168.

Presbitero P, Somerville J, Revel-Chion R, Ross D. Open aortic valvotomy for congenital aortic stenosis: Late results. Br Heart J 1982; 47:26.

Rupprath G, Neuhaus KL. Percutaneous balloon valvuloplasty for aortic valve stenosis in infancy. Am J Cardiol 1985; 55:1655.

Sanchez GR, Mehta AV, Ewing LL, et al. Successful percutaneous balloon valvuloplasty of the aortic valve in an infant. Pediatr Cardiol 1985; 6:103.

Sandor GGS, Olley PM, Trusler GA, et al. Long term follow up of patients after valvotomy for congenital valvular aortic stenosis in children: A clinical and actuarial follow up. J Thorac Cardiovasc Surg 1980; 80:171.

Sholler GF, Keane JF, Perry SB, Sanders SP, Lock JE. Balloon dilation of congenital aortic valve stenosis. Results and influence of technical and morphologic features on outcome. Circulation 1988; 78:351.

Sink JD, Smallhorn JF, Macartney FJ, et al. Management of critical aortic stenosis in infancy. J Thorac Cardiovasc Surg 1984; 87:82.

Van Praagh R, Bano-Rodrigo A, Smolinsky A, et al. Anatomic variations in congenital valvar, subvalvar and supravalvar aortic stenosis: A study of 64 post mortem cases. In Takahashi M, ed. Challenge in the treatment of congenital cardiac anomalies. New York: Futura Publishing, 1986:p 13.

Waller BF, Girod DA, Dillon JC. Transverse aortic wall tears in infants after balloon angioplasty for aortic valve stenosis: Relation of aortic wall damage to diameter of inflated angioplasty balloon and aortic lumen in seven necropsy cases. J Am Coll Cardiol 1986; 4:1235.

Wren C, Sullivan I, Ball C, Deanfield J. Percutaneous balloon dilatation of aortic valve stenosis in neonates and infants. Br Heart J 1987; 58:608.

Zeevi B, Keane JF, Castaneda AR, Perry SB, Lock JE. Neonatal critical valve aortic stenosis. A comparison of surgical and balloon dilation therapy. Circulation 1989; 80:831.

10

The Management of Subaortic Stenosis in Children

Davis C. Drinkwater, Jr., and Hillel Laks

The entity of subaortic stenosis in children has several basic configurations, which may be either isolated or combined with other lesions. Correspondingly this may be relatively straightforward or one of the more difficult problems in pediatric open-heart surgery. The management of the more complex obstructions may be challenging with regard to timing of intervention and in providing a complete and safe repair that does not have long-term adverse results. There may also be associated specific cardiac and extracardiac lesions that need to be considered at the time of repair.

CLINICAL EVALUATION

Symptoms may vary greatly both within and between groups of patients and are usually related to the degree and duration of left ventricular outflow stenosis from mild and moderate to severe. Symptoms may include those of congestive heart failure in general, such as shortness of breath, easy fatigability, and even chest pain and syncope in some instances. The percentage of patients who are asymptomatic, however, is in the range of 25% to 30%, and therefore careful physical examinations and diagnostic evaluations are necessary to identify and follow this important subset of patients.

Signs of subaortic stenosis may include a systolic ejection murmur with or without a diastolic murmur of aortic insufficiency. If the stenosis is severe, the signs may be typical of aortic stenosis. Mitral insufficiency may also be associated and detected in patients with either intrinsic mitral disease or, more commonly, secondary mitral regurgitation.

LABORATORY EVALUATION

The chest film is generally nonspecific for these lesions. The ECG may show left ventricular hypertrophy as well as occasionally arrhythmias of the supraventricular and ventricular types.

Echocardiography is an important component of the evaluation; both 2D-echocardiography and Doppler echocardiography are employed. The ability to distinguish between isolated or predominately discrete and tunnel subaortic stenosis is often best achieved through a subcostal four-chamber view by echocardiography. Certainly for repeat evaluations, the echocardiogram is the test of choice in the majority of patients, particularly the smaller patients.

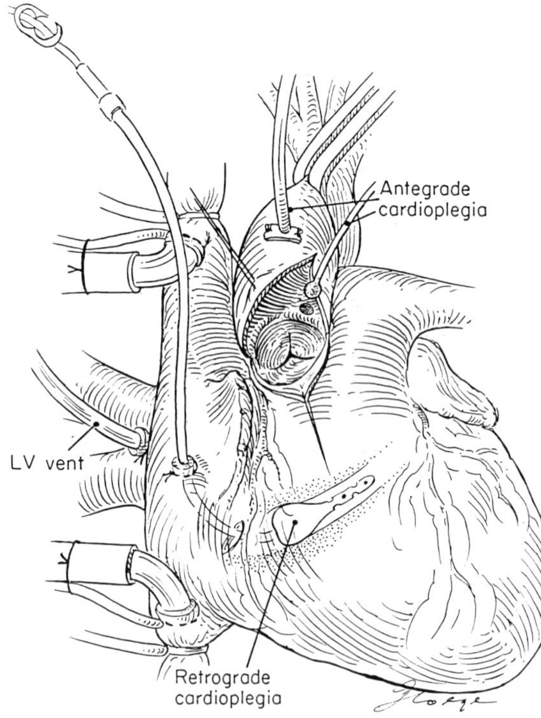

Figure 10.1 Surgical approach to aortic root surgery. Arterial cannulation of the femoral artery (or distal ascending aorta) and either single or double venous cannulation, depending on the presence of right-sided lesions. The left ventricular vent passed through the right pulmonary veins provides optimum visualization of the subaortic area and decompresses the left ventricle if aortic insufficiency is present. Cardioplegia is provided by either antegrade (aortic or coronary ostia) or a combination of antegrade and retrograde routes in cases of aortic valve insufficiency and left ventricular hypertrophy.

The more invasive cine angiogram is useful to define the anatomy further using the LAO view and may be helpful in the larger patient in whom the echo "window" is less optimal. Catheter pullback pressure tracings may also further define the level(s) and extent of the obstruction. If an isolated subaortic membrane is present, echocardiography alone may be adequate for diagnosis. In the future, tests such as cine magnetic resonance imaging or fast computed tomography may provide some additional anatomic data.

DISCRETE FIBROMUSCULAR STENOSIS

One of the more common causes of subaortic stenosis is a discrete fibromuscular membrane, which may or may not be circumferential (ring). The membrane is typically located anteriorly, 1 to 2 mm below the aortic valve cusps, although infrequently it may be attached to the base of one or more of the aortic cusps, in particular the right cusp. The gradient across these membranes may vary widely and in fact be relatively low (30 mmHg) initially; however, over time this gradient increases in the majority of patients. It is also clear that the turbulence created by even mild stenosis is capable of damaging the aortic valve, resulting in aortic insufficiency or in producing endocarditis (Wright et al. 1983). If the membrane (and stenosis) is completely resected, the aortic insufficiency remains mild on long-term follow-up, with a recurrence rate less than 3% to 4% (Ashraf et al. 1985). Thus if a definite membrane in association with even mild stenosis is identified, patients should be referred for surgery.

□ Surgery

APPROACH TO AORTIC ROOT SURGERY IN GENERAL

The basic surgical approach shown in Figure 10.1 is through a transverse aortotomy, using single or double venous cannulae, depending on the presence of associated right-sided defects. A left ventricular vent passed through the right superior pulmonary vein can be useful in providing good visualization throughout the procedure. We tend to use retrograde (coronary sinus) cardioplegia along with antegrade (aortic) cardioplegia to protect the myocardium if the left ventricular outflow tract surgery is complex or particularly if there is concomitant aortic valve insufficiency. Both antegrade and retrograde infusions of blood cardioplegia are monitored for pressure and flow to ensure adequate myocardial protection, which is particularly important in hearts in which left ventricles are often hypertrophied.

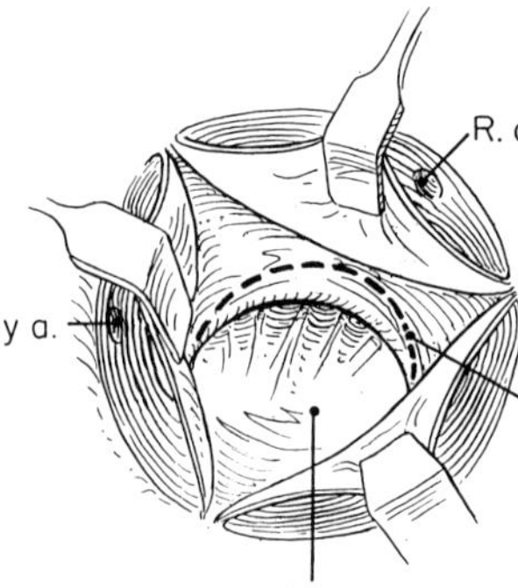

Figure 10.2 Resection of discrete subaortic membrane. View through the aortotomy showing resection margins of a typical discrete membrane, which may be close to the base of the right coronary cusp. Once the plane is developed, the membrane may be dissected from the underlying endocardium, the area of conduction, and possible attachments to the anterior leaflet of the mitral valve.

□ Discrete Subaortic Membrane

The subaortic membrane is dissected away from the endocardium, while great care is taken to avoid damage to either the aortic valve cusps or the conduction bundle (Figure 10.2). The latter lies in the membranous septum subadjacent to the rightward aspect of the right coronary cusp. The membrane may be attached to the septal leaflet of the mitral valve, and care should be taken in peeling it away not to damage the leaflet itself. If any significant septal hypertrophy is appreciated, an additional myomectomy may be needed to abolish the obstruction, using care not to create a ventricular septal defect (VSD) or heart block (Figure 10.3). Intraoperative pressures are obtained by both direct needle measurements and Doppler echocardiography. Temporary pacing wires are placed routinely at surgery regardless of rhythm at the end of the procedure because of possible transient heart block from edema. Operative mortality rate is approximately 2% for the repair of discrete (membrane) subaortic stenosis.

□ Follow-up

Long-term follow-up includes regular 6-month examinations and echo Doppler measurements of the gradient if indicated. This is so because subaortic membranes may recur to a variable degree in up to 20% of patients, depending on the extent of resection at the first operation. An adequate myomectomy in addition may decrease the recurrence rate by changing the left ventricular outflow tract ge-

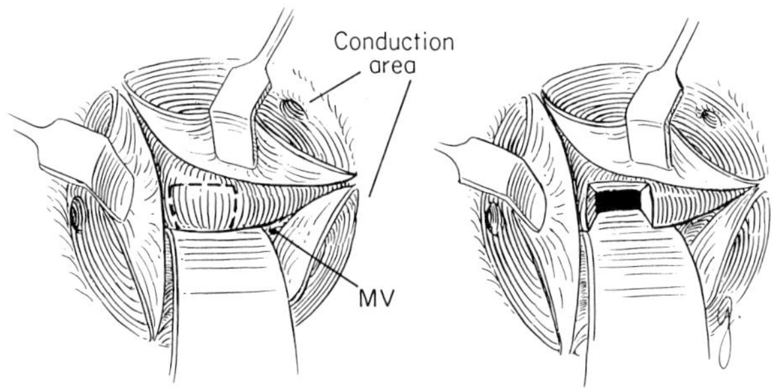

Figure 10.3 Septal myomectomy for hypertrophic obstructive cardiomyopathy. The resection area is shown beneath the base of the right coronary cusp extending to the depth (1.5 to 3 cm) of the hypertrophic segment. Avoidance is mandatory of the conduction area (membranous septum), rightward of the right coronary ostium. Compression of the anterior myocardium using a sponge stick may provide improved exposure of the septal area. A thin ribbon retractor is useful to protect the anterior mitral valve leaflet during the long parallel incisions.

ometry and turbulence. It is also prudent to provide endocarditis prophylaxis to the postsurgical patient, with the incidence of late endocarditis almost 5% in some series (Brown et al. 1988).

□ Associated Anomalies

The entity of Shone's syndrome, in which there is frequently coarctation of the aorta, supramitral stenosis, and subaortic stenosis, must be recognized and excluded. Occasionally malaligned VSDs may have a similar membrane in the left ventricular outflow tract (in addition to the more common septal obstruction) located on the crest of the defect and causing minimal to mild obstruction and turbulence. Usually an additional aortotomy approach is required to perform an adequate resection should it be necessary.

HYPERTROPHIC OBSTRUCTIVE CARDIOMYOPATHY

Hypertrophic obstructive cardiomyopathy is a primary myocardial defect that produces left ventricular outflow tract obstruction because of isolated septal hypertrophy. The pathophysiology of the obstruction to outflow is a subsequent

Venturi effect at the point of hypertrophy, which draws the anterior mitral valve leaflet forward toward the septum, causing both obstruction and possible mitral valve regurgitation. This lesion may frequently be familial or found less frequently as an isolated form. Along with systolic dysfunction, there is a diastolic component that results in a delayed ventricular relaxation and abnormal filling compliance. The condition is first treated with inotropic depressant agents such as beta-blockers or calcium channel blockers. However, if symptoms, including presyncope, chest pain, and fatigability, persist in the presence of measured gradients greater than 50 mmHg, surgery may be indicated (Maron et al. 1987).

□ Surgery

The procedure for repair of hypertrophic obstructive cardiomyopathy is resection of a portion of the septal muscle as demonstrated in Figure 10.3. The resection of an adequate amount of muscle to abolish both the resting and the dynamic outflow gradient requires care in avoiding some of the associated complications. Parallel incisions are made for the length of the septal hypertrophy, leftward of the right coronary ostium at the level of the nadir of the right coronary cusp. These are then connected, removing the muscle as intact as possible. Additional trimming may be facilitated using a small angled rongeur. Complications include complete heart block, VSD creation, and injury to either aortic or mitral valve leaflets; such complications are rare. Unless there is intrinsic mitral valve pathology, its replacement should be avoided. Mortality rate for the septal myomectomy procedure varies from 2% to 5% (Williams et al. 1987; Rephael et al. 1989).

TUNNEL SUBAORTIC STENOSIS

This lesion, although less common than other lesions, is more problematic in its ultimate treatment and surgery. As mentioned previously, patients may have both lesions and therefore require a more complex procedure to relieve completely the obstruction after removal of a subaortic membrane. The circumferential and diffuse nature (1 to 3 cm) of this lesion generally requires more extensive enlargement of the outflow tract than a septal myomectomy. The aortoventriculoplasty or modification (with or without an aortic valve replacement) is usually necessary to relieve the obstruction completely and avoid early recurrences. A thorough preoperative evaluation of the aortic valve is a prerequisite to plan the appropriate procedure, when, for example, the aortic valve is deformed and incompetent or the annulus is inadequate and would therefore need replacement. The most significant variation once a valve replacement is indicated includes the use of either mechanical aortic valve or aortic allograft as a root replacement. The choice is based largely on experience as well as availability of allografts, while the individual patient's needs may also mitigate toward a homograft. For example, if a patient is female and potentially child-bearing, or there is evidence of recent or ongoing endocarditis, a homograft valve would be indicated whenever possible.

□ Surgery

If the aortic valve is abnormal or hypoplastic, as is frequently the case with tunnel subaortic stenosis, the operation of aortoventriculoplasty (Konno) is performed.

The surgical approach, as demonstrated in Figure 10.4, is by means of longitudinal incisions through the abnormal aortic valve, leaving the right coronary artery rightward and avoiding the area of conduction. The right ventricular free wall incision is joined, staying inferior to the pulmonic valve and finally completing the septal incision as a continuation of the aortic opening. The septum is patched with dacron or allograft tissue and the aortic valve sutured into both the old annulus posteriorly and the septal patch anteriorly. Frequently an oversized aortic valve can easily be placed. To complete the operation, a right ventricular patch is used to close the defect in the free wall. If an allograft is used in the pediatric patient, it is usually as a root replacement and the coronary arteries are reimplanted. The mortality rate of the operation varies from 6% to 12%, and complications are infrequent (1% to 2%) but include complete heart block, bleeding, and mitral valve injury (Fleming and Sarafian 1987; Clarke 1989). There is also an early experience with the so-called Ross procedure, whereby the pulmonary autograft replaces the aortic valve and a pulmonary allograft the resected pulmonic valve (Randolph et al. 1989). This operation is generally limited to those stenoses primarily valvar or immediately subvalvar. Over time it remains to be demonstrated whether the autograft will be free of failure significantly longer than the allograft. The additional mortality and extent of this procedure probably restricts its use to the more straightforward left ventricular outflow tract obstructions.

If the aortic valve is adequate in size and functioning normally, a modified ventriculoplasty is performed as depicted in Figure 10.5. This procedure involves preservation of the aortic valve while enlarging the ventricular septal area below the valve with a dacron patch similar to the above-mentioned operation. The right ventricular incision may be placed transversely and closed primarily.

□ Left Ventricle to Aortic Conduit

An alternative procedure is the placement of an apical left ventricular valved conduit to either the ascending or the descending aorta (Figure 10.6). The choice of the configuration depends on a number of factors, including the relative size of the aortic portions, the aortic arch sidedness, and probably most importantly the experience of the operating team. The use of an aortic homograft for the valve portion has added a measure of convenience and efficacy in avoiding anticoagulants

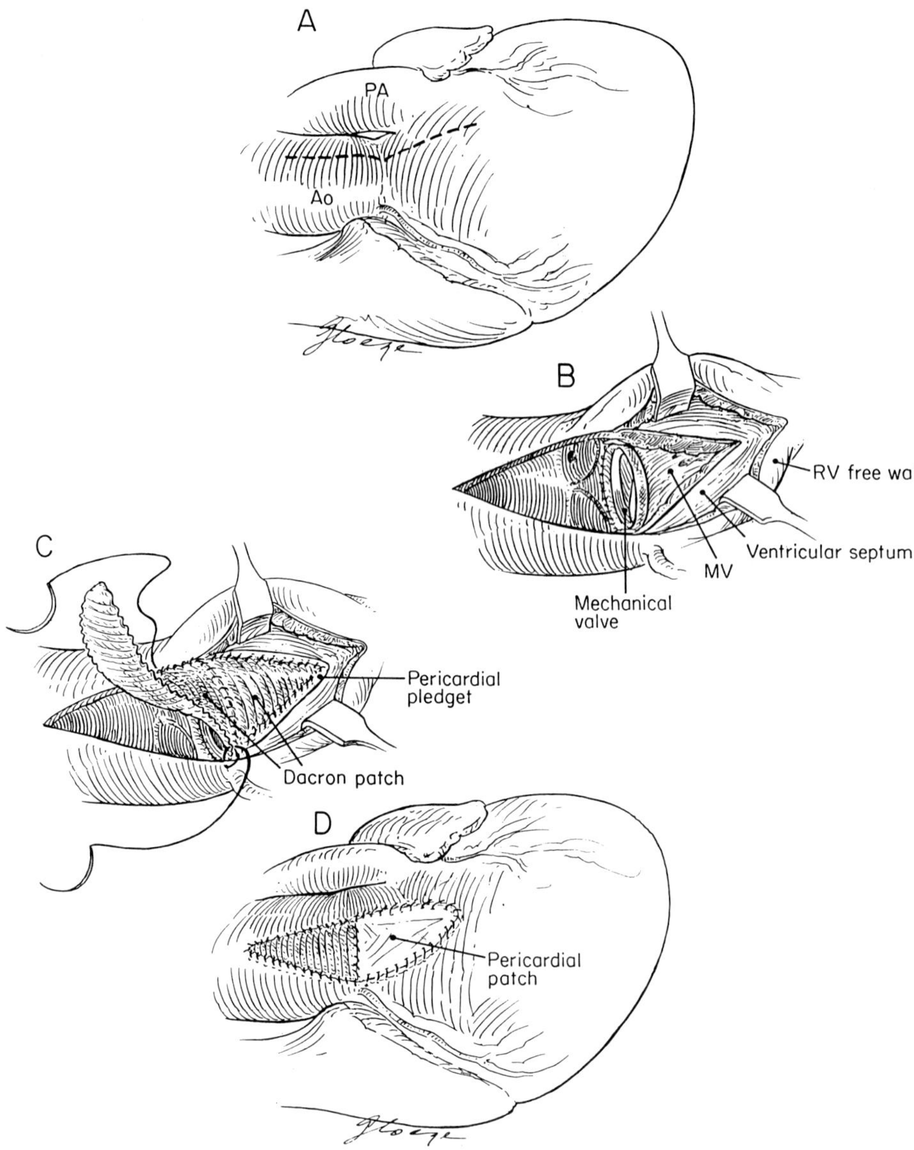

Figure 10.4 Aortoventriculoplasty (Konno procedure). (A) The first incision is longitudinally through the aorta and connected to the right ventricular free wall incision, below the pulmonic valve. (B) The ventricular septum has been opened to connect with the aortotomy and the abnormal aortic valve cusps resected. A mechanical valve, in this case, has been partially sutured in place posteriorly along the old true annulus. (C) An enlargement of the ventricular septum using dacron also provides the anterior fixation of the prosthetic valve. (D) The aortotomy closure is completed followed by the right ventricular closure using glutaraldehyde-treated pericardium.

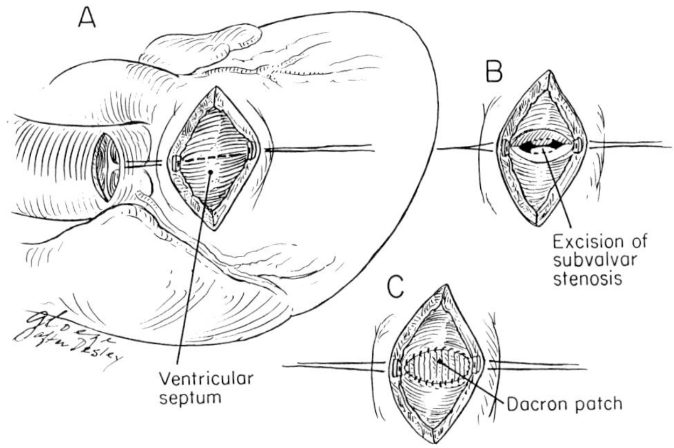

Figure 10.5 Modified ventriculo(septo)plasty. (A) Transverse counterincisions are made in both the aorta and the right ventricular free wall. (B) Guided by palpation through the aortic valve, the left ventricular outflow tract is entered through the septum and the hypertrophic segment resected in part. (C) The septectomy and left ventricular outflow tract are augmented using dacron patch, closing the right ventricular free wall primarily.

Figure 10.6 Left Ventricular apical-aorta conduit. A composite homograft and dacron conduit are depicted between the left ventricular apex and the descending aorta to bypass a severe left ventricular outflow tract obstruction. The ascending aorta is also used if of adequate size and positioned to avoid compression with the chest closed.

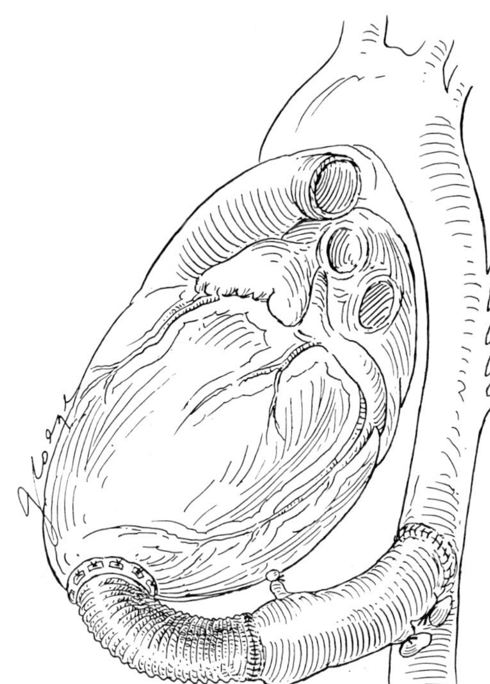

and in ease of implantation and positioning in the closed chest. The major drawback is the probable need for replacement for either size or failure considerations, perhaps one or more times. The projected longevity of a tissue valve conduit (most prior information is from the porcine valved conduit) is less than that of an aortoventriculoplasty in this condition and is therefore generally a second choice option. The mortality rate of the conduit operation is similar at 3% to 5% (DiDonato et al. 1984; Brown et al. 1988).

COEXISTING ANOMALIES WITH SUBAORTIC OBSTRUCTION

There are a number of cardiac conditions that may predispose to subaortic stenoses. Their management may include alternate techniques based on the unique anatomic configuration as well as the techniques previously discussed.

□ Interrupted Aortic Arch and Ventricular Septal Defect

A significant number of patients with interrupted aortic arch (IAA) and VSD may have an associated subaortic stenosis as high as one quarter to one third of the cases. This stenosis is secondary to malalignment of the infundibular septum, resulting in "crowding" of the left ventricular outflow tract. This entity can also be seen with isolated malaligned VSD as well as the more typical subpulmonic VSD associated with IAA. In the case of IAA, the aortic annulus can also be hypoplastic and its leaflets dysplastic. These conditions then require left ventricular outflow enlarging procedures, which may vary from simple resection to aortoventriculoplasty (Konno) to conduit procedures. A one-stage operation combining IAA repair is preferable in these cases. Patients with this lesion should be carefully followed to rule out development of significant subaortic stenosis in the postoperative period (Scott et al. 1988; Sell et al. 1988).

□ Single Ventricle Morphology

Single ventricles with left ventricular outflow chambers (bulboventricular foramen) may become obstructed as a result of the narrowing between the infundibular septum and the hypertrophied ventricle. The outflow through a VSD can also become restrictive in conditions with an atretic atrioventricular valve such as DORV or tricuspid atresia with transposition, resulting in another form of subaortic stenosis. Pulmonary artery banding may further exacerbate this condition over

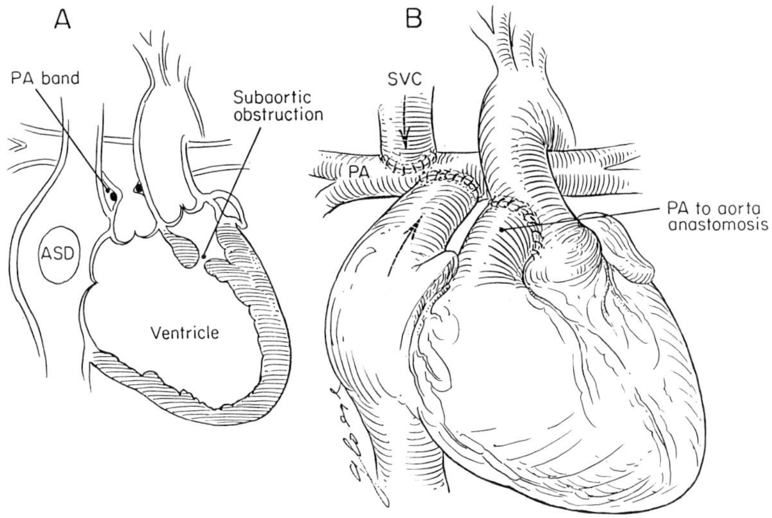

Figure 10.7 Aortopulmonary connection for subaortic stenosis. An aortopulmonary connection (Damus-Kaye Stansel procedure) is depicted, bypassing the subaortic stenosis from a restrictive bulboventricular foramen after pulmonary artery banding. In this condition, a modified Fontan procedure is also carried out in a concomitant or staged fashion. A competent pulmonary valve is a prerequisite.

the long term. The resultant obstruction can be approached, if feasible, by enlarging the VSD, a procedure associated with a significant incidence of complete heart block (12%). More frequently, an aortopulmonary artery connection (Damus-Kaye-Stansel or Norwood procedure) is carried out to correct this condition, with concomitant or staged Fontan repair (Figure 10.7). The pulmonic valve must be normal in function and uninjured from a previously placed pulmonary artery band for this procedure to be effective. There is a significant mortality recognized with surgical procedures in these very challenging patients (Jonas et al. 1985; DeLeon et al. 1986; Cheung et al. 1990).

DISCUSSION

Subaortic stenosis is prone to develop in a number of cardiac lesions, as discussed here, with subsequent management that may vary depending on the intracardiac anatomy. The long-term satisfactory outcome of these patients is dependent on both the early recognition and the adequate relief of the subaortic obstruction without injuring important adjacent structures.

REFERENCES

Ashraf H, Cotronea J, Dhar N, et al. Long-term results after excision of fixed subaortic stenosis. J Thorac Cardiovasc Surg 1985; 90:864.

Brown JW, Stevens LS, Holly S, et al. Surgical spectrum of aortic stenosis in children: A thirty-year experience with 257 children. Ann Thorac Surg 1988; 45(4):393.

Cheung HC, Lincoln C, Anderson RH, et al. Options for surgical repair in hearts with univentricular atrioventricular connections and subaortic stenosis. J Thorac Cardiovasc Surg 1990; 100:51.

Clarke DR. Cryopreserved valve conduits for outflow tract reconstruction in pediatric patients. Ann Thorac Surg 1989; 48:S85.

DeLeon SA, Idriss FS, Ilbawi MN, et al. The Damus-Stansel-Kaye procedure. J Thorac Cardiovasc Surg 1986; 91:747.

DiDonato RM, Danielson GK, McGoon DC, et al. Left ventricle-aorta conduits in pediatric patients. J Thorac Cardiovasc Surg 1984; 88:82.

Fleming WH, Sarafian LB. Aortic valve replacement with concomitant aortoventriculoplasty in children and young adults: Long-term follow-up. Ann Thorac Surg 1987; 43:575.

Jonas RA, Castaneda AR, Lang P: Single ventricle (single or double-inlet) complicated by subaortic stenosis: Surgical options in infancy. Ann Thorac Surgery 1985; 39:361.

Maron BJ, Bonow RO, Cannon RO, Leon MB, Epstein SE: Hypertrophic cardiomyopathy, interrelations of clinical manifestations, pathophysiology, and therapy. N Engl J Med 1987; 316:780 (Part 1), 844 (Part 2).

Randolph JD, Toal K, Stelzer P, Elkins RC: Aortic valve and left ventricular outflow tract replacement using allograft and autograft valves: A preliminary report. Ann Thorac Surg 1989; 48:345.

Rephael M, Schaff HV, Danielson GK, et al. The outcome of surgical treatment of hypertrophic obstructive cardiomyopathy, experience over 15 years. J Thorac Cardiovasc Surg 1989; 97:666.

Scott WA, Rocchini AP, Bove EL, et al. Repair of interrupted arch in infancy. J Thorac Cardiovasc Surg 1988; 96:564.

Sell JE, Jonas RA, Mayer JE, et al. The results of a surgical program for interrupted aortic arch. J Thorac Cardiovasc Surg 1988; 96:864.

Williams WG, Wigle ED, Rakowski H, et al. Results of surgery for hypertrophic obstructive cardiomyopathy. Circulation 1987; 76(suppl V):104.

Wright GB, Keane JF, Nadas AS, Bernhard W, Castaneda AR: Fixed subaortic stenosis in the young: Medical and surgical course in 83 patients. Am J Cardiol 1983; 52:830.

11

Surgical Techniques for Relief of Complex Left Ventricular Outflow Tract Obstruction

David R. Clarke

Fifteen years ago, the resources and techniques available to pediatric cardiac surgeons were limited and often experimental. Anomalies that required closed cardiac surgery were repaired or palliated with relative ease, and simple anomalies that necessitated open cardiac procedures could often be incised, sutured, patched, or reconstructed. Complex cardiac anomalies were an almost insurmountable problem that afforded little hope for the patient's survival. Complex cardiac anomalies remain a challenge but one that is being met with innovative new surgical tools and techniques.

Left ventricular outflow tract obstruction (LVOTO) is associated with a wide range of complexity and severity. The obstruction may occur at one or any combination of three levels and may be of many diverse types. It can be associated with multiple congenital cardiac anomalies. Optimal techniques for surgical repair must be extremely versatile, to allow the surgeon to accommodate varied complex anatomies.

VALVAR AORTIC STENOSIS

Aortic valvar disease is often a simple problem but can become complex in a young child when it is recurrent stenosis with or without regurgitation or aortic insufficiency following valvotomy. Aside from repeat valvotomy, which is frequently ineffective because the annulus diameter is inadequate, several surgical options are available. If aortic regurgitation is absent or minimal, a left ventricle to aortic conduit is advocated by some surgeons. The procedure allows placement of an adult size prosthetic aortic valve and adequately relieves even severe transaortic gradients. These positive features may be outweighed by a high incidence of late failure in both the native aortic and the conduit valve. In addition, the myocardial damage produced by direct ventricular insertion and the physiologically abnormal direction of blood flow may be detrimental to long-term ventricular function (DiDonato et al. 1984).

Infants and small children who undergo prosthetic aortic valve replacement may require a concomitant procedure to enlarge the annulus. Several methods are available for surgical management of such a situation. One option is the Manouguian procedure (Manouguian and Seybold-Epting 1979). This technique, in which the annulus is enlarged posteriorly, allows a maximum of approximately 4 mm implantation diameter enlargement. The aortic annular diameter is enlarged when an incision is made into the base of the anterior leaflet of the mitral valve and the V-shaped defect is filled by a fusiform patch. The resultant increase in aortic implantation diameter allows placement of a prosthesis that is one to two sizes larger than originally would have been accommodated.

An alternative approach is aortoventriculoplasty. The procedure was devised for the treatment of complex LVOTO secondary to subvalvar tunnel, idiopathic hypertrophic subaortic stenosis (IHSS), hypoplastic aortic annulus, or replacement of a small valve prosthesis. The concept was proposed concurrently by Konno and Rastan in 1970 (Konno et al. 1975; Rastan and Koncz 1976). A longitudinal incision is made in the aorta and carried caudally to the aortic annulus, to the left of the right coronary orifice. A transverse incision is made in the right ventricular outflow tract and is extended medially to the aortic annulus. Just beneath the pulmonary valve, a ventricular septal defect is created by extension of the aforementioned incisions across the aortic annulus into the infundibular septum. An elliptical, double-layer patch is sewn into the septal incision up to the aortic level. The aortic valve is then implanted, followed by repair of both the aortic and the right ventricular outflow tract incisions with the leaflets of the double-layer patch.

If aortic valve allograft conduits are available, an aortic root replacement (ARR) may be used to relieve complex LVOTO. More extensive left ventricular outflow tract resection is needed with the ARR than is involved in aortoventriculoplasty. Therefore the risk of heart block is increased. ARR includes interposition of an allograft with subsequent reimplantation of the coronary arteries and was designed jointly by Somerville and Ross (1982).

The ARR technique was further modified with the introduction of the extended aortic root replacement (EARR). The concept of EARR evolved from the aortoventriculoplasty and ARR techniques and employs the anterior leaflet of the donor mitral valve to enlarge the left ventricular outflow tract (Clarke 1988). Both ARR and EARR can be used for the repair of valvar LVOTO. They are discussed in detail later.

SUBVALVAR AORTIC STENOSIS

Subvalvar LVOTO occurs in different forms. Anatomy below the aortic valve may consist of an isolated, fibrous ridge; hypertrophied septal muscle that causes dynamic narrowing; or a fibromuscular, tunnel narrowing. When the anomaly presents as an isolated lesion, surgery is relatively simple. As an alternative to sharp excision of a portion of a subvalvar aortic membrane, Ross postulated a technique for blunt dissection of the fibrous tissue (McKay and Ross 1982). The revised procedure is intended to reduce the incidence of operative complications, such as aortic or mitral valve injury, heart block, or late recurrence of subvalvar aortic stenosis. The operation is initiated with an oblique incision into the aortic root, which extends into the noncoronary sinus. A plane of separation between the fibrous tissue and the left ventricular endocardium is exposed, and the ridge of membrane is peeled away. A myectomy is advised if septal muscle hypertrophy is present.

Diffuse subvalvar aortic stenosis caused by IHSS can be surgically managed as proposed by Morrow (1978). He advises removal of a 1-cm block of muscle from below the base of the right coronary leaflet of the aortic valve. This is accomplished with two myotomies, which extend at least 4 cm into the ventricular septum, succeeded by a transverse incision to excise the cube. The Morrow procedure is executed through an ascending aortotomy. One must exercise caution to prevent conduction tissue injury, accidental creation of a ventricular septal defect, or aortic valve leaflet injury during excision of the hypertrophic muscle.

When a fibromuscular tunnel or truly hypoplastic left ventricular outflow tract is encountered, the pathway may be enlarged with a technique devised by Vouhe (Vouhe et al. 1984). The Vouhe procedure is applicable when diffuse subvalvar stenosis is accompanied by an aortic valve of normal or near normal size and function. The operation is performed through a right ventriculotomy and includes an incision beginning below the right coronary, left coronary commissure of the aortic valve, which is carried as far as necessary into the interventricular septum. The left ventricular outflow tract is enlarged by resecting fibrous or muscular tissue from the septotomy edges and applying an elliptical patch to close the septal incision.

When a patient with recurrent subvalvar aortic stenosis and fibromuscular tunnel stenosis presents for surgery, the aortic valve is often severely deformed and regurgitant. In such situations, the valve must be replaced. Aortoventriculoplasty and EARR provide suitable alternatives for repair of combined valvar and subvalvar disease.

Subvalvar aortic stenosis is often associated with other cardiac anomalies. In most instances, the obstruction in these situations can be surgically managed with one of the previously described techniques or a variation thereof. When subvalvar stenosis is concurrent with atrioventricular septal defect, the Vouhe procedure provides excellent relief since the associated stenosis is usually tunnel type with a normal aortic valve.

Nikaidoh (1984) has proposed the aortic translocation to replace the conventional Rastelli baffle technique used to repair transposition of the great arteries with concomitant ventricular septal defect and LVOTO. The aorta is detached from the right ventricle beneath the valve and with coronaries intact and is moved posteriorly in the left ventricular outflow tract. Right ventricle to pulmonary artery continuity can then be restored with a patch or cardiopulmonary allograft.

Rastan has devised a technique for double valve replacement secondary to complex aortic stenosis and severe mitral valve deformity (Rastan et al. 1981). The mitral and aortic annuli are each incised at their point of continuity. Prosthetic valves are implanted, which are partially supported by a patch. The patch extends from the area of valve continuity onto the left atrium posteriorly and the ascending aorta anteriorly.

Interrupted aortic arch is occasionally accompanied by a severely deformed left ventricular outflow tract. A modification of the ARR was used for cardiac reconstruction in one such case and is discussed later.

SUPRAVALVAR AORTIC STENOSIS

Supravalvar aortic stenosis occurs infrequently as an isolated anomaly usually associated with Williams syndrome. It can also occur at the site of aortotomy following other left ventricular outflow tract repair or reconstructive procedures. It commonly presents as part of multilevel aortic obstruction. Supravalvar stenosis is usually in one of two forms: An isolated hourglass-shaped deformity immediately distal to the coronary sinus or a diffuse hypoplasia of the entire ascending, and sometimes more distal, aorta. Additionally, if the entry to the sinuses of Valsalva is stenosed, there is a potential for compromised coronary blood flow. This potential must be kept in mind when considering surgical options.

Discrete supravalvar aortic stenosis as a primary lesion can sometimes be repaired by a simple patch aortoplasty (McGoon et al. 1961). A lateral aortotomy is extended across the supravalvar stenosis and into the noncoronary sinus of Valsalva. An elliptical patch is sutured into the aortotomy.

More often, a degree of valvar stenosis is associated with the supravalvar component. In approximately 30% of primary supravalvar aortic stenoses, there are thickened leaflets, coaptation of the commissures is distorted, or both occur. It is often necessary to extend the patch into more than one of the coronary sinuses to provide complete surgical repair of the stenosis. The extended aortoplasty technique suggested by Doty more symmetrically reconstructs the left ventricular outflow tract, resulting in a more anatomically correct anatomy (Doty et al. 1977). The supravalvar aortic ring is incised into both the noncoronary and the right coronary sinuses of Valsalva as an extension of a vertical aortotomy. An inverted Y-shaped patch is used to fill the incision and enlarge the area. Postoperative obstruction of the coronary arteries is less prevalent, and left ventricular outflow tract pressure gradients are more adequately relieved. The three-prong patch approach suggested by Szarnicki (personal communication 1989) is an alternative when fibrosis or obstruction of all the coronary sinuses complicates the anatomy. In such a situation, it might be simpler technically to use a tubular prosthesis that has been scalloped across the proximal end to replace the ascending aorta. This procedure has been successfully accomplished in an 11-year-old boy with valvar and supravalvar aortic stenosis.

RELIEF OF LEFT VENTRICULAR OUTFLOW TRACT OBSTRUCTION WITH CRYOPRESERVED AORTIC VALVE ALLOGRAFTS

Cryopreserved aortic valve allografts have developed a reputation as a versatile tool for intracardiac repair. The story of allograft valve conduits and their use in the surgical repair of cardiac anomalies began in the 1950s (Murray 1956). In 1972, Ross began using aortic valve allografts in aortic root replacements secondary to endocarditis and concomitant annular abscess (Donaldson and Ross 1982). Application of the procedure was then expanded to include repair of tunnel LVOTO and small aortic annulus. The technique was further modified with the introduction of the EARR.

In Denver, 34 aortic root replacements have been performed since June 1985 using cryopreserved aortic valve allografts. Allografts offer several advantages over the use of mechanical or other biologic prostheses. Cryopreserved allograft valves obviate the need for anticoagulation in the pediatric population. Surgical implantation can be performed with minimal bleeding and little or no intraoperative gradient. Of particular importance is the decreased incidence of reoperation since large valves can often be placed in small children.

□ Extended Aortic Root Replacement

EARR is indicated for the repair of LVOTO complicated by aortic insufficiency, hypoplastic annulus, or multilevel obstruction. No definite contraindications to the procedure have been ascertained thus far. From September 1985 to September 1989, 26 children have undergone 27 EARR procedures at The University of Colorado Health Sciences Center and The Childrens Hospital. EARR recipients

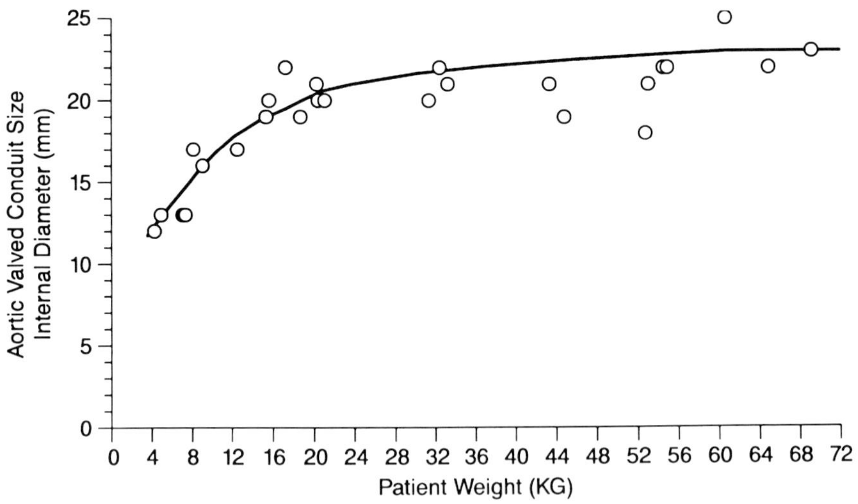

Figure 11.1 Extended aortic root replacement. The relationship between patient weight and allograft size.

ranged in age from 11 days to 15 years (mean 7.3 years). With the exception of one, each patient had undergone prior cardiac surgery. Indication for operation was multilevel aortic stenosis in 13 children, recurrent subvalvar aortic stenosis in nine, aortic stenosis with hypoplastic annulus in three, and isolated aortic insufficiency in two.

□ Surgical Procedure

In preparation for EARR, an aortic valve allograft of appropriate size is chosen. Conduit size is estimated by patient weight (Figure 11.1). After completion of a median sternotomy, standard preparations are made for cardiopulmonary bypass. Total bypass is instituted by first cannulating the ascending aorta near the origin of the innominate artery. Right angle cannulae are then inserted into the superior and inferior vena cavae. After cooling the child to 20°C, the myocardium is preserved by antegrade or retrograde infusion of blood cardioplegia. As cardiopulmonary bypass preparations are begun, the allograft is removed from liquid nitrogen storage. Still enclosed in the three plastic pouches, it is thawed in a 37°C to 42°C water bath for up to 16 minutes. The tissue is removed from its two outer pouches and is passed onto the sterile field. After removal from the innermost pouch, it is rinsed sequentially in three basins of increasing concentrations of Dulbeccos medium to dilute the dimethyl sulfoxide concentration. The allograft undergoes a final rinse in lactated Ringer's solution. A small piece of distal conduit is sent to microbiology for culture, and the tissue is ready for implantation.

An oblique incision is carried across the right ventricular outflow tract, and a vertical one similar to that performed in aortoventriculoplasty is made along the

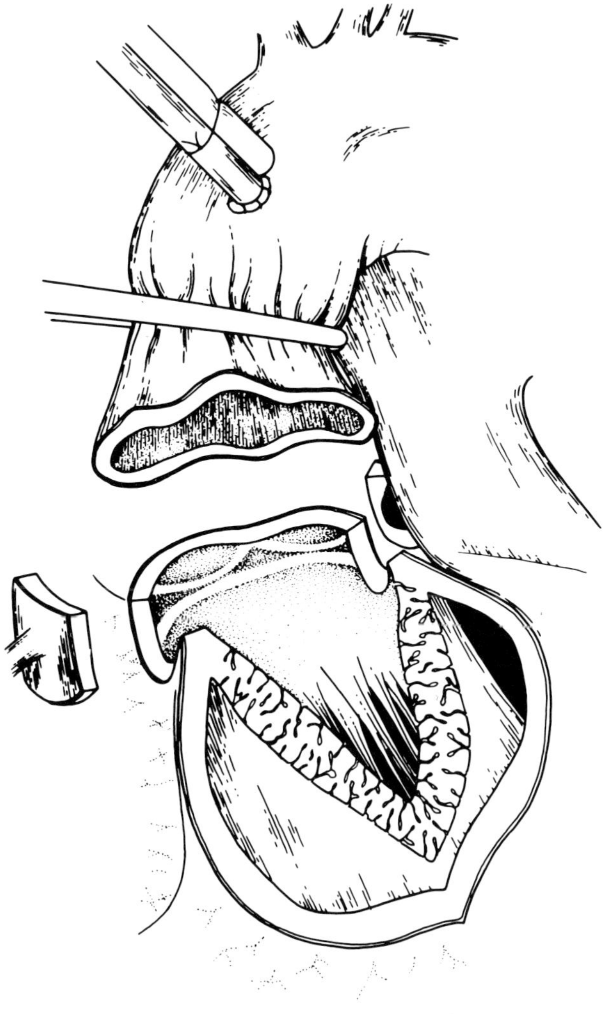

Figure 11.2 An oblique incision across the right ventricular outflow tract and a vertical incision along the ascending aorta intersect between the left and right coronary cusps. The incision is carried across the aortic annulus and into the infundibular interventricular septum. The ascending aorta is transected and buttons of aortic wall and aortic valve leaflets are excised. (Clarke DR. Extended aortic root replacement for treatment of left ventricular outflow tract obstruction. J Cardiac Surg 1987;1(suppl):121. By permission.)

ascending aorta. The two incisions meet at the aortic annulus between left and right coronary ostia. From the point of intersection, an incision is carried across the annulus into the infundibular interventricular septum. After transecting the ascending aorta, the coronary ostia with attached buttons of aortic wall are excised (Figure 11.2). The native valve leaflets are resected, and the aortic annulus is then ready for conduit insertion.

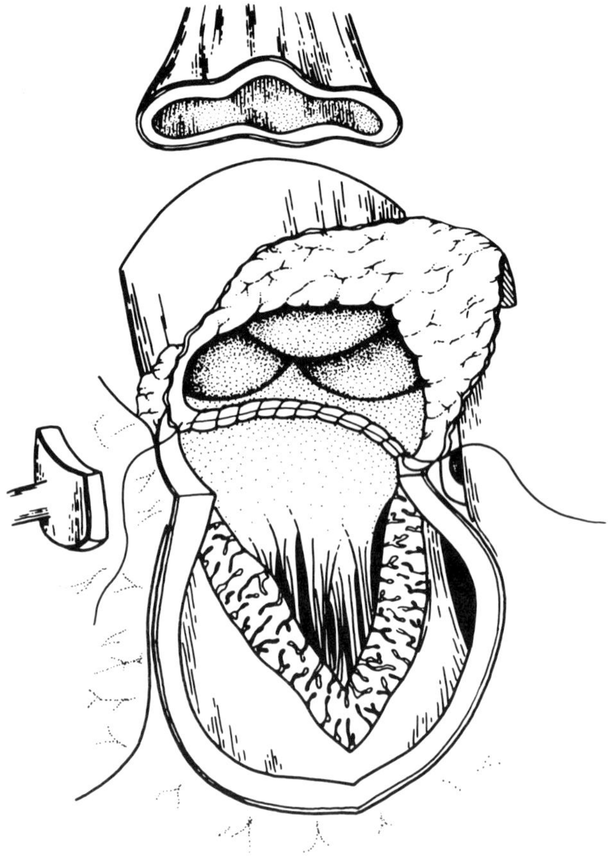

Figure 11.3 Excess muscle is trimmed from the allograft, and the valve annulus is thinned. Proximal anastomosis is begun posteriorly and continued left and right to the interventricular septum. (Clarke DR. Extended aortic root replacement for treatment of left ventricular outflow tract obstruction. J Cardiac Surg 1987;1(suppl):121. By permission.)

The allograft is tailored by trimming excess muscle to within a few millimeters of the annulus. The remaining area is thinned to avoid creation of a bulky proximal suture line. The proximal anastomosis between the allograft annulus and the recipient's annulus and proximal aortic wall is performed first. Suture lines are begun posteriorly and continued right and left to the interventricular septum (Figure 11.3). After trimming, the donor mitral valve leaflet is used to fill the septal incision and enlarge the area (Figure 11.4). The suture line, reinforced by horizontal mattress sutures with Teflon felt pledgets, is continued around the right ventricular edge of the septal incision.

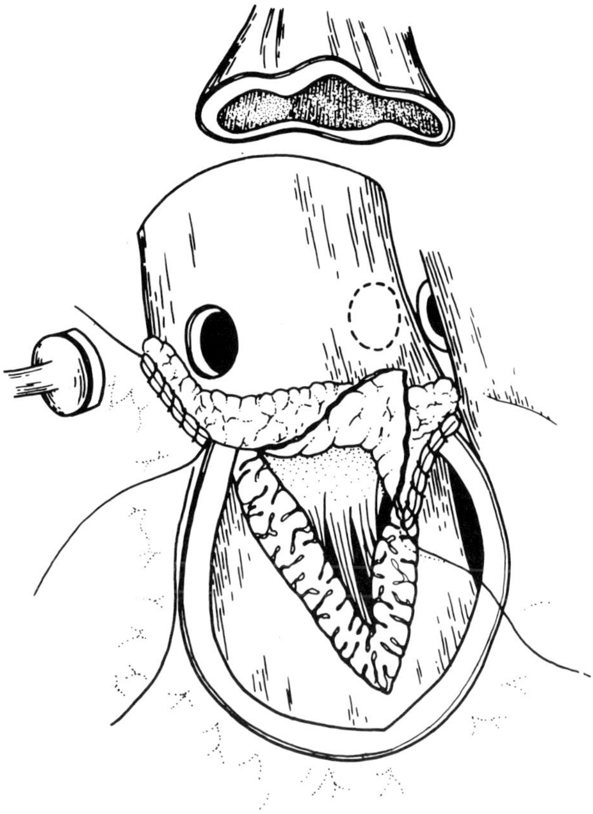

Figure 11.4
The anterior leaflet of the donor mitral valve is used to fill the septal incision and enlarge the area. (Clarke DR. Extended aortic root replacement for treatment of left ventricular outflow tract obstruction. J Cardiac Surg 1987;1(suppl):121. By permission.)

In preparation for the distal anastomosis, the allograft is cut to the precise length necessary to complete its connection to the ascending aorta. A 5- or 6-mm diameter aortic punch is used to create holes in the donor aortic root while protecting the easily visible valve leaflets. Each coronary ostial button is sewn into its corresponding hole, and the distal anastomosis is subsequently begun. The suture line is initiated posteriorly from inside the lumen with running stitches. The anterior and lateral connection is completed from the outside. The aortic cross clamp is released.

A triangular shaped patch constructed of distal allograft conduit is used to mend the right ventricular outflow tract. The base of the tissue is sutured to the donor aortic root at the annulus. Corners between the right ventricular myocardium, allograft conduit, and patch free edges are carefully sutured to avoid bleeding (Figure 11.5). With the heart beating, the right ventricular suture line is completed. Temporary pacemaker wires are attached for postoperative management. The patient is weaned from cardiopulmonary bypass and decannulated, and surgery is completed in the standard manner.

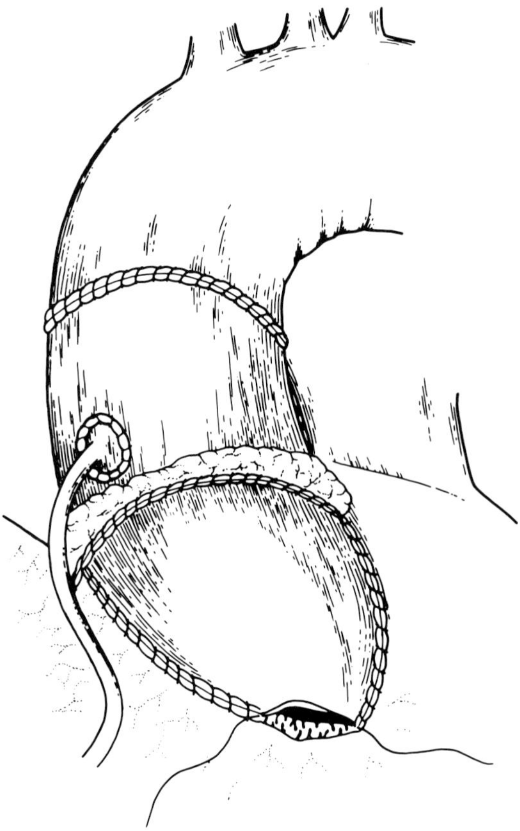

Figure 11.5
Coronary ostial buttons are sutured into the allograft. The distal anastomosis is completed, and a piece of distal allograft is used to patch the right ventricular outflow tract. (Clarke DR. Extended aortic root replacement for treatment of left ventricular outflow tract obstruction. J Cardiac Surg 1987;1(suppl):121. By permission.)

□ Operative Results and Follow-Up

Internal diameter of the implanted aortic valve allografts ranged from 12 to 23 mm (mean 19 mm). Eighteen (67%) allografts were 19 mm or larger. There were three early deaths. Two patients could not be weaned from cardiopulmonary bypass secondary to biventricular cardiac failure. Left and right ventricular failure was the cause of death in a 9-year-old patient with recurrent valvar and subvalvar aortic stenosis and associated mitral stenosis. EARR and concomitant mitral valvuloplasty was complicated by coagulopathy. The child succumbed 1 week after surgery.

Seven (29%) patients experienced a benign postoperative recovery. There was a diverse compilation of early postoperative complications (Table 11.1). Four children developed transient heart block, one of whom had a pacemaker implanted but is currently in sinus rhythm. Cardiac transplantation secondary to left ven-

Complication	No. of Patients
Transient heart block	4
Arrhythmias	2
Bleeding which required reoperation	2
Postpericardiotomy syndrome	2
Left ventricular failure (cardiac transplantation)	1
Pleural effusion	1
Pericardial effusion	1
Atelectasis	1
Right phrenic palsy	1
Dialysis and ventilatory support	1
Serratia marcescens mediastinitis	1
Superficial wound infection	1
Incisional ventral hernia	1

Table 11.1 Early Postoperative Complications Following Extended Aortic Root Replacement

tricular incompetence was ultimately necessary in a 5-year-old boy who underwent EARR and concurrent mitral valve replacement.

Allograft recipients have been followed 2 months to 4 years (mean 25 months). Six months after aortic allograft placement, coronary bypass was necessary in a 14-year-old boy with familial hyperlipidemia. A 22-month-old girl underwent repeat EARR when she developed severe aortic allograft regurgitation. At reoperation, findings were compatible with rejection. Cyclosporine was begun with implantation of the second allograft valve. After 10 months of follow-up, the child continues to thrive. The 22 (85%) survivors of EARR are clinically asymptomatic. Echocardiographic evaluation in 21 of 22 patients reveals favorable operative results (Table 11.2).

	< 6 mo Postop. (N = 5 Pts.)	6 mo–1 yr Postop. (N = 3 Pts.)	> 1 yr Postop. (N = 13 Pts.)
Left ventricular function	Normal—4	Normal—3	Normal—12
	Poor—1		Mildly decreased—1
Aortic stenosis	None—3	None—3	None—11
	Mild—2		Mild—2
Aortic insufficiency	None—2	Mild—3	None—6
	Mild—2		Mild—4
	Moderate—1		Moderate—3

Table 11.2 Most Recent Echocardiographic Evaluation in 21 of 22 Survivors of Extended Aortic Root Replacement

AORTIC ROOT REPLACEMENT

Since June 1985, six patients have undergone seven aortic root replacements using cryopreserved aortic allograft valves. The techniques can be significantly different than those described for EARR as dictated by anatomic variation. Indications for ARR include repair of complex LVOTO and the presence of endocarditis with abscess (Lau et al. 1984).

Children undergoing ARR have ranged from 1 day to 12 years (mean 2.5 years) of age. Hemodynamic indication for operation was complex aortic stenosis and insufficiency in three cases, complex aortic stenosis in two, and isolated severe insufficiency in two. Five patients had undergone prior cardiac surgery. Cryopreserved aortic valve allografts of 11 to 23 mm (mean 14 mm) internal diameter were used for the left ventricular outflow tract repairs. Five (71%) patients required a concomitant cardiac surgical procedure.

□ Operative Results and Follow-Up

Two (29%) children experienced an uncomplicated postoperative course. Minor complications were resolved by discharge. There were two (29%) hospital deaths. Intraoperative death secondary to myocardial dysfunction occurred in a neonate. The second perioperative death occurred in a 3-year-old patient who had combined mitral valve replacement and ARR. The child succumbed 11 days following surgery secondary to *Candida albicans* sepsis.

Survivors of ARR have been followed for 13 months to 4.2 years (mean 2.7 years). Echocardiography reveals mild aortic insufficiency to be prevalent but physiologically inconsequential. A 2-year-old boy with interrupted aortic arch, small aortic annulus and root, and ventricular septal defect has done exceptionally well. He had undergone pulmonary artery banding and construction of a main pulmonary artery to descending thoracic aorta conduit as a neonate. Two years later, he underwent a complex ARR. The repair was begun with removal of the graft conduit followed by pulmonary artery band resection and reanastomosis of the pulmonary artery. The small ascending aorta was transected proximal to the coronary arteries and closed (Figure 11.6). A long aortic valve allograft was then used to create a new left ventricular outflow tract and aortic arch. The conduit was anastomosed side to side, to the detached ascending aorta to revascularize the carotid and coronary arteries (Figure 11.7). After 14 months of follow-up, the child is active, asymptomatic, and quickly recompensing his preoperatively retarded development.

One late death has occurred in a child who received three successive aortic allografts, two of which were used in ARR procedures. The child was born with aortic root hypoplasia and aortic valvar atresia. The initial allograft that replaced

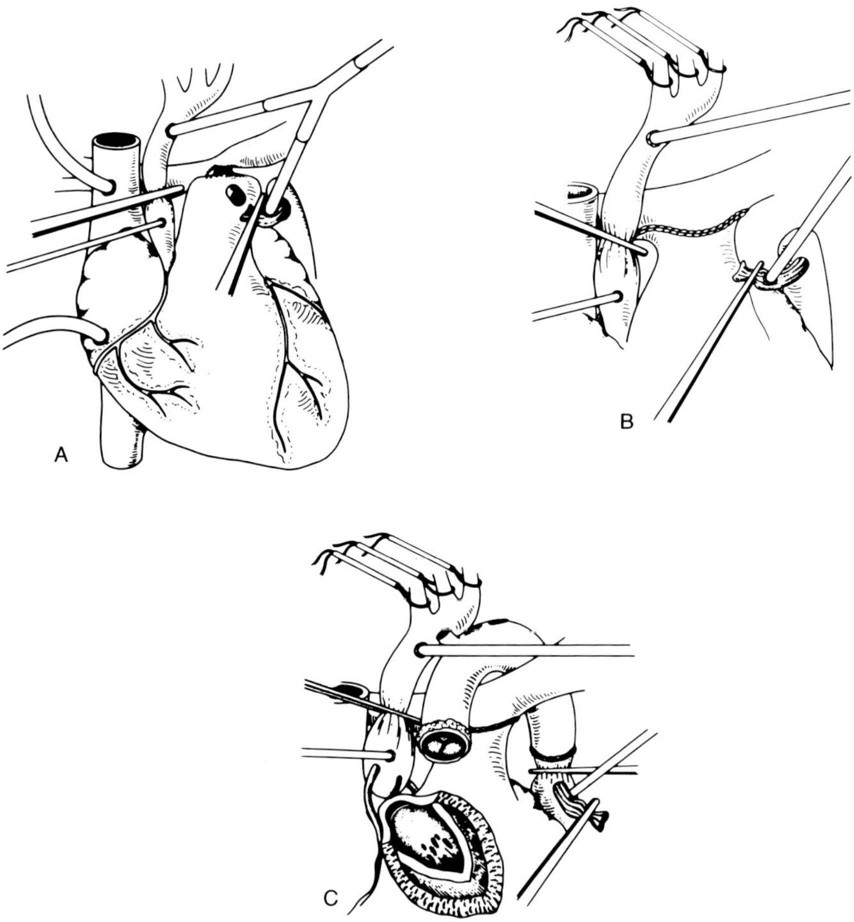

Figure 11.6 (A) The graft conduit is taken down. (B) The pulmonary artery band is resected, and the artery is reanastomosed. (C) The ascending aorta is transected and closed below the coronary arteries. The distal aortic allograft is attached to the descending thoracic aorta. (Clarke DR, Campbell DN, Bishop DA. Homografts for congenital heart disease. In Cardiac surgery: State of the art reviews. Philadelphia: Hanley & Belfus, 1989:p363. By permission.)

the aortic root rapidly became regurgitant. A second allograft placed in the descending thoracic aorta underwent similar degeneration, and rejection was suspected. A third allograft was used to replace the first and within a few weeks became regurgitant. The progression of allograft insufficiency was interrupted when azathioprine therapy was initiated. Following an asymptomatic respite, the child expired with irreversible myocardial failure secondary to an infectious car-

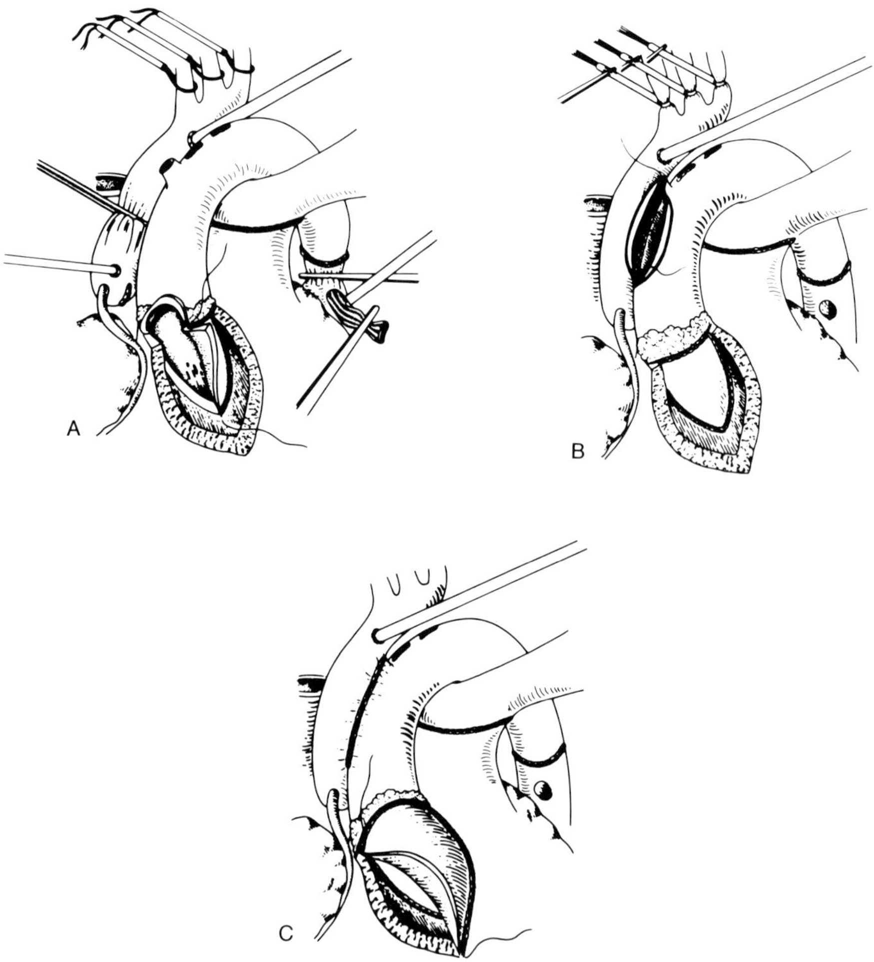

Figure 11.7 (A, B) Side to side anastomosis between the ascending aorta and aortic allograft is performed. (C) A new left ventricular outflow tract is created using the allograft in a technique similar to extended aortic root replacement. (Clarke DR, Campbell DN, Bishop DA. Homografts for congenital heart disease. In Kron IL, Mavroudis C, eds. Cardiac surgery: State of the art reviews. Philadelphia: Hanley & Belfus, 1989:p363. By permission.)

diomyopathy at 1 year of age. These instances of allograft tissue rejection, combined with the suspected rejection that resulted in a repeat EARR, have prompted the use of donor-recipient, ABO-compatible allograft valves in all ensuing cases.

DISCUSSION

In an age in which the impossible is being realized daily, the field of pediatric cardiac surgery is certainly no exception. Complex LVOTO no longer carries the ominous and often fatal prognosis it once did. A variety of options are available for the surgical relief of complex congenital aortic outflow stenoses at all levels. This chapter has presented a brief synopsis of the possibilities. Limited only by our imagination, the struggle to improve existing techniques and devise new ones is never ending. Although the search for improved patch, conduit, and valve replacement materials has been rewarding, it is also perpetual. The techniques and tools described herein offer increased hope to children born with these complex cardiac anomalies.

REFERENCES

Clarke DR. Extended aortic root replacement in 12 patients with complex left ventricular outflow tract obstruction. In Yankah AC, Hetzer R, Miller DC, et al, eds. Cardiac valve allografts 1962–1987: Current concepts on the use of aortic and pulmonary allografts for heart valve substitutes. New York: Springer-Verlag, 1988:p 157.

DiDonato RM, Danielson GK, McGoon DC, et al. Left ventricle–aortic conduits in pediatric patients. J Thorac Cardiovasc Surg 1984;88:82.

Donaldson RM, Ross DN. Homograft aortic root replacement for complicated prosthetic valve endocarditis. Circulation 1982;70(suppl I):78.

Doty DB, Polansky DB, Jenson CB. Supravalvular aortic stenosis. Repair by extended aortoplasty. J Thorac Cardiovasc Surg 1977;74:362.

Konno S, Imai J, Iida Y, et al. A new method for prosthetic valve replacement in congenital aortic stenosis associated with hypoplasia of the aortic valve ring. J Thorac Cardiovasc Surg 1975;70:909.

Lau JKH, Robles A, Cherian A, et al. Surgical treatment of prosthetic endocarditis: Aortic root replacement using a homograft. J Thorac Cardiovasc Surg 1984;87:712.

Manouguian S, Seybold-Epting W. Patch enlargement of the aortic valve ring by extending the aortic incision into the anterior mitral leaflet. New operative technique. J Thorac Cardiovasc Surg 1979;78:402.

McGoon DC, Mankin HT, Vlad P, et al. The surgical treatment of supravalvular aortic stenosis. J Thorac Cardiovasc Surg 1961;41:125.

McKay R, Ross DN. Technique for the relief of discrete subaortic stenosis. J Thorac Cardiovasc Surg 1982;84:917.

Morrow AG. Hypertrophic subaortic stenosis. Operative methods utilized to relieve left ventricular outflow obstruction. J Thorac Cardiovasc Surg 1978;76:423.

Murray G. Homologous aortic valve segment transplants as surgical treatment for aortic and mitral insufficiency. Angioplasty 1956;7:466.

Nikaidoh H. Aortic translocation and biventricular outflow tract reconstruction. A new surgical repair for transposition of the great arteries associated with ventricular septal defect and pulmonary stenosis. J Thorac Cardiovasc Surg 1984;88:365.
Rastan H, Atai M, Hadi H, et al. Enlargement of mitral valvular ring. New technique for double valve replacement in children or adults with small mitral anulus. J Thorac Cardiovasc Surg 1981;81:106.
Rastan H, Koncz J. Aortoventriculoplasty: A new technique for the treatment of left ventricular outflow tract obstruction. J Thorac Cardiovasc Surg 1976;71:920.
Somerville J, Ross D. Homograft replacement of aortic root with reimplantation of coronary arteries. Results after one to five years. Br Heart J 1982;47:473.
Szarnicki RJ. Personal communication, 1989.
Vouhe PR, Poulain H, Bloch G, et al. Aortoseptal approach for optimal resection of diffuse subvalvular aortic stenosis. J Thorac Cardiovasc Surg 1984;87:887.

12

Extracardiac Valved Conduits in Congenital Heart Surgery

Richard A. Jonas

At the simple end of the spectrum of congenital heart disease are a number of anomalies that can be corrected by elimination of a shunt (patent ductus arteriosus [PDA], atrial septal defect [ASD], ventricular septal defect [VSD]) or removal of a gradient (coarctation, pulmonary valve stenosis, aortic valve stenosis). At the middle of the spectrum, exemplified by tetralogy of Fallot, both a shunt and a gradient must be corrected. The more complex end of the spectrum involves anomalies that require a reconstructive operation to create great vessels that have failed to develop. These anomalies range from tetralogy of Fallot with pulmonary atresia (also known as pulmonary atresia with VSD) to Dextro- and Levo- loop transposition of the great arteries with VSD and pulmonary stenosis, double outlet right ventricle with VSD and pulmonary stenosis, and truncus arteriosus. At the most complex end of the spectrum is hypoplastic left-heart syndrome, in which not only must a neo-aorta be constructed but in addition there is only one effective ventricle. Most of these more complex anomalies require use of an extracardiac conduit for satisfactory reconstruction.

HISTORY OF ARTERIAL SUBSTITUTES

Early this century, Alexis Carrell carefully investigated the use of transplanted allograft (homograft) arteries and veins in an experimental setting using canine models (Carrel 1907, 1908, 1912; Guthrie 1910). He developed a number of the surgical techniques and instruments that remain in use today. He was many years ahead of his time, so that it was not until the development of antibiotics that his ideas could be clinically applied.

Surgery for congenital heart disease began at The Children's Hospital, Boston, in 1938 when Gross ligated a PDA (Gross and Hubbard 1939). Having conquered the simplest of the persistent shunts, his thoughts were next directed to the simplest anomaly involving a persistent gradient: coarctation of the aorta. Although the elasticity of the aorta would allow resection and direct anastomosis in most cases, this was not universally so. He needed a safe arterial substitute and like Carrel looked first to an aortic homograft. In laboratory studies investigating methods of preparation and storage of aortic homografts, Gross found that some methods of storage could result in frequent catastrophic failure, namely death by homograft rupture (Gross et al. 1949). Nine of 12 dogs that received abdominal aortic homografts that had been frozen to −72°C (CO_2), without a cryoprotectant agent, died within 2 weeks of surgery from homograft rupture. In contrast, none of 25 homografts that had been stored in a balanced salt solution at 4°C failed by rupture.

Crafoord undertook the first repair of coarctation in 1944 (Crafoord and Nylin 1945), followed shortly thereafter by Gross (Gross and Hufnagel 1945). Over the next decade, many aortic homografts were implanted for coarctation with no widely known reports of failure, although undoubtedly aneurysms, aorto–left bronchial fistulae, and rupture occurred sporadically (Hagland et al. 1959; DeWeese and Fry 1962; Gerber and Rubaum 1966).

Arterial homografts were subsequently applied to other peripheral vascular problems such as abdominal aortic aneurysms and iliac and femoral arterial occlusive disease. This clinical experience in the early 1950s suggested that peripheral arterial homografts such as the femoral artery had a higher risk of aneurysm formation or thrombosis than proximal, more elastic arteries such as the ascending aorta (Meade et al. 1966; Brock 1968). In addition, the logistical and legal problems of collection and storage led to general dissatisfaction with homografts.

The explosion of knowledge in the field of plastics technology led to numerous durable synthetic fabrics appearing in the late 1940s and early 1950s. These fabrics were soon used by DeBakey and others to construct synthetic tube grafts or conduits. Dacron (polyester) was recognized as more stable and resistant to degradation when in a biologic milieu relative to some of its polymer cousins such as nylon and ivalon (Voorhees et al. 1952; Deterling and Bhonslay 1955; Edwards and Tapp 1955; Sauvage and Wesolowski 1955).

Edwards (1957) emphasized in an early report that the porosity of fabric tubes was an advantage over nonporous alternatives. A totally impervious conduit, such as a Silastic tube, showed progressive accumulation of an inert capsule (both inner and outer), with no adhesion of that capsule to the prosthesis, much like the thick capsule surrounding a pacemaker generator (Andrade 1973).

Wesolowski pursued the relationship between synthetic conduit porosity and healing with a wide range of laboratory studies (Wesolowski et al. 1961; Wesolowski 1965). He concluded that optimal healing occurred with a water porosity of 5000 ml/cm^2/min at a pressure of 120 mmHg. In fact, most of the higher porosity knitted dacron grafts in use today have a porosity of approximately 2000 ml/cm^2/min. In the nonheparinized patient undergoing peripheral vascular surgery, this high porosity can be controlled at the time of implantation by preclotting the graft with the patient's own blood. This is not adequate in the fully heparinized patient undergoing cardiac surgery. Numerous attempts have been made over the last

25 years to achieve temporary porosity control with biologic sealants. However, early investigators had persistent problems with cracking and dissection of sealant material (Bascom 1961; Humphries et al. 1961; Jordan et al. 1963). An alternative approach was simply to use less porous fabric. This led to the introduction of woven fabric tubes with a baseline porosity of 100 to 250 ml/cm²/min such as the Cooley Veri-Soft graft (Meadox Medical Inc., Newark, NJ). Since acceptable blood loss in the heparinized patient requires a porosity of less than 50 ml/cm²/min, even these grafts required preclotting. Another technique that has become popular has been to bake such tube grafts after soaking them in heparinized blood or albumin (Wuerflein and Campbell 1963; Bethea and Reemtsma 1979). To avoid the need for any graft preparation, very tightly woven grafts such as the Cooley Lo-Por graft[2] were introduced. Such grafts have a porosity of approximately 50 $ml/cm_2/min$. Such grafts are difficult to handle because of their rigidity and difficulty of needle penetration. In addition, Edwards and Wesolowski's predictions about the healing of such grafts proved to be correct. These grafts accumulate a poorly adherent thick pseudointima with areas of hemorrhagic dissection between the luminal surface of the graft and the pseudointima. Although this may not be of clinical significance in a large diameter (greater than 20 mm) straight tube graft (for example, used for replacement of an abdominal aortic aneurysm), it is certainly of significance in smaller grafts and particularly when placed in growing children.

Another approach, as popularized by Sauvage, has been to introduce velour, either internally, externally, or both. The velour fibers form loops that project above or below the basic framework of the prosthesis. These loops are said to encourage fibrous and vascular ingrowth and thus anchor the pseudointima (Sauvage et al. 1971; Holub et al. 1978; Mitchell et al. 1980). At the same time, the velour loops decrease the porosity of the fabric but only to a limited degree. Therefore the search has continued for a suitable technique of incorporating a biologically degradable component within the graft.

One approach initiated by an intensive study by Wesolowski in 1963 (Wesolowski et al. 1963) was to incorporate biologically degradable material within a composite fabric. He also further studied the "sealant" concept with a number of materials including aldehyde cross-linked collagen. He concluded from this study that delayed resorption of the absorbable component, as for example with strongly cross-linked collagen, actually accelerated pseudointima formation and graft occlusion. Wesolowski concluded that the absorbable component should be organized at the rate of autologous fibrin.

Work has continued through this decade to find a biologic sealant suitable for commercial preparation. A knitted Dacron graft sealed with human albumin was released briefly in the early 1980s (Domurado et al. 1978; Guidoin et al. 1984) but was subsequently withdrawn from the market in the United States because of manufacturing and packaging difficulties. The graft is currently being resubmitted for approval by the Food and Drug Administration. The Tascon knitted graft (Tascon Medical Technology Corp., Irvine, CA) was presealed with a thin, luminal coating of glutaraldehyde cross-linked collagen. Laboratory studies at Boston Children's Hospital revealed that resorption of the collagen was very slow, and because the coating was on the luminal surface, there was poor adhesion of pseudointima to the graft (Jonas et al. 1986, 1987). In a small clinical trial, the graft was confirmed to fail early in a number of cases because of rapid pseudointima accumulation (Jonas et al. 1987). Collagen can be less strongly cross linked by using formaldehyde rather than glutaraldehyde. This is the basis of the Hemashield (Meadox Medical Inc., Newark, NJ) process, which has recently become commercially available in the United States. Laboratory studies using subcutaneous implants of treated dacron in the rat as well as circulatory implants in sheep have suggested that this material has little effect on the normal healing process of dacron. Porosity studies have confirmed excellent porosity control to less than 10 ml/cm^2/min (Jonas et al. 1986, 1987).

Another approach currently undergoing FDA scrutiny is to use the tropocollagen subunits of collagen as found in gelatin. This material is highly water soluble and has been used as a plasma expander for many years. The collagen subunits are weakly aldehyde cross linked. The degree of cross linking can be controlled by chemically converting some of the amino groups that take part in the cross link to carboxyl groups. Laboratory studies undertaken at Boston Children's Hospital suggest that this approach also does not significantly impede the normal healing process of knitted dacron (Jonas et al. 1988).

Fibrin glue is basically a human fibrinogen, bovine thrombin two-component material, which can be applied to porous vascular prostheses (Haverich et al. 1981). Although appropriate resorption is likely, the material suffers from the risk of potential for viral transmission as well as the disadvantage of a tedious dissolving, mixing, and application process.

A number of workers continue to pursue the concept of a composite fabric in which one of the yarns incorporated in the weave is bioresorbable (Bowald et al. 1980; Galletti et al. 1984; Van der Lei 1985). Careful assessment must be made of the rate of decay of fabric strength, and the fabric must have sufficient long-term strength to resist aneurysm formation.

Another important area of contemporary research is focused on seeding endothelial cells onto dacron or polytetrafluoroethylene (PTFE) grafts (Herring et al. 1978; Zamora et al. 1986). Such cells can be mechanically or enzymatically debrided from a suitable dispensable autologous vessel and are then suspended in the patient's blood, which is used to preclot the prosthesis. Cell culture techniques can be used to increase the number of cells. Despite promising early results, these techniques present logistical difficulties.

ARTERIAL PROSTHESES FOR RECONSTRUCTIVE CARDIAC SURGERY

The first conduit used in a cardiac reconstructive procedure was constructed from the patient's own pericardium. It was interposed between the right ventricle and pulmonary artery for tetralogy with pulmonary atresia by Kirklin in 1965 (Rastelli

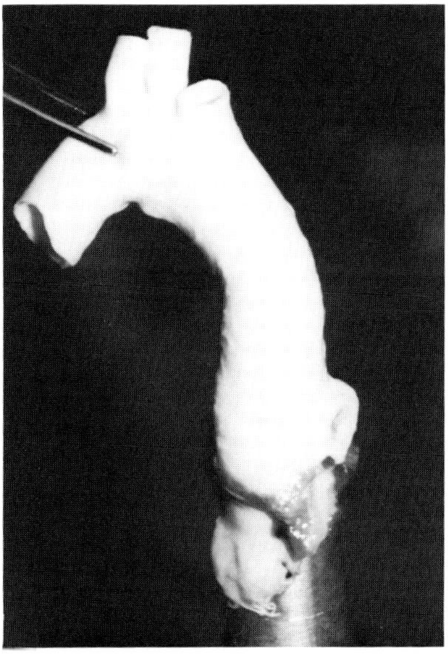

Figure 12.1
Valved aortic homograft conduit is harvested to include the anterior leaflet of the mitral valve as well as the aortic arch.

et al. 1965). Because adequate pericardium is often not available in these patients, Ross and Somerville (1966) in Britain introduced the concept of an aortic homograft conduit (Figure 12.1). Unlike Gross' homograft conduits for coarctation, Ross included the aortic valve with the aortic root and ascending aorta, thus reconstructing the normal valved right ventricular outflow tract. Ross' homografts were collected from cadavers, generally within 24 to 48 hours of death. Following dissection, the homografts were treated with an antibiotic solution for a few days and were then stored either in a balanced salt solution or in tissue culture medium at 4°C for up to 4 weeks. When homografts were introduced in the United States, at least two important changes to Ross' original method were made. First, instead of a weak antibiotic solution to "sterilize" the homografts, high-power irradiation was employed. Second, rather than wet storage at 4°C, many homografts were freeze-dried. Both these techniques alone and particularly in combination led to death of cells and severe damage to the collagen within the valve leaflets. Although Ross had observed calcification in the wall of this conduit, valve leaflet calcification was extremely rare (Saravalli et al. 1980). In contrast, the irradiated freeze-dried homografts rapidly developed valvar stenosis, and homografts fell into general disrepute in the United States (McGoon et al. 1982).

At about this time, the very low porosity woven dacron conduits became available (Bowman et al. 1973). Such conduits were combined with the glutaraldehyde-treated pig valve as pioneered by Carpentier. The immense logistical advantage of such conduits, which could be stocked with a complete range of sizes, proved very attractive, and over the next decade many thousands of these Hancock and Carpentier-Edwards conduits were implanted.

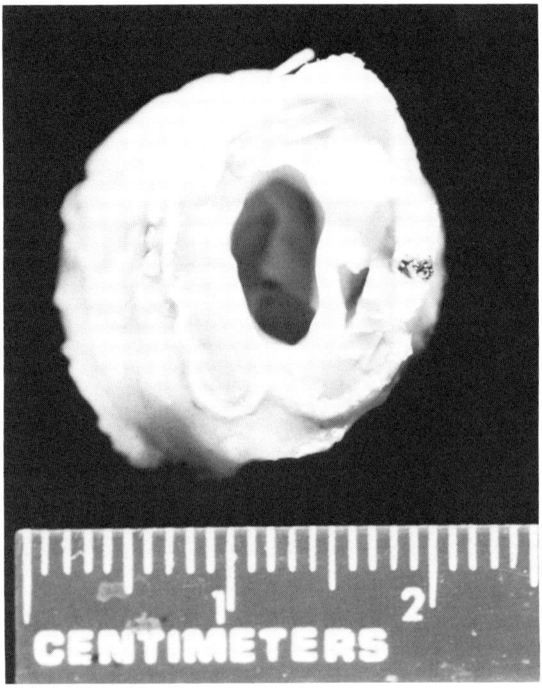

Figure 12.2
Low porosity dacron conduits can rapidly accumulate a thick pseudointima ("peel"). This 14-mm dacron conduit needed replacement within 15 months of implantation.

Within just 5 years, reports of unsatisfactory performance of these conduits appeared (Bailey et al. 1976; Norwood et al. 1977; Alfieri et al. 1978). As could have been predicted by Wesolowski in 1963, a thick pseudointima frequently rapidly accumulated (Figure 12.2). In addition, others noted that glutaraldehyde tanning of pig valves resulted in rapid calcification in children (Geha et al. 1979; Williams et al. 1982). Thus a combination of pseudointima formation and valvar stenosis resulted in a less than 50% freedom from conduit replacement within 9 years of implantation (Jonas et al. 1985). In their favor, however, it should be noted that the mode of failure of these conduits was only very rarely catastrophic. Simple monitoring of the systolic murmur and right ventricular hypertrophy on ECG allowed for elective replacement of these conduits at very low risk.

Addition of a valve to the conduit appeared to accelerate pseudointima formation (Fiore et al. 1983), so one response to the problem was a more liberal use of nonvalved conduits. By this time, however, the outstanding very long-term results of Ross and others (DiCarlo et al. 1984; Kay and Ross; 1985) became widely appreciated, and in the mid 1980s, the homograft once again became the conduit of first choice for cardiac reconstruction within the United States.

CURRENT METHODS OF HOMOGRAFT PREPARATION

Homografts stored at 4°C gradually loose their tissue integrity and are discarded within 4 to 6 weeks of collection. This presents a major logistical problem, particularly for the management of smaller children, where the number of appropriate sized donors is limited. Major advances in cryopreservation technology now allow the preservation of many cells, such as sperm and red cells, and even complete embryos can be preserved, possibly indefinitely. Unlike the dry ice temperatures of −72° employed by Gross with such disastrous results, liquid nitrogen at −196°C is currently employed. In addition, a cryoprotectant such as dimethyl sulfoxide (DMSO) prevents intracellular ice crystal formation during the freezing process. The specific antibiotics employed can also influence the long-term performance of homografts (Armiger et al. 1983). Currently, CLPVA (cefoxitin, lincomycin, polymixin B, vancomycin, and amphotericin) is used in most centers. The organization of regional organ banks has facilitated the collection of homografts. Until now, most donors in the United States have been brain dead/heart beating multiple organ donors. The collection has been undertaken in the sterile setting of an operating room. To supply the rapidly increasing demand for a wide range of homograft sizes, it will be important in the coming years to expand collection to cadavers, as has been the practice in Britain, New Zealand, and other countries for more than 25 years.

FAILURE OF HOMOGRAFT CONDUITS

Catastrophic failure of homograft conduits used for cardiac reconstruction has not yet been reported. However, based on the clinical experience of vascular surgeons of the 1950s (Hagland et al. 1959; DeWeese and Fry 1962; Gerber and Rubaum 1966; Meade at al. 1966; Brock 1968), it seems likely that with more widespread application of this biologic material there will be failure by homograft rupture, pseudoaneurysm formation, and conduit to bronchial fistula formation. Enthusiasm has developed for the use of pulmonary homografts to maximize the pool of available homograft sizes. The pulmonary artery is much thinner than the aorta and, particularly when applied in a situation in which it will be exposed to systemic pressure or greater, can show rapid dilation. Because the pulmonary valve lacks a fibrous annulus, there is a significant risk of pseudoaneurysm formation at the proximal anastomosis. In fact, such pseudoaneurysms have already necessitated more than six reoperations in more than 100 pulmonary homografts inserted at Boston Children's Hospital over the last 5 years. We have also experienced rupture of a pulmonary homograft exposed to systemic pressure as part of the reconstruction of a neo-aorta for hypoplastic left-heart syndrome. It would therefore seem prudent to limit the use of pulmonary homografts to sites where the predicted intrahomograft pressure will be substantially subsystemic. In addition, any children receiving a homograft conduit must be carefully followed for life for early detection of the potential complications already enumerated.

THE FUTURE:

□ (A) Living Blood Vessel Equivalent?

The "living skin equivalent" has been an important advance in the treatment of extensive skin loss due to burns. Using cell culture methods, the various layers of the dermis are built up, resulting in skin that is histologically and functionally similar to normal skin (Bell et al. 1981). Concerted efforts are currently underway to fabricate a living blood vessel equivalent employing the same technology. Vessels are grown on glass mandrils with an intima, media, and adventitia being reproduced. If such a vessel could ever be imbued with appropriate growth potential, it would represent a tremendous leap forward for the child with great vessel atresia undergoing reconstructive cardiac surgery in early life.

□ (B) Arterial Autograft

Sawatari et al. have recently demonstrated in a laboratory study and in a clinical case report that incorporation of a longitudinal strip of arterial autograft within a pericardial or homograft conduit allows for growth of the conduit. Potential autologous arterial tissue available through a median sternotomy includes a segment of the ascending aorta as well as the subclavian arteries. The neonatal arterial switch experience has confirmed the very low risk of late stenosis following circumferential anastomosis of the great vessels in the neonate.

CLINICAL INDICATIONS FOR CONDUIT INSERTION

The classic indications for conduit insertion have been tetralogy with long segment pulmonary atresia (pulmonary atresia with VSD); the so-called Rastelli procedure for transposition, VSD, and pulmonary stenosis; and the repair of truncus arteriosus. Double outlet right ventricle with subpulmonary VSD represents part of the spectrum between tetralogy and transposition and is a rarer indication for conduit placement. L-loop transposition (corrected transposition with VSD and pulmonary stenosis) requires conduit placement because of the course of the right coronary artery across the right-sided left ventricular outflow tract.

In the early years of ready availability of the porcine valved dacron conduit before its high rate of failure was suspected, conduits were freely applied to a number of reconstructive problems in which they can in fact clearly be avoided. For example, children with moderately severe hypoplasia of the main pulmonary artery as part of simple tetralogy had conduits placed for the perceived benefit of a competent valve in the right ventricular outflow tract.

Availability of the Hancock conduit also coincided with the introduction of the Fontan procedure (Fontan and Baudet 1971) for children with a single functional ventricle. These children clearly demonstrated within a short time that the gradient resulting from the pseudointima accumulation and porcine valve stenosis was a major hemodynamic disadvantage. Accordingly innovative techniques were devised by Kreutzer et al. (1973), Bjork et al. (1979), and others to eliminate the need for a conduit as part of the Fontan procedure. The need to perform a direct anastomosis as part of the systemic venous (or atrial) pulmonary connection has also substantially decreased the enthusiasm for the classic Glenn shunt as a preliminary to the Fontan procedure. Division of the right pulmonary artery as part of the classic Glenn shunt frequently results in the need for conduit reconstruction as part of the Fontan operation and is therefore to be avoided. The bidirectional Glenn shunt in contrast provides excellent palliation before the Fontan and sets the stage for a direct anastomotic Fontan procedure (Hopkins et al. 1985).

Other operations that have fallen into disrepute with the recognition of the unsatisfactory long-term performance of conduits include the Damus-Stansel-Kaye procedure and the left ventricular–apical aortic conduit. Damus (1975), Stansel (1975), and Kaye (1975) described an operation for transposition with intact ventricular septum based on the premise that it was desirable to use the left ventricle as the systemic ventricle as part of a more physiologic correction of transposition than was achieved by the atrial inversion procedures such as the Mustard or Senning operations. The main pulmonary artery is divided, and the proximal main pulmonary artery is anastomosed end to side to the aorta. A conduit is placed between the right ventricle and distal divided main pulmonary artery. Not only did this carry the late complication of a high reoperation rate for conduit obstruction, but in addition the early mortality was high (Ceithaml et al. 1984). Although the concept of a pulmonary aortic anastomosis has been preserved (for the bypass of subaortic obstruction with single ventricle), the Damus-Stansel-Kaye operation has otherwise become of little more than historical significance.

Long severe tunnel subaortic stenosis or left ventricular outflow tract obstruction has always been and continues to be a major surgical challenge. After a brief period of enthusiasm for the placement of a valved conduit from the left ventricular apex to the descending thoracic aorta (Norwood et al. 1983), it soon became clear that this was not a satisfactory long-term solution. It was frequently difficult to achieve an unobstructed proximal anastomosis to the very hypertrophied left ventricle. Stents only partially solved this problem and were highly susceptible themselves to pseudointima accumulation. Probably the most compelling reason why surgeons have largely abandoned this procedure was the tremendous difficulty in reoperating and replacing such conduits (in contrast to the relative ease of replacing a right ventricular to pulmonary artery conduit). Today various left ventricular outflow tract enlarging procedures, such as the Konno operation (Konno et al. 1975) or extended aortic root replacement with a homograft (Schaffer et al. 1986), have replaced the apical aortic conduit.

Not only have conduits been used less frequently for the Fontan procedure and left ventricular outflow tract obstruction, but in addition a concerted effort has been made to minimize their use in the more traditional setting of tetralogy with pulmonary atresia. If there is some development of the main pulmonary artery, wide mobilization of the branch pulmonary arteries allows the proximal main pulmonary artery to be anastomosed directly to a right ventricular infundibular incision. The anterior wall of the pulmonary artery and ventriculotomy can be supplemented with an autologous pericardial patch. The appreciation of the elasticity and consequent mobility of the pulmonary arteries has in part developed from the widespread application of the Lecompte pulmonary arteriopexy procedure performed as part of the arterial switch procedure for transposition (Lecompte et al. 1981).

SURGICAL TECHNIQUE OF HOMOGRAFT INSERTION

The cryopreserved homograft must be thawed for approximately 10 minutes in a water bath at 37°C. The DMSO is rinsed out by serial dilution. A small segment must be sent for bacteriologic culture. The walls and valve tissue are carefully examined, and the coronary arteries are suture ligated. The homograft is cut to length. When the homograft is used to establish continuity between the right ventricle and the pulmonary arteries, the distal anastomosis is fashioned with a continuous prolene suture. The homograft should be oriented so that the mitral valve, which should be left attached to the homograft aortic valve during the dissection, lies mainly posteriorly and slightly rightward. In the case of tetralogy with pulmonary atresia, for example, this allows the natural curve of the homograft to lie appropriately. It also avoids the bar of ventricular septal muscle lying in the line of the right ventricular outflow. A direct anastomosis is fashioned between the homograft anterior mitral leaflet and the right ventricular incision over its superior half. The anastomosis is completed with a hood or roof of autologous pericardium treated with 0.6% glutaraldehyde for 30 minutes. Particularly in the case of the pulmonary homograft, it is important that this suture line catch the collagenous vessel wall and not be limited to the muscle below the valve.

A pulmonary artery monitoring line should be placed through a mattress suture just inferior to the anastomosis in the right ventricular free wall. It should be directed into the distal pulmonary artery under vision. This allows monitoring of pulmonary artery pressure in the early postoperative period as well as giving a pullback gradient between the distal pulmonary artery and right ventricle across both anastomoses when it is withdrawn, generally on the day following surgery (Gold et al. 1986). As discussed previously, it is probably not wise to use pulmonary artery homografts, particularly in children beyond infancy, in whom the homograft will be exposed to systemic pressure.

RESULTS OF SURGERY

Use of rigid prosthetic conduits containing a porcine valve carried a relatively high early mortality. Undoubtedly this in part reflects the complex underlying anatomy and physiology of many of these children. However, in addition, there was clearly technical difficulty in suturing rigid low porosity woven dacron to thin friable small pulmonary arteries. The rigid metal valve stent often lay over the left coronary artery and could cause coronary compression and ischemia. Thus in our analysis of 12 years experience with prosthetic conduits, there was a 22% early mortality among 201 patients (Jonas et al. 1985). Long-term actuarial survival was 83% at 9 years. No patient was free of the need for conduit replacement by 10 years from the time of surgery (Figure 12.3). Postoperative catheterization frequently revealed significant right ventricular to pulmonary artery gradients. In an early study at Children's Hospital of 19 patients with Hancock conduits catheterized a mean of 1.6 years after surgery, five had gradients greater than 75 mm and only four had gradients less than 20 mm (Norwood et al. 1977). Repeat cardiac catheterization revealed rapid progression of these high early gradients (Figure 12.4). At the time of replacement surgery, the cause of obstruction was found to be a combination of valve calcification and pseudointima peel accumulation in most patients.

There have been many reports over the years (Shabbo et al. 1980; DiCarlo et al. 1984; Fontan et al.; Kay and Koss 1985) documenting superior performance of antibiotic treated nonfrozen aortic homografts stored at 4°C. To date, there are only early data with respect to cryopreserved homografts (Kirklin et al. 1987; Lamberti et al. 1988; McGrath et al. 1988). However, there are laboratory data to suggest that there is unlikely to be a significant difference in the long-term performance of wet stored and frozen aortic homografts (Jonas et al. 1988). At Children's Hospital, 274 aortic and pulmonary homografts have been placed over

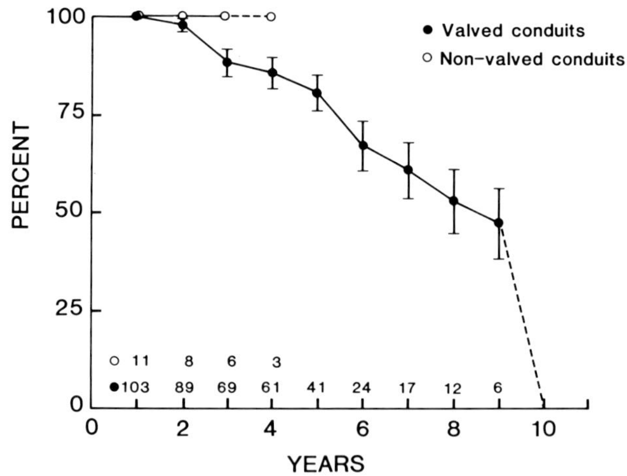

Figure 12.3 Actuarial freedom from need for conduit replacement among 201 patients receiving low porosity dacron extracardiac conduits at Children's Hospital, Boston, 1971 through 1983.

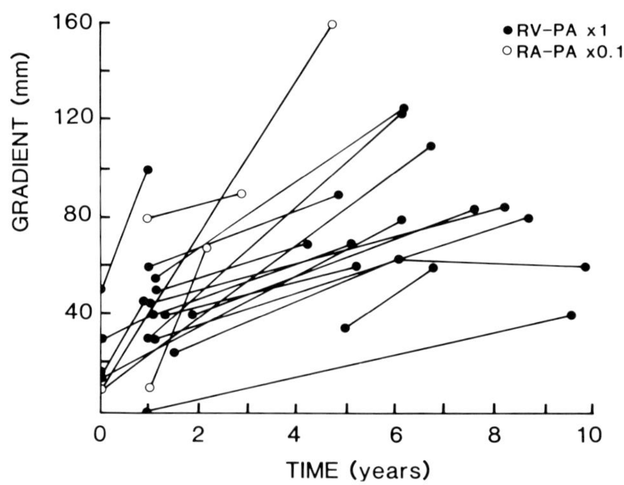

Figure 12.4 Serial transconduit gradients for right ventricular (RV)–pulmonary arterial (PA) (× 1) and right atrial (RA)–PA (× 0.1) low porosity dacron conduits. Note high early postoperative gradients and rapid progression of gradients.

the last 4½ years. Two children have required reoperation for obstruction due to simple outgrowth of the conduit. Significant gradients of greater than 20 mm have been seen rarely, unlike the prosthetic conduit experience, where they were the rule. Six of the 105 children with pulmonary homografts have developed false aneurysms necessitating reoperation in all. One child with hypoplastic left-heart syndrome died following rupture of an 11-mm pulmonary homograft. In each of these cases, the pulmonary homograft was exposed to at least systemic pressure. No child with an aortic homograft of the 169 inserted has developed a false or true aneurysm, although most aortic homografts show evidence of heavy conduit wall calcification within 6 to 12 months of insertion. True valve leaflet calcification has not been observed in 4½ years of follow-up. This is consistent with the "fresh" homograft experience and laboratory data.

INDICATIONS FOR CONDUIT REPLACEMENT

Right ventricular hypertension is frequently well tolerated for many years. However, review of the experience with simple tetralogy suggests that patients with right ventricular hypertension and a right ventricular scar have a definite risk of ventricular ectopy and sudden death. Our policy has been to undertake conduit replacement if right ventricular pressure approaches systemic pressure or if there are symptoms or signs of right ventricular failure. Balloon dilation of conduit obstruction has rarely been of benefit other than over the very short term.

With the widespread current application of homografts, it is important once again to note that, similar to any biologic material, there is likely to be an incidence of tissue failure. This is likely to result in false aneurysm formation, true aneurysm formation, and conduit to bronchial fistulae. Unlike the failure mode of synthetic conduits, which is progressive but predictable, allowing timely elective replacement, it seems likely that at least some late homograft failures will be of a more catastrophic nature unless very careful follow-up has occurred. In spite of this, it is hoped, very small, very long-term risk, homografts continue to represent a tremendous step forward over prosthetic alternatives with a lower early mortality risk, markedly decreased incidence of transconduit gradients, and decreased incidence of need for conduit replacement procedures.

REFERENCES

Alfieri O, Blackstone EH, Kirklin JW, Pacifico AD, Bargeron LM. Surgical treatment of tetralogy of Fallot with pulmonary atresia. J Thorac Cardiovasc Surg 1978; 76:321.

Andrade JD. Interfacial phenomena and biomaterials. Med Instrum 1973; 7:110.

Armiger LC, Gavin JB, Barratt-Boyes HG. Histological assessment of orthotopic aortic valve leaflet allografts: Its role in selecting graft pretreatment. Pathology 1983; 15: 67.

Bailey WW, Kirklin JW, Bargeron LM, Pacifico AD, Kouchoukos NT. Late results with synthetic valved external conduits from venous ventricle to pulmonary arteries. Circulation 1976; 56(suppl II):73.

Bascom JU. Gelatin sealing to prevent blood loss from knitted arterial grafts. Surgery 1961; 50:504.

Bell E, Ehrlich HP, Buttle DJ, Nakatsuji T. Living tissue formed in vitro and accepted as skin equivalent tissue of full thickness. Science 1981; 211:1052.

Bethea MC, Reemtsma K. Graft hemostasis: An alternative to preclotting. Ann Thorac Surg 1979; 27:374.

Bjork VO, Olin CL, Bjarke BB, Thoren CA. Right atrial–right ventricular anastomosis for correction of tricuspid atresia. J Thorac Cardiovasc Surg 1979; 77:452.

Bowald S, Busch C, Eriksson I. Absorbable material in vascular prostheses. A new device. Acta Chir Scan 1980; 146:391.

Bowman FO, Hancock WD, Malm JR. A valve containing dacron prosthesis. Arch Surg 1973; 107:724.

Brock L. Longterm degenerative changes in aortic segment homografts, with particular reference to calcification. Thorax 1968; 23:249.

Carrel A. Heterotransplantation of blood vessels preserved in cold storage. J Exp Med 1907; 9:226.

Carrel A. Results of the transplantation of blood vessels, organs and limbs. JAMA 1908; 51:1662.

Carrel A. Ultimate results of aortic transplantations. J Exp Med 1912; 15:389.

Ceithaml EL, Puga FJ, Danielson GK, McGoon DC, Ritter DC. Results of the Damus-Stansel-Kaye procedure for transposition of the great arteries and for double outlet right ventricle with subpulmonary ventricular septal defect. Ann Thorac Surg 1984; 38:433.

Crafoord C, Nylin G. Congenital coarctation of the aorta and its surgical treatment. J Thorac Surg 1945; 14:347.

Damus PS. A proposed operation for transposition of the great vessels [correspondence]. Ann Thorac Surg 1975; 20:724.

Deterling RA, Bhonslay SB. An evaluation of synthetic materials and fabrics suitable for blood vessel replacement. Surgery 1955; 38:71.

DeWeese MS, Fry WJ. Small-bowel erosion following aortic resection. JAMA 1962; 179:142.

DiCarlo D, de Leval MR, Stark J. "Fresh" antibiotic sterilized aortic homografts in extracardiac valved conduits. Long-term results. Thorac Cardiovasc Surgeon 1984; 32:10.

Domurado D, Guidoin R, Marois M, et al. Albuminated Dacron prostheses as improved blood vessel substitutes. J Bioeng 1978; 2:79.

Edwards WS. The effect of porosity in solid plastic artery grafts. Surg Forum 1957; 8:446.

Edwards WS, Tapp JS. Chemically treated nylon tubes as arterial grafts. Surgery 1955; 38:61.

Fiore AC, Peigh PS, Robison RJ, et al. Valved and nonvalved right ventricular-pulmonary arterial extracardiac conduits. J Thorac Cardiovasc Surg 1983; 86:490.

Fontan F, Baudet E. Surgical repair of tricuspid atresia. Thorac 1971; 26:240.

Fontan F, Choussat A, Deville C, et al. Aortic valve homografts in the surgical treatment of complex cardiac malformations. J Thorac Cardiovasc Surg 1984; 87:649.

Galletti PM, Ip TK, Chiu TH, et al. Extending the functional life of bioresorbable yarns for vascular grafts. Trans Am Soc Artif Intern Organs 1984; 30:399.

Geha AS, Laks H, Stansel HC, et al. Late failure of porcine valve heterografts in children. J Thorac Cardiovasc Surg 1979; 78:351.

Gerber A, Rubaum N. Gastrointestinal hemorrhage due to rupture of an aortic homograft. Calif Med 1966; 105:377.

Gold JP, Jonas RA, Lang P, et al. Transcutaneous intracardiac monitoring lines in pediatric surgical patients: A 10 year experience. Ann Thorac Surg 1986; 42:185.

Gross RE, Bill AH, Peirce EC. Methods for preservation and transplantation of arterial grafts. Surg Gyn Obstet 1949; 88:689.

Gross RE, Hubbard JP. Surgical ligation of a patent ductus arteriosus. Report of first successful case. JAMA 1939; 112:729.

Gross RE, Hufnagel CA. Coarctation of the aorta: Experimental studies regarding its surgical correction. N Engl J Med 1945; 233:287.

Guidoin R, Snyder R., Martin L, et al. Albumin coating of a knitted polyester arterial prosthesis: An alternative to preclotting. Ann Thorac Surg 1984; 37:457.

Guthrie CC. Survival of engrafted tissues. III. Blood vessels. Heart 1910; 2:115.

Hagland LA, Sweetman WR, Wise RA. Rupture of an abdominal aortic homograft with ileal fistula. Am J Surg 1959; 98:746.

Haverich A, Walterbusch G, Borst HG. The use of fibrin glue for sealing vascular prostheses of high porosity. Thorac Cardiovasc Surg 1981; 29:252.

Herring M, Gardner A, Glover J. A single staged technique for seeding vascular grafts with autogenous endothelium. Surgery 1978; 84:498.

Holub DA, Trono R, Klima T, Norman JC. Macroscopic, microscopic, and mechanical analyses of prototype double velour vascular grafts. Bull Texas Heart Inst 1978; 5:365.

Hopkins RA, Armstrong BE, Serwer GA, et al. Physiological rationale for a bidirectional cavopulmonary shunt. J Thorac Cardiovasc Surg 1985; 90:391.

Humphries AW, Hawk WA, Cuthbertson AM. Arterial prosthesis of collagen impregnated Dacron tulle. Surgery 1961; 50:947.

Jonas RA, Freed MD, Mayer JE, Castaneda AR. Longterm followup of patients with synthetic right heart conduits. Circulation 1985; 72(suppl II):77.

Jonas RA, Mayer JE, Castaneda AR. Unsatisfactory clinical experience with a collagen sealed knitted dacron extracardiac conduit. J Cardiac Surg 1987; 2:257.

Jonas RA, Schoen FJ, Levy RJ, Castaneda AR. Biological sealants and knitted dacron: Porosity and histological comparisons of vascular graft materials with and without collagen and fibrin glue pretreatments. Ann Thorac Surg 1986; 41:657.

Jonas RA, Schoen FJ, Ziemer G, Britton L, Castaneda AR. Biological sealants and knitted Dacron conduits: Comparison of collagen and fibrin glue pretreatments in circulatory models. Ann Thorac Surg 1987; 44:283.

Jonas RA, Ziemer G, Britton L, Armiger LC. Cryopreserved and fresh antibiotic sterilized valved aortic homograft conduits in a longterm sheep model. J Thorac Cardiovasc Surg 1988; 96:746.

Jonas RA, Ziemer G, Schoen FJ, Britton L, Castaneda AR. A new sealant for knitted Dacron prostheses: Minimally cross-linked gelatin. J Vasc Surg 1988; 7:414.

Jordan GL, Stump MM, Allen J, et al. Gelatin impregnated prosthesis implanted into porcine thoracic aorta. Surgery 1963; 53:45.

Kay PH, Ross DN. Fifteen years' experience with the aortic homograft: The conduit of choice for right ventricular outflow tract reconstruction. Ann Thorac Surg 1985; 40:360.

Kaye MP. Anatomic correction of transposition of the great arteries. Mayo Clin Proc 1975; 50:638.

Kirklin JW, Blackstone EH, Maehara T, et al. Intermediate term fate of cryopreserved allograft and xenograft valved conduits. Ann Thorac Surg 1987; 44:598.

Konno S, Imai Y, Iida Y, Nakajima M, Tatsuno K. A new method for prosthetic valve replacement in congenital aortic stenosis associated with hypoplasia of the aortic valve ring. J Thorac Cardiovasc Surg 1975; 70:909.

Kreutzer G, Galindez E, Bono H, dePalma C, Laura JP. An operation for the correction of tricuspid atresia. J Thorac Cardiovasc Surg 1973; 66:613.

Lamberti JJ, Angell WW, Waldman JD, et al. The cryopreserved homograft valve in the pulmonary position: Early results and technical considerations. J Cardiac Surg 1988; 3:247.

Lecompte Y, Zannini L, Hazan E. Anatomic correction of transposition of the great arteries: New technique without use of a prosthetic conduit. J Thorac Cardiovasc Surg 1981; 82:629.

McGoon DC, Danielson GK, Puga FJ, et al. Late results after extracardiac conduit repair for congenital cardiac defects. Am J Cardiol 1982; 49:1741.

McGrath LB, Gonzalez-Lavin L, Graf D. Pulmonary homograft implantation for ventricular outflow tract reconstruction: Early phase results. Ann Thorac Surg 1988; 45:273.

Meade JW, Linton RR, Darling RC, Menendez CV. Arterial homografts. Arch Surg 1966; 93:392.

Mitchell RS, Miller CD, Billingham ME, et al. Comprehensive assessment of the safety, durability, clinical performance, and healing characteristics of a double velour knitted Dacron arterial prosthesis. Vasc Surg 1980; 14:197.

Norwood WI, Freed MD, Rocchini AP, Bernhard WF, Castaneda AR. Experience with valved conduits for repair of congenital cardiac lesions. Ann Thorac Surg 1977; 24:223.

Norwood WI, Lang P, Castaneda AR, Murphy JD. Management of infants with left ventricular outflow obstruction by conduit interposition between the ventricular apex and thoracic aorta. J Thorac Cardiovasc Surg 1983; 86:771.

Rastelli GC, Ongley PA, Davis GD, Kirklin JW. Surgical repair for pulmonary valve atresia with coronary-pulmonary artery fistula: Report of case. Mayo Clin Proc 1965; 40:521.

Ross DN, Somerville J. Correction of pulmonary atresia with a homograft aortic valve. Lancet 1966; 2:1446.

Saravalli OA, Somerville J, Jefferson KE. Calcification of aortic homografts used for reconstruction of the right ventricular outflow tract. J Thorac Cardiovasc Surg 1980; 80:909.

Sauvage LR, Berger K, Wood SJ, et al. An external velour surface for porous arterial prostheses. Surgery 1971; 70:940.

Sauvage LR, Wesolowski SA. The healing and fate of arterial grafts. Surgery 1955; 38:1090.

Sawatari K, Kawata H, Armiger LC, Jonas RA. Growth of composite conduits utilizing longitudinal arterial autograft. Submitted to Journal of Thoracic and Cardiovasc Surgery.

Schaffer MS, Campbell DN, Clarke DR, Wiggins JW, Wolfe RR. Aortoventriculoplasty in children. J Thorac Cardiovasc Surg 1986; 92:391.

Shabbo FP, Wain WH, Ross DN. Right ventricular outflow reconstruction with aortic homograft conduit: Analysis of the longterm results. Thorac Cardiovasc Surg 1980; 28:21.

Stansel HC. A new operation for d-loop transposition of the great arteries. Ann Thorac Surg 1975; 19:565.

Ven der Lei B, Darius H, Schror K, et al. Arterial wall regeneration in small caliber vascular grafts in rats. J Thorac Cardiovasc Surg 1985;90:378.

Voorhees AB, Jaretzki A, Blakemore AH. The use of tubes constructed from Vinyon "N" cloth in bridging arterial defects: A preliminary report. Ann Surg 1952; 135:332.

Wesolowski SA. The healing of vascular prostheses. Surgery 1965;57:319.

Wesolowski SA, Fries CC, Domingo RT, et al. The compound prosthetic vascular graft: A pathologic survey. Surgery 1963; 53:19.

Wesolowski SA, Fries CC, Karlson KE, et al. Porosity: Primary determinants of ultimate fate of synthetic vascular grafts. Surgery 1961; 50:91.

Williams DB, Danielson GK, McGoon DC, et al. Porcine heterograft valve replacement in children. J Thorac Cardiovasc Surg 1982; 84:446.

Wuerflein RD, Campbell GS. Analysis of preclotting technics for prosthetic arterial grafts. Am Surg 1963; 29:179.

Zamora JL, Navarro LT, Ives CL, et al. Seeding of arteriovenous prostheses with homologous endothelium. A preliminary report. J Vasc Surg 1986; 3:860.

13

Autografts and Cryopreserved Allografts for Valve Replacement in Children

Ronald C. Elkins

One of the more exciting applications of cryopreserved allografts is their use in correction of congenital cardiac defects. One of their earliest uses was in the treatment of congenital aortic stenosis, when in 1976 Ross replaced the aortic valve in an 11-year-old using a fresh allograft (Somerville and Ross 1982). Since that time an ever-widening array of congenital cardiac defects have been repaired using allograft tissue. This tissue has been used as a valved conduit, nonvalved conduit, and patch or onlay graft. The use of allograft tissue for valve replacement in children has been relatively slow in evolving because the availability of a large number of allografts was limited as well as because of difficulties associated with early attempts at sterilization with betapropriolactone (Malm et al. 1967), irradiation (Beach et al. 1972), ethyline oxide (Bodnar et al. 1979), or buffered formalin (Barratt-Boyes 1971). Those valves sterilized with antibiotics and stored at 4°C in a nutrient medium had a limited "shelf life," and it was only with the advent of cryopreservation that an increasing number of valves and conduits of suitable size have become available. Ross in London, Barrett-Boyes of Auckland, New Zealand, and O'Brien in Brisbane, Australia have contributed to the development of the technical expertise to use these valves in large numbers of patients. The operative techniques became reproducible with an acceptable risk, such that their use has rapidly expanded. With the development of cryopreservation techniques pioneered by O'Brien and the development of commercial laboratories and valve banks within the United States, their use has rapidly expanded. As of July 1989, 5316 valves have been prepared, sterilized with antibiotics, and cryopreserved before implantation by a single commercial laboratory (McNally et al. 1989). This experience has demonstrated the increasing acceptance of these valves as a useful modality in the management of patients with critical valvular dysfunction.

In 1967, Ross (1967) extended his work with allografts to include replacement of the aortic valve with the patient's pulmonary valve, a valve with all the characteristics that would make it an ideal substitute for the deformed aortic valve (Matsuki et al. 1988). This effort has been developed almost entirely by Ross.

Perhaps the magnitude of the operative procedure, that is, converting a single valve replacement to a double valve replacement and the lack of a suitable replacement for the pulmonary artery and valve, led most cardiac surgeons not to consider this procedure in children with aortic valve disease. The availability of cryopreserved allografts for replacement of the transplanted pulmonary valve (most often a pulmonary allograft) and the demonstration of excellent long-term success (80% at 16 years) have eliminated one of these objections (Gerera et al. 1989). This, coupled with dissatisfaction with all other available valve substitutes, prosthetic and bioprosthetic, has led to expanding interest and acceptance of the operation and the possibility of performing one operation that might provide the patient with a life-lasting substitute for the aortic valve.

The ensuing discussion deals with allograft replacement of the aortic, pulmonary, and atrioventricular valves as well as the use of the pulmonary valve as an autograft in the aortic position and its reported use as an alternative for the severely abnormal atrioventricular valve.

AORTIC VALVE REPLACEMENTS

□ Pulmonary Valve Autograft

The pulmonary valve is an ideal substitute for the diseased aortic valve. It is viable tissue that does not cause the development of thrombi, it can repair itself, it is the appropriate size, it can withstand infection, it does not damage circulating cellular elements in the blood, and when used as a root replacement it may grow appropriate to the child's growth.

The autograft may be implanted intra-aortic as a cylinder or as a root replacement. My choice would be to implant it as a cylinder in children older than 7 who have had normal growth and whose primary cardiac lesion is valvular stenosis or insufficiency without marked dilatation or asymmetry of the aortic annulus. In younger patients or patients with small aortic roots, a dysplastic annulus, or tunnel aortic stenosis, we use the root replacement techniques. These techniques have been previously reported but are summarized here briefly (Figures 13.1–13.3).

As of December 1990 (Santangelo et al. In press), we have used the autograft in 23 patients 21 years of age or less. The youngest is 2 years of age, and the average age is 12 years. Twenty-two have been done as cylinder and 15 have been as root replacements. Twenty have had predominantly valvular aortic stenosis and 17 had predominantly aortic insufficiency. The length of postoperative evaluation has been limited in these patients; however, all but two patients have excellent aortic valve function. One patient required replacement of his pulmonary autograft valve with a homograft 6 months after the original procedure. This failure was due to technical error of malalignment early in our experience. A second patient had significant aortic insufficiency by echocardiography and cardiac catheterization

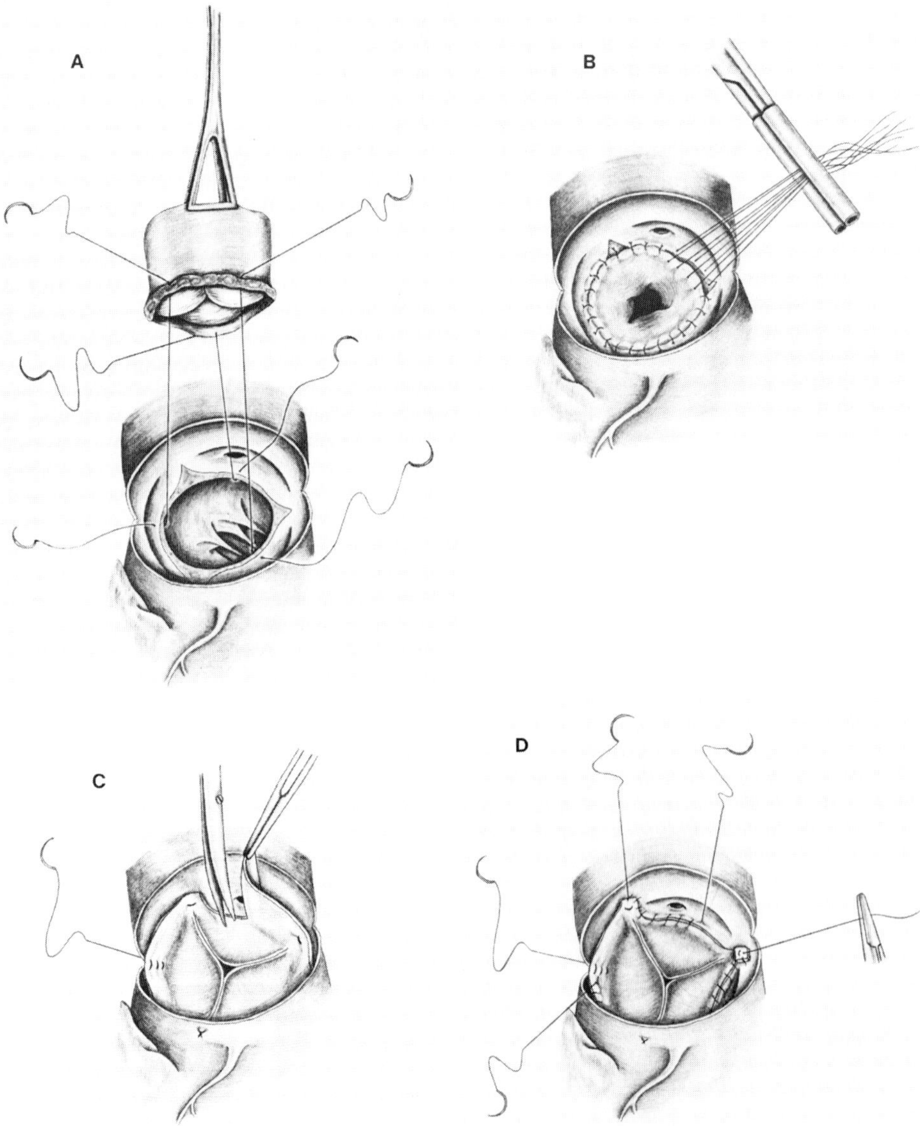

Figure 13.1 Free-hand aortic valve replacement with allograft or autograft. (A) Proximal suture line begins with sutures at the midpoint of each sinus of Valsalva. (B) The inverted valve is sewn below the native annulus with interrupted 4–0 polypropylene. (C) Everting the valve, the commissures are anchored and two sinuses are scalloped beneath the coronary ostia. (D) The noncoronary sinus is left intact, and the distal suture line is a running suture below the coronary orifices. (Randolph JD, Toal K, Stelzer P, et al. Aortic valve and left ventricular outflow tract replacement using allograft and autograft valves. Ann Thorac Surg 1989; 48:345. By permission.)

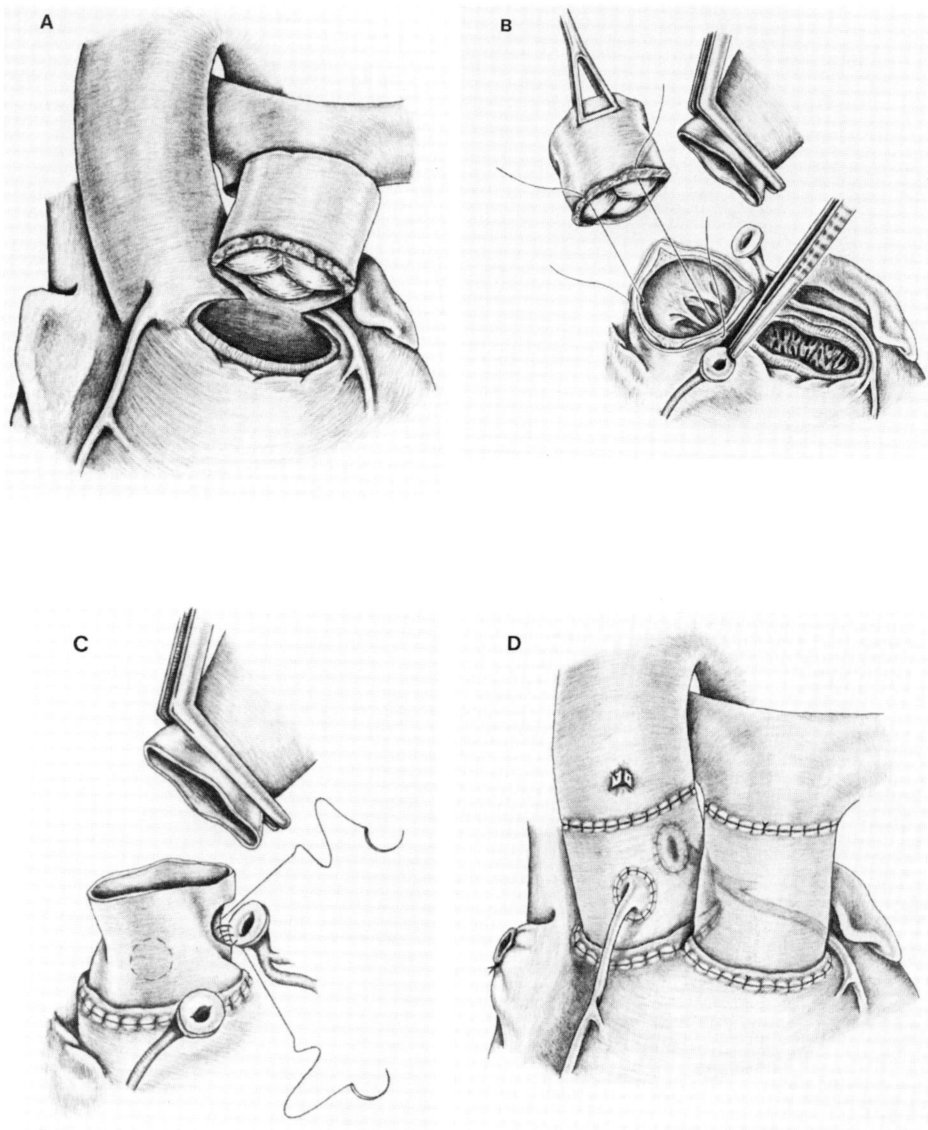

Figure 13.2 Pulmonary autograft root replacement of aortic valve. (A) Harvesting of pulmonary artery with its valve from right ventricular outflow tract. (B) The proximal suture line begins attaching the pulmonary root to the residual aorta and aortic annulus. (C) The left coronary is implanted with a running suture of 5–0 polypropylene using a button of aorta. (D) The distal suture line is completed, the pulmonary root distended, and the right coronary implanted. The pulmonary root is replaced with a pulmonary allograft. (Stelzer P, Jones DJ, Elkins RC. Aortic root replacement using pulmonary autograft. Circulation 1989; 80:5. By permission.)

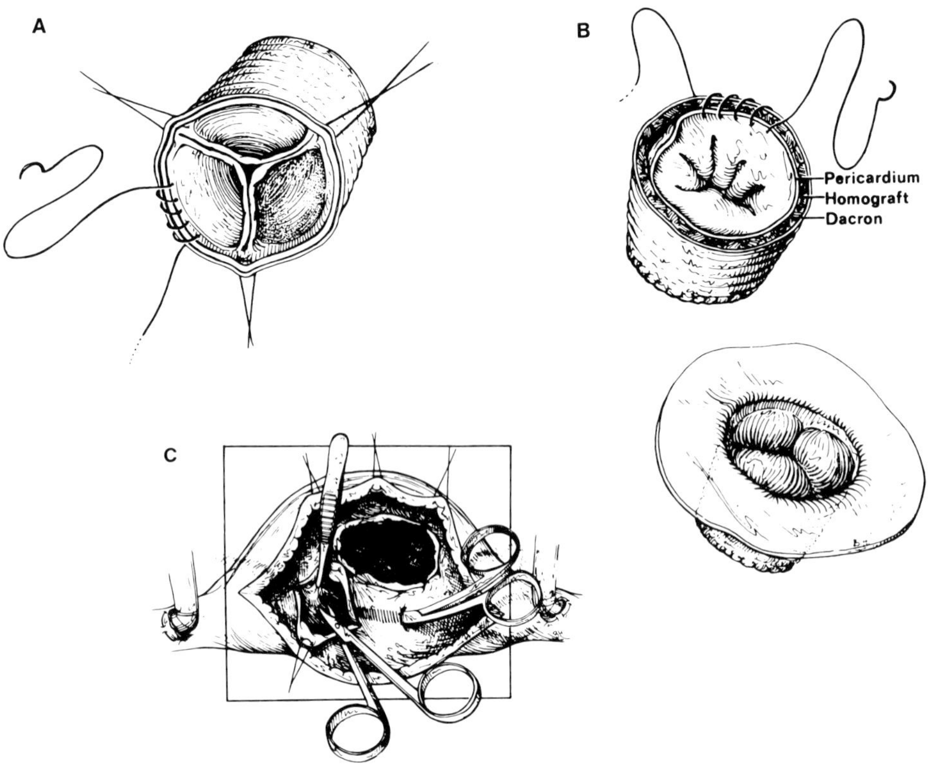

Figure 13.3 Tricuspid valve replacement with a pulmonary allograft. (A) The distal end of a homograft is attached to a Dacron sleeve 3 to 4 mm larger than the allograft. (B) The proximal anastomosis between the allograft and a Dacron sleeve includes an autologous pericardial flange. (C) The tricuspid valve is excised, and the coronary sinus is unroofed through an atrial septal incision. (D) The atrial defect is closed, and the distal end of the

and underwent allograft replacement of his autograft valve. Three years following the autograft procedure associated with patch closure of a ventricular septal defect, the right coronary leaflet became adherent to the patch and progressively prolapsed with significant insufficiency.

Ross reported his initial experience with pulmonary autograft replacement in children (<18 years of age), and it was associated with a relatively high operative mortality ($>10\%$) (Gerera et al. 1989). However, recent experience would suggest that this can be accomplished with a very low mortality; Ross and colleagues reported no deaths since 1971 and our experience of 37 patients with one death. In Ross' series there has been no thromboembolism, and the incidence of endocarditis has been 1.8% per patient year. The freedom from reoperation in this series of 34 children has been 74% ± 11% at 16 years. The actuarial functional

D

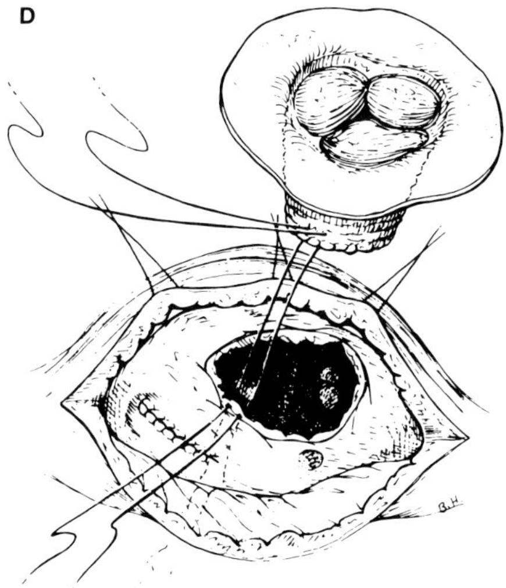

E

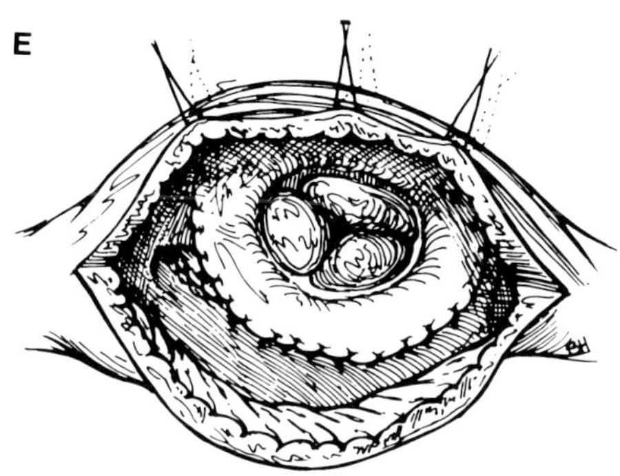

valve is attached to the tricuspid annulus with everting sutures. (E) The pericardial flange is sutured to the right atrial wall, covering the coronary sinus and avoiding the conduction system to produce a smooth inflow to the valve. (McKay R, Sono J, Arnold RM. Tricuspid valve replacement using an unstented pulmonary homograft. Ann Thorac Surg 1988; 46:58. By permission.)

life free from all valve-related complications including late death is 55% ± 12% at 16 years.

□ Allograft Replacement of Aortic Valve

Because of our strong preference for the pulmonary valve autograft, our experience with homograft replacement of the aortic valve is more limited. However, it is our valve of choice in any patient requiring aortic valve or aortic root replacement when the patient's pulmonary valve is abnormal or in the patient who requires replacement of the ascending aorta because of localized pathology. The pulmonary artery autograft has limited length and is therefore not suited for those patients requiring extensive replacement of the ascending aorta or transverse arch.

We have used homografts primarily as root replacements in 19 patients, including six patients with truncus arteriosus and truncal valve stenosis and insufficiency. The patients' ages ranged from 14 days to 21 years. Thirteen patients survived their operative procedure, and their aortic valve function is normal.

Late results of homograft replacement of the aortic valve in children has been reported by Ross and associates (Gerosa et al., in press). Eighty-eight patients, 18 years of age or younger with the youngest being 18 months, underwent replacement of the aortic valve. Forty-four of these were done as a valve replacement and 44 as a root replacement. The actuarial patient survival curve was 55.1% ± 14.5% at 20 years. The incidence of bacterial endocarditis was 0.8% per patient year. Thromboembolism or anticoagulant-related hemorrhage has not been reported in these patients. Valve-related complications appear to be secondary to the development of aortic regurgitation, and this lesion has been the primary mode of valve failure. The freedom from reoperation for all causes in these patients has been 43.3% ± 12.9% at 20 years.

These data, although limited in patient numbers, strongly support the use of the pulmonary autograft or the aortic allograft for replacement of the aortic valve or root in patients with severe deformity of the left ventricular outflow tract.

O'Brien et al. (1987) have reported a comparison of viable cryopreserved and fresh allograft valves in which the survival of the two groups of patients was the same. The fresh allograft valves are sterilized with antibiotics and are comparable to those used by Ross (Matsuki et al. 1988) and others (Khaghani et al. 1986; Barratt-Boyes et al. 1987). Of more importance is the freedom from reoperation in the cryopreserved, viable allograft group of 92% at 10 years as compared with 84% for the fresh allograft group. Freedom from reoperation for valve degeneration was 89% at 10 years and 59% at 15 years for the fresh allograft and 99% at 10 years for the viable cryopreserved allograft. These data suggest that successful valve replacement with a viable cryopreserved allograft may provide even greater freedom from reoperation and a more lasting satisfactory result in children. The hope of increased survival of patients requiring aortic valve replacement may be realized because patient-related determinants of survival (Mitchell et al. 1986) are less operative in children.

Clark and co-workers (McKowen et al. 1987) have used aortic allografts in 27 patients (23 long-term survivors) with complicated left ventricular outflow tract obstruction as an "extended root replacement." The early results in this series of patients are very encouraging. The possibility of using the techniques of Konno (Konno et al. 1975), Rastan (Rastan and Koncz 1976), and their associates to reconstruct the left ventricular outflow tract as well as allograft replacement of the aortic valve, thereby avoiding the risk of thromboembolism or anticoagulant-related hemorrhage, is very appealing. One would anticipate that the allografts' durability is less than a prosthetic valve, but the freedom from sudden valve failure, thromboembolism, and anticoagulant-related hemorrhage should allow the patient a better quality of life with improved life expectancy.

□ Pulmonary Valve

Many children have undergone right ventricular outflow tract reconstruction for stenosis or atresia of the outflow tract. In many of these patients, the original operation consisted of resection of obstructing tissue, including on occasion the pulmonary valve, with placement of a transannular outflow tract patch. Many of these patients have pulmonary insufficiency, and some have residual obstruction or distal pulmonary artery branch stenosis that may contribute to right ventricular dysfunction.

It has been our recommendation that patients with signs or symptoms of failure or evidence of increasing right ventricular dysfunction by echocardiography or cardiac catheterization undergo pulmonary valve replacement. Our choice has been to use allograft tissue for this replacement, and in general we have used the pulmonary homograft. There are several characteristics of a pulmonary homograft, which include a decreased incidence of calcification of the allograft wall (Kay et al. 1986). These properties would suggest that the valve and conduit's longevity should be increased over that of an aortic homograft used for replacement of the pulmonary outflow tract. There are special situations in which we have noted early failure of the pulmonary homografts. These include the patient with increased pulmonary vascular resistance and the patient with elevated pulmonary artery pressure due to distal branch stenosis. In these patients we have used an aortic homograft and have been very pleased with our short-term results.

Saravelli et al. (1980) have reported their experience with replacement of the pulmonary valve and demonstrated a 27% incidence of radiologically proved calcification when the procedure was done for replacement of the transplanted pulmonary valve. The actuarial freedom from reoperation rate for the right ventricular outflow tract is 80% ± 10% at 16 years in those children who have undergone a pulmonary autograft procedure (Gerera et al. 1989).

When reconstructing the right ventricular outflow tract, dacron tube extensions of the allograft should not be used. These have been associated with early restenosis in the patients reported by Ross (Kay and Ross 1985) and by Start (Bull et al. 1987). The site of restenosis appeared to be the dacron tube with proliferation of a neo-intimal peal in this tube. If a longer allograft is needed, an aortic allograft can be used or the outflow tract can be reconstructed with a tube of autologous pericardium and a pulmonary allograft. The technical aspects of replacement of the pulmonary valve have been described by Ross (Moore et al. 1976), Stark (Bull et al. 1987), and Stelzer (Stelzer and Elkins 1989).

ATRIOVENTRICULAR VALVES

In management of the patient with atrioventricular valve dysfunction, operative repair, with salvage of the patient's valve whenever possible, is preferred. In patients with mitral valve dysfunction, initial attempts involved closed commissurotomy, open commissurotomy, and more recently annuloplasty and valvuloplasty as championed by Carpentier (Murray et al. 1956; Carpentier 1983). Numerous ingenious surgical techniques have evolved, including annuloplasty without encircling prosthetic material to "fix" annulus size permanently, rectangular resection of segments of the posterior leaflet, chordal transfer for flail segments of the anterior leaflet, and shortening of chordae for those patients with prolapse secondary to chordal elongation. However, in many patients these techniques have been inadequate to provide satisfactory valve function, and replacement has been the only alternative.

In 1956, Murray et al. (1956) successfully replaced the mitral valve using an homologous aortic valve segment in a patient with mitral insufficiency. The first replacement of the mitral valve using extracorporeal circulation was by Heimbecker et al. (1962) in 1962. This patient survived 1 month, and at autopsy the donor aortic cusps appeared normal. In 1967, Ross (1967) began using preserved aortic homografts and pulmonary autografts for replacement of the mitral valve. A later report included stent-mounted homografts and homografts wrapped in a Dacron or Teflon sleeve to provide commissural support and four inserted without support. This initial experience with 46 patients involving new techniques was associated with a high operative mortality (8/46) and 10 late deaths. Three of the four unsupported valves failed early, and four of the five patients with a stented valve developed early regurgitation. The best results were obtained in those patients in whom the valve was supported with a Dacron sleeve. This series demonstrated the difficulties associated with early preservation techniques and led to the use of fresh, antibiotic-sterilized homografts and the recommendation that they not be supported with stents.

Yacoub and co-workers (O'Dell 1986) began to use antibiotic-sterilized aortic homografts in 1968 and by June 1977 had replaced the mitral valve in 379 patients, aged 18 to 71 years. These valves were placed in a large Dacron tube graft and fixed at each end. The ventricular aspect of the valve and Dacron sleeve was sutured to the mitral annulus with interrupted sutures, and the atrial end had a collar of autogenous pericardium attached. This collar was then sewn to the left atrial wall, excluding the left atrial appendage and creating a new left atrial floor such that the Dacron sleeve was excluded from normal pulmonary venous flow into the aortic homograft.

This series of patients had an actuarial survival rate of 52% at 15 years, a freedom from valve degeneration of 55% at 15 years, and freedom from thromboembolism of 96% at 15 years. The clinical course of these patients was very similar to groups with other tissue valves used in the mitral position, with a slightly decreased incidence of early valve degeneration but an increasing incidence of valve failure after 8 years. The incidence of thromboembolism was less than with other valves, and because most of these patients were not anticoagulated, anticoagulant-related hemorrhage was not a problem. This experience and improved results with prosthetic valve replacement in adults led the authors to discontinue their use of this technique in adults. However, they continue to use antibiotic-sterilized homografts and fresh homografts obtained under sterile conditions in children to avoid the use of anticoagulants and because there is no accelerated degeneration as is seen with other bioprosthetic valves.

O'Dell (1986) has reported the use of stent-mounted homografts in the mitral position in 106 patients under 15 years of age. There were eight operative deaths, and 38 patients have required reoperation for valve degeneration in the more than 20 years of this series. These authors recognize that the results are suboptimal but believe that it is the best tissue valve for use in the mitral position primarily because of its lower incidence of calcification.

Although the experience with aortic homograft replacement of the mitral valve in children has been limited and there are obvious difficulties with durability, many cardiac surgeons continue to believe that it is the best available biologic valve and preferable to the bioprosthetic or prosthetic valve alternatives. Certainly their use, particularly the viable cryopreserved aortic homograft, should continue to be cautiously explored based on the experience of Yacoub (Mankad et al. 1986), Ross (Oh et al. 1973), and others, in which an unstented homograft provided better durability than other alternatives.

Occasional reports of the use of antibiotic-sterilized mitral valve homografts have appeared. Most of these have been associated with early chordal degeneration and early valve failure. The possibility of transferring inferences about improved viability with present cryopreservation biology that has been demonstrated in aortic allografts (O'Brien et al. 1987) to the mitral valves warrants further investigation.

□ Tricuspid Valve

Replacement of the tricuspid valve with a stent-mounted semilunar homograft valve has been evaluated by Barratt-Boyes et al. (1988). Ninety-one patients underwent tricuspid valve replacement. In 74 patients the homograft valve was a pulmonary valve and in 17 an aortic valve. The actuarial freedom from tricuspid valve dysfunction was 92% at 3 years postoperative and 76% at 8 years postoperative. The freedom from reoperation was 83% at 8 years and 70% at 10 years. In this series of patients, aged 7 to 77, mean 36 years, annuloplasty was the preferred technique for management of significant tricuspid regurgitation. When this was unsuccessful in correcting the regurgitation or when stenosis was present, tricuspid valve replacement using a stent-mounted, antibiotic-sterilized homograft was a more suitable alternative. These data have been acquired in adult patients and are not specific for the management of children requiring tricuspid valve replacement and also involve the use of stent-mounted homografts, which have been functionally less satisfactory on the left side; however, the data encourage a new look at the use of allografts for replacement of the tricuspid valve.

McKay et al. (1988) have reported the use of unstented pulmonary homografts in two infants. Both patients had severe tricuspid regurgitation and were operated on, one at 4 years of age and one at 3 years of age, using the techniques described by Yacoub (Mankad et al. 1986). The valve is mounted in a Dacron sleeve with the distal end attached to the tricuspid annulus and remaining valve remnant along the area of the atrioventricular node and bundle of His. The coronary sinus is unroofed into the left atrium. An autologous cuff of pericardium is sutured to the proximal end of the allograft and sleeve and then fixed to the right atrial wall to create a smooth pathway to the orifice of the valve (see Figure 13.3).

This technique, which was successful in both patients, offers several practical advantages over other available prosthetic or bioprosthetic valves and avoids the use of a stent, which may impinge on the ventricular myocardium and which has been associated with a high incidence of heart block in children (Yacoub et al. 1986). The pulmonary allograft, which is available in larger sizes and which has a number of theoretical advantages over aortic allografts, may prove to be an effective alternative for the child requiring a tricuspid valve replacement.

DISCUSSION

Autograft and allograft valves have been shown to be effective and safe alternatives for use in those patients requiring an aortic valve replacement. With experience, the autograft has proved to be the most durable valve replacement and avoids the major complications of thromboembolism and anticoagulant-related hemorrhage. It does have a risk of bacterial endocarditis, and this complication continues to be a major cause of reoperation. Failure is never sudden, and therefore the slow progression of regurgitation allows elective replacement when necessary. In those patients in whom the pulmonary valve is abnormal or in whom the anatomic defect does not lend itself to autograft replacement, the aortic allograft is a very acceptable alternative. The availability of viable allografts makes this a more attractive choice because it appears that this valve has a slower rate of degeneration than fresh allografts or those prepared with alternative methods of sterilization. The cryopreserved allograft lends itself to use as a free-hand, cylinder implant or as a root replacement. Although the free-hand technique has an early incidence of technical failure, its late failure rate appears similar to that of a root replacement. Failure of the allograft is due to slow degeneration, and many authors believe that this is due to chronic immunologic rejection (Yankah 1986). Certainly the autograft and allograft valve replacement experience strongly supports their continued use and warrants strong consideration as the valve of choice in children. Pulmonary valve replacement should be accomplished with the use of a pulmonary allograft whenever possible.

Atrioventricular valve replacement in children continues to be a very difficult, high-risk procedure with less satisfactory results than semilunar valve replacement. Present available experience suggests continued cautious use of cryopreserved allografts when replacement is the only alternative for the patient. The technique of Yacoub appears to provide better results than any of the other alternatives and may provide a functional valve without major complication in up to 70% of patients at 10 years. Further investigation and careful longitudinal evaluation should, it is hoped, provide more meaningful data and an acceptable choice for the young infant or child requiring valve replacement.

REFERENCES

Barratt-Boyes BG. Long-term follow-up of aortic valvular grafts. Br Heart J 1971; 33(suppl):60.

Barratt-Boyes BG, Roche AHG, Subramanyan R, et al. Long-term follow-up of patients with the antibiotic sterilized homograft inserted free hand in the aortic position. Circulation 1987; 75:768.

Barratt-Boyes BG, Rutherford JD, Whitlock RML, et al. A review of surgery for acquired tricuspid valve disease, including an assessment of the stented semilunar homograft valve and the results of operation for multivalvular heart disease. Aust NZ J Surg 1988; 58:23.

Beach PM Jr, Bowman FO Jr, Kaiser GA, et al. Aortic valve replacement with frozen irradiated homografts. Circulation 1972; 45(suppl I):29.

Bodnar E, Wain WH, Martelli V, Ross DN: Long-term performance of 580 homograft and autograft valves used for aortic valve replacement. J Thorac Cardiovasc Surg 1979; 27:31.

Bull C, McCartney FJ, Horvath P, et al. Evaluation of long-term results of homograft and heterograft valves in extracardiac conduits. J Thorac Cardiovasc Surg 1987; 94:12.

Carpentier A. Cardiac valve surgery: The "French correction." J Thorac Cardiovasc Surg 1983; 86:323.

Clark DR. Extended aortic root replacement with cryopreserved nomografts, do they hold up? Paper presented at: Current Controversies and Techniques in Congenital Heart Surgery, 1989, September 8–9; Baltimore, MD. Ann Thorac Surg 1991, in press.

Gerera G, McKay R, Ross DN. Replacement of the aortic valve or root with a pulmonary autograft in children. Ann Thorac Surg 1991;51(3):424.

Gerosa G, McKay R, Davies J, et al. Two decades' of experience of aortic homograft replacement in children. Circulation, in press.

Heimbecker RO, Baird RJ, Lajos TZ, et al. Homograft replacement of the human mitral valve. A preliminary report. Can Med Assoc J 1962; 86:805.

Kay PH, Livi U, Robles A, et al. Pulmonary homografts. In Bodnar E, Yacoub M, eds: Biologic and bioprosthetic valves. New York: Yorke Medical Books, 1986:p 58.

Kay PH, Ross DN: Fifteen years' experience with the aortic homograft: The conduit of choice for right ventricular outflow tract reconstruction. Ann Thorac Surg 1985; 40:360.

Khaghani A, Dhalla N, Penta A, et al. Patient status 10 years or more after aortic valve replacement using antibiotic sterilized homografts. In Bodnar E, Yacoub M, eds. Biologic and bioprosthetic valves. New York: Yorke Medical Books, 1986:p 38.

Konno S, Imai Y, Iada Y, et al. A new method for prosthetic valve replacement in congenital aortic stenosis associated with hypoplasia of the aortic valve ring. J Thorac Cardiovasc Surg 1975; 70:909.

Malm JR, Bowman FO Jr, Harris PD, et al. An evaluation of aortic valve homografts sterilized by electron beam energy. J Thorac Cardiovasc Surg 1967; 54:471.

Mankad PS, Khaghani A, Esposito G, et al. Late results of mitral valve replacement using unstented antibiotic-sterilized aortic homografts. In Bodnar E, Yacoub M, eds. Biologic and bioprosthetic valves. New York: Yorke Medical Books, 1986:p 47.
Matsuki O, Okita Y, Almeida JP, et al. Two decades' experience with aortic valve replacement with pulmonary autograft. J Thorac Cardiovasc Surg 1988; 95:705.
Matsuki O, Robles A, Gibbs S, et al. Long-term performance of 555 aortic homografts in the aortic position. Ann Thorac Surg 1988; 46:187.
McKay R, Sono J, Arnold RM. Tricuspid valve replacement using an unstented pulmonary homograft. Ann Thorac Surg 1988; 46:58.
McKowen RH, Campbell DN, Woelfel GF, et al. Extended aortic root replacement with aortic allografts. J Thorac Cardiovasc Surg 1987; 93:366.
McNally RT, Barwick RA, Morse BS. 54 month results of a uniform and reliable preservation method for heart valve allografts. Marietta, GA, Cryolife Cardiovascular, Inc., 1989.
Mitchell RS, Miller DC, Stinson EB. Significant patient-related determinants of prosthetic valve performance. J Thorac Cardiovasc Surg 1986; 91:807.
Moore CH, Martelli V, Ross DN. Reconstruction of right ventricular outflow tract with a valved conduit in 75 cases of congenital heart disease. J Thorac Cardiovasc Surg 1976; 71:11.
Murray G, Roschlou W, Lougheed W. Homologous aortic-valve-segment transplants as surgical treatment for aortic and mitral insufficiency. Angiology 1956; 7:466.
O'Brien MF, Stafford EG, Gardner MAH. A comparison of aortic valve replacement with viable cryopreserved and fresh allograft valves, with a note on chromosomal studies. J Thorac Cardiovasc Surg 1987; 94:812.
O'Brien MF, Stafford G, Gardner M, et al. The viable cryopreserved allograft aortic valve. J Cardiac Surg 1987; 1(suppl I):153.
O'Dell JA. Comments. In Bodnar E, Yacoub M, eds. Biologic and bioprosthetic valves. New York: Yorke Medical Books, 1986:p 64.
Oh W, Somerville J, Ross DN, et al. Mitral valve replacement with preserved cadaveric aortic homografts. J Thorac Cardiovasc Surg 1973; 65:712.
Randolph JD, Toal K, Stelzer P, et al. Aortic valve and left ventricular outflow tract replacement using allograft and autograft valves. Ann Thorac Surg 1989; 48:345.
Rastan H, Koncz J. Aortoventriculoplasty: A new technique for the treatment of left ventricular outflow tract obstruction. J Thorac Cardiovasc Surg 1976; 71:920.
Ross DN. Replacement of aortic and mitral valves with a pulmonary autograft. Lancet 1967; 2:956.
Sanders SP, Levy RJ, Freed MD, et al. Use of Hancock porcine xenografts in children and adolescents. Am J Cardiol 1980; 46:429.
Santangelo K, Elkins RC, Stelzer P, et al. Normal left ventricular function following pulmonary autograft replacement of the aortic valve in children. J Cardiac Surg, in press.
Saravalli OA, Sommerville J, Jefferson KE. Calcification of aortic homografts used for reconstruction of the right ventricular outflow tract. J Thorac Cardiovasc Surg 1980; 80:909.
Somerville J, Ross DN. Homograft replacement of aortic root with reimplantation of coronary arteries. Results after one to five years. Br Heart J 1982; 47:473.
Stelzer P, Elkins RC. Homograft valves and conduits: 2 applications in cardiac surgery. Curr Probl Surg 1989; 26:437.
Stelzer P, Jones DJ, Elkins RC. Aortic root replacement using pulmonary autograft. Circulation 1989; 80:5.

Yacoub M, Suitters A, Khaghani A, et al. Localization of major histocompatibility complex (HLA, ABC, and DR) antigens in aortic homografts. In Bodnar E, Yacoub M, eds. Biologic and bioprosthetic valves. New York: Yorke Medical Books, 1986:p 65.

Yankah AC, Dreyer W, Wottge HU, et al. Kinetics of endothelial cells of preserved aortic valve allografts used for heterotropic transplantation in inbred rat strains. In Bodnar E, Yacoub M, eds. Biologic and bioprosthetic valves. New York: Yorke Medical Books, 1986:p 71.

14

Hypoplastic Left-Heart Syndrome

Marshall L. Jacobs and William I. Norwood

Hypoplastic left-heart syndrome is the fourth most common congenital cardiac anomaly presenting in the first year of life. It is the most common form of congenital cardiac malformation, in which there is only one fully developed ventricle. It represents fully 9% of those heart defects of infants with critical heart disease and has been reported to cause 23% of the deaths due to congenital heart disease in the newborn period (Watson and Rowe 1962; Fyler 1980).

The central anatomic features are aortic valve atresia or severe stenosis with associated marked hypoplasia or absence of the left ventricle (Noonan and Nadas 1958). The aortic arch and ascending aorta are functionally a branch of the ductus arteriosus–thoracic aorta continuum with retrograde flow through the aortic arch into a diminutive ascending aorta, which is usually 2 to 3 mm in diameter. There is associated mitral valve hypoplasia or atresia. Twenty-five percent of children with hypoplastic left-heart syndrome have either double outlet right ventricle with aortic valve atresia and left ventricular hypoplasia or complete common atrioventricular canal malaligned over the right ventricle with associated left ventricular hypoplasia and aortic valve atresia or hypoplasia. The principal physiologic consequence of hypoplastic left-heart syndrome is that systemic blood flow is provided virtually in its entirety from the right ventricle through a patent ductus arteriosus. The fetus is generally well and unaffected by the anatomic abnormality. The transition from fetal life to newborn physiology, however, is associated with two life-threatening alterations. As the ductus arteriosus begins to close, systemic perfusion is impaired. Additionally, the decrease in pulmonary vascular resistance that accompanies birth results in a volume shift from the systemic to the pulmonary circulation, also impairing systemic perfusion. Satisfactory systemic perfusion and oxygenation can be maintained in the newborn by ensuring patency of the ductus arteriosus, ensuring adequate intravascular volume, and avoiding large differences between systemic and pulmonary vascular resistance.

DIAGNOSIS

Neonates with hypoplastic left-heart syndrome typically exhibit tachypnea and tachycardia within the first few days of life. Mild cyanosis is usually present. Depending on the degree of patency of the ductus arteriosus at the time of evaluation, peripheral pulses may be normal, diminished, or absent. A soft systolic murmur is often heard, and one third of patients may have a gallop rhythm. The ECG often reflects the underlying pathology. Right atrial enlargement and right ventricular hypertrophy are frequently present. In patients with a malaligned common atrioventricular canal defect, the QRS axis is to the left and superior. The findings on the chest film in hypoplastic left-heart syndrome are nonspecific but often include cardiomegaly and increased vascular markings. In the occasional patient with a severely restrictive atrial septal defect, the appearance of the lung fields on chest film may resemble that seen in total anomalous pulmonary venous connection with pulmonary venous obstruction.

2D-echocardiography is diagnostic in this lesion. A diminutive ascending aorta is characteristic of this malformation. After the anatomic details have been determined by 2D-echocardiographic imaging, pulse Doppler, continuous wave Doppler, and color flow imaging are used to evaluate physiology. Of primary concern is the assessment of the tricuspid or common atrioventricular valve for regurgitation (Barber et al. 1988). Routine cardiac catheterization is no longer necessary or appropriate in the evaluation of infants with hypoplastic left-heart syndrome. Furthermore, because some degree of obstruction to pulmonary venous return limits pulmonary overcirculation in patients with this syndrome, performance of a balloon atrial septostomy during cardiac catheterization may result in hemodynamic deterioration and should be avoided.

PREOPERATIVE MANAGEMENT

Preoperative management of all infants with hypoplastic left-heart syndrome includes continuous infusion of prostaglandin E_1 to maintain patency of the ductus arteriosus. In general, the infant's condition is influenced by the principle that the distribution of blood flow to the systemic and pulmonary vascular beds is determined by the relative resistances of those beds. Only rarely, when there is virtual absence of an interatrial communication, does hypoxemia as a consequence of a low pulmonary to systemic blood flow ratio occur. Rather, the baby is most often threatened not by metabolically important hypoxemia but by decreased systemic perfusion as a consequence of a low pulmonary vascular resistance or increased systemic vascular resistance. In such circumstances, a relative degree of hypoventilation may have a stabilizing influence because it will be associated with an increased PCO_2 and, thus, pulmonary vascular resistance. This is generally sufficient to ensure adequate systemic perfusion. Occasionally, a continuous infusion of sodium nitroprusside may be used to decrease abnormally elevated systemic vascular resistance. The use of catecholamines in the preoperative period is almost never necessary or appropriate. Although the vast majority of infants with hypoplastic left-heart syndrome can be stabilized for a period of time by ensuring the patency of the ductus arteriosus, prolonged association of the pulmonary circulation with the systemic circulation ultimately results in either intractable congestive heart failure or development of pulmonary vascular obstructive disease. As with other single ventricle complexes, the management of hypoplastic left-heart syndrome includes eventual separation of the pulmonary and systemic circulations by application of a modification of Fontan's procedure (Pigott et al. 1988). The pulmonary vascular resistance of the newborn is prohibitively high for a Fontan procedure, and therefore staged surgical therapy is necessary (Norwood et al. 1983).

SURGERY

As for other cardiac malformations characterized by the presence of only one effective ventricle, a staged surgical approach to the management of hypoplastic left-heart syndrome has been devised, leading eventually to a modification of Fontan's procedure. The initial palliative procedure is embodied by three basic principles. (1) The aorta must be associated directly with the right ventricle in a fashion that guarantees unobstructed flow from the right ventricle to the systemic circulation with growth potential obviating further aortic surgery. (2) Pulmonary blood flow must be regulated for proper growth and development and maturation of the pulmonary vasculature to avoid the development of pulmonary vascular obstructive disease and to minimize the volume load on the ventricle. (3) A large interatrial communication is necessary to avoid pulmonary venous hypertension.

The infant is transported to an operating room that has been maintained at 20°C; thus, surface cooling begins immediately. General anesthesia is achieved by administration of a narcotic (fentanyl, 10 μg/kg) and a muscle relaxant (pancuronium, 0.2 mg/kg). Additional narcotic is administered after the establishment of cardiopulmonary bypass. Preparation of the patient includes establishment of arterial and venous access and the placement of a urinary drainage catheter; a nasogastric tube; and temperature probes in the nasopharynx, the esophagus, and the rectum. By this time, the rectal temperature has generally lowered to within the range of 30°C to 34°C. Surgery commences with a conventional midline sternal

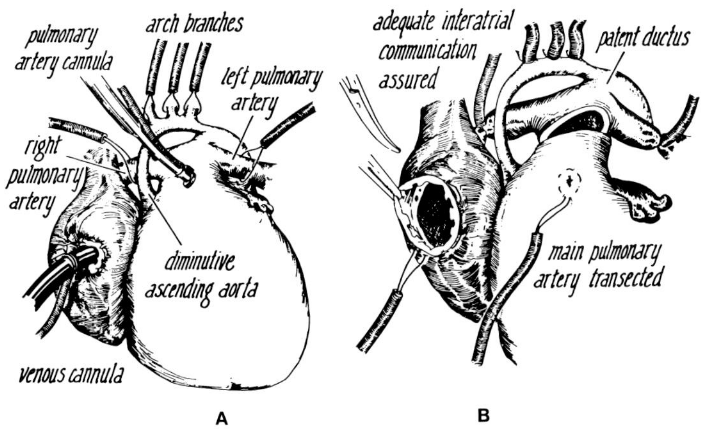

Figure 14.1 (A) The heart as seen through a median sternotomy incision and after cannulation of the main pulmonary artery and the right atrium. Tourniquets around the branch vessels of the pulmonary artery are occluded as soon as cardiopulmonary bypass has been established. Those around the branch vessels of the aortic arch are occluded at the onset of hypothermic circulatory arrest. (B) Septum primum is inspected through the right atrial cannulation site and is excised. The main pulmonary artery is transected immediately proximal to the takeoff of the right branch pulmonary artery.

splitting incision. Most of the thymus is excised, and the pericardium is then opened in the midline. The heart is disturbed as little as possible at this point, so as not to disrupt the fragile hemodynamic balance. Pursestring sutures are placed in the anterior wall of the large main pulmonary artery, immediately above the sinuses of Valsalva, and in the appendage of the right atrium. Heparin is administered directly into the right atrium. A partially occluding vascular clamp (C-clamp) is used to control the anterior portion of the main pulmonary artery while a short incision is made within the pursestring and a 10 Fr straight arterial cannula is introduced. The cannula is introduced to a depth of 3 or 4 mm within the lumen of the main pulmonary artery. This may be controlled by a rubber bumper placed near the tip of the cannula. No attempt is made to advance the tip of the cannula into or through the ductus arteriosus because this is unnecessary and such manipulation may be destabilizing. A 16 Fr venous cannula is then placed in the right atrial appendage, and hypothermic bypass is commenced (Figure 14.1A). The right and left pulmonary artery branches are rapidly exposed and occluded with 2–0 Tevdek tourniquets to ensure systemic perfusion through the ductus arteriosus. While further cooling is achieved, the diminutive ascending aorta is dissected away from the large main pulmonary artery. The branch vessels of the aortic arch are exposed and are looped with 2–0 Tevdek tourniquets in preparation for circulatory arrest. Dissection is extended around the aortic arch

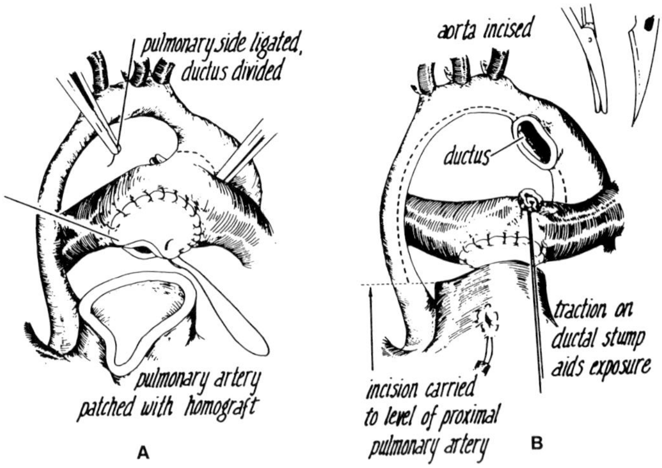

Figure 14.2 (A) The distal pulmonary artery is closed with a small patch of pulmonary artery homograft, and the ductus arteriosus is ligated. (B) The ductus arteriosus is transected beyond the ligature; the opening into the thoracic aorta is extended distally by incision into the descending thoracic aorta and proximally along the lesser curvature of the aortic arch and the medial aspect of the ascending aorta.

onto the thoracic aorta in the posterior mediastinum. The infant is cooled to 20°C, while nasopharyngeal, esophageal, and rectal temperatures are monitored.

At this point, tourniquets are used to occlude the branch vessels of the aortic arch. The circulation is discontinued, and blood is drained into the venous reservoir. The arterial and venous cannulae are removed. The first assistant occludes the descending thoracic aorta with forceps, while cold cardioplegic solution is infused into the cannulation site in the main pulmonary artery, thus perfusing the myocardium by passing retrograde through the diminutive ascending aorta. Septum primum is inspected through the right atrial cannulation site and is excised (Figure 14.1B). Only occasionally, in instances when there might be significant posterior deviation of the superior attachment of septum primum or a very restrictive interatrial communication, is a right atriotomy necessary to facilitate exposure for an adequate atrial septectomy. The main pulmonary artery is then transected just beyond the arterial cannulation site and immediately proximal to the takeoff of the right branch pulmonary artery. The distal pulmonary artery is closed with a small patch of pulmonary arterial homograft tissue, which is used to ensure an unobstructed confluence of the right and left branch pulmonary arteries (Figure 14.2).

The ductus arteriosus is then exposed. It is ligated near its pulmonary artery end and transected just beyond this. The opening of the ductus into the thoracic aorta is inspected. From here, an incision in the aorta is extended distally for 1 or 2 cm into the descending thoracic aorta and then proximally along the lesser

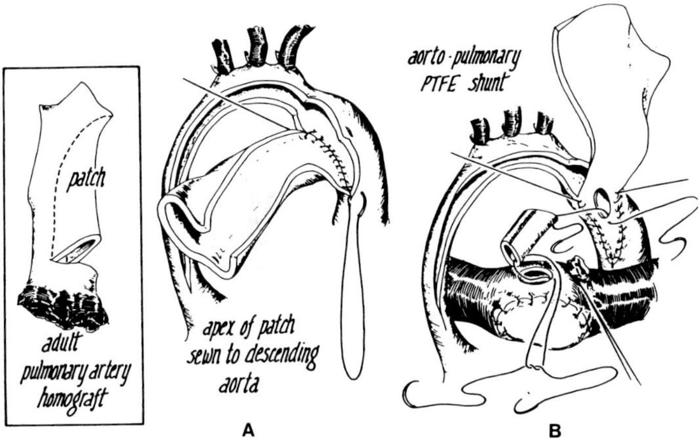

Figure 14.3 (A) The aorta is augmented with a gusset of pulmonary artery homograft. (B) A central aortopulmonary shunt is constructed using a segment of polytetrafluoroethylene (PTFE) graft, which is interposed between the inferior aspect of the augmented aortic arch and the confluence of the branch pulmonary arteries.

curvature of the aortic arch and down the medial aspect of the ascending aorta to a point adjacent to the rim of the transected proximal main pulmonary artery (Figure 14.2B). Because the isthmus of the aorta and the aortic arch actually function as a branch of the main pulmonary artery–ductus–thoracic aorta continuum, the junction of the isthmus and thoracic aorta should be gusseted with a patch and the intimal ridge excised to minimize the development of distal aortic arch obstruction (Figure 14.3A). We favor the use of cryopreserved pulmonary artery homograft for this patch because it has the advantage of being thin, pliable, and hemostatic. Fine monofilament running suture technique is used.

A short central aortopulmonary shunt is constructed using a segment of 4-mm polytetrafluoroethylene (PTFE) tube graft, which is interposed between the inferior aspect of the augmented aortic arch and the confluence of the branch pulmonary arteries (Figure 14.3B). The use of a central shunt is associated with more even distribution of flow and, thus, more symmetric growth and development of the right and left pulmonary arteries. The remaining pulmonary artery homograft is then anastomosed to the edges of the incision in the ascending aorta to a point approximately 5 mm above the most proximal extent of the incision (Figure 14.4A). The proximal anastomosis of the main pulmonary artery to the ascending aorta is then begun and may be accomplished with multiple interrupted fine monofilament sutures to avoid pursestringing of the inlet into the diminutive aortic root (Figure 14.4B). The reconstruction is completed by anastmosis of the ascending aorta, main pulmonary artery, and pulmonary homograft, thus creating outflow from the right ventricle through the pulmonary valve into the augmented aorta (Figure 14.5). Saline is instilled into the heart through the right atrial can-

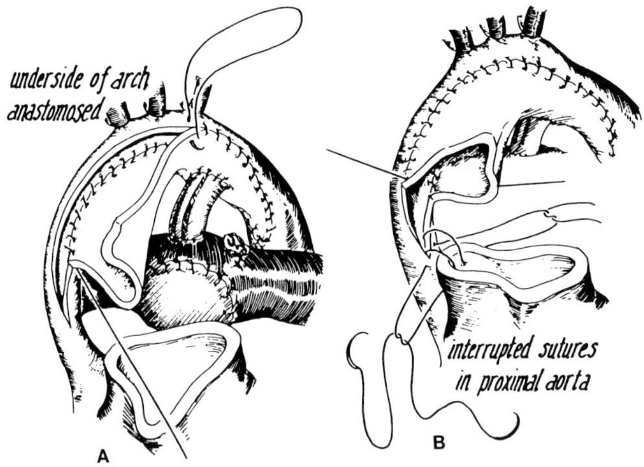

Figure 14.4 (A) The pulmonary artery homograft gusset is anastomosed to the edges of the incision in the ascending aorta to a point approximately 5 mm above the most proximal extent of the incision. (B) The anastomosis of the main pulmonary artery to the ascending aorta is accomplished with interrupted fine monofilament sutures to avoid pursestringing of the inlet into the diminutive aortic root.

nulation site, to displace air from within the cardiac chambers. The aortic and venous cannulae are then reinserted. Cardiopulmonary bypass is recommenced. The tourniquets are released from the branch vessels of the aortic arch, but those on the branch pulmonary arteries remain occluded while rewarming continues.

After the completion of rewarming, the tourniquets are removed from the branch pulmonary arteries and the infant is weaned from cardiopulmonary bypass. Cannulae are removed from the heart, and heparin is reversed with protamine. An atrial pressure monitoring line is placed through the pursestring suture in the right atrial appendage. Ventilation is maintained using the lowest possible mean airway pressure, and the PCO_2 is maintained at a level between 20 and 30 mmHg to minimize pulmonary vascular resistance. Arterial PO_2 is generally in the range of 40 to 45 mmHg. An arterial PO_2 of 50 mmHg or greater is suggestive of a large pulmonary to systemic flow ratio, which may result in inadequate systemic perfusion. Should this be the case, ventilation may be adjusted to influence the pulmonary to systemic flow ratio by rapidly decreasing the fraction of inspired of oxygen (FIO_2) and by maintaining the PCO_2 in a slightly higher range. Pharmacologic support of any type is rarely necessary in the postoperative period.

As before palliative surgery, the right ventricle supports both the systemic and the pulmonary circulations and thus is subjected to both a volume and a pressure load. The majority of these infants are maintained on anticongestive therapy consisting of digoxin and a diuretic. With a goal of long-term preservation of ventricular function, assessment of suitability for Fontan's procedure is done at 12 to 18 months

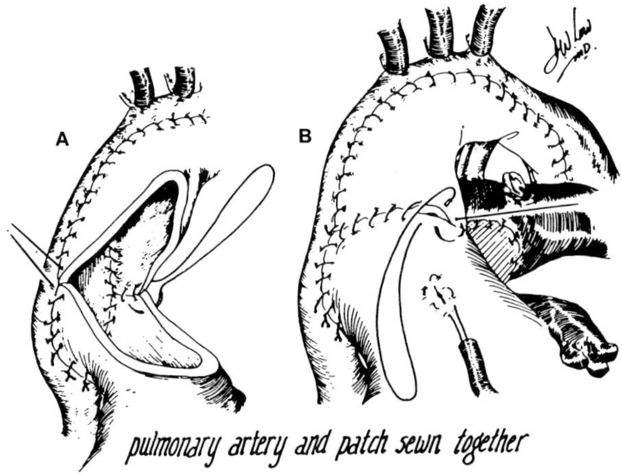

Figure 14.5 Aortic reconstruction is completed by anastomosis of the ascending aorta, main pulmonary artery, and pulmonary homograft, thus creating outflow from the right ventricle through the pulmonary valve into the augmented aorta.

of age. At this age, the pulmonary resistance is likely to be low (less than 2.5 Wood's units) and ventricular end diastolic pressure normal (less than 7 to 8 mmHg), and surgery to separate the previously parallel systemic and pulmonary circulations may be undertaken.

The heart is exposed through a midline sternotomy. Arterial cannulation can generally be accomplished at or near the site that was used for the first palliative procedure. A single venous cannula is inserted through the right atrial appendage. The systemic to pulmonary artery shunt is identified and is occluded as cardiopulmonary bypass is established. Again, nasopharyngeal, esophageal, and rectal temperatures are monitored, and the infant is cooled to 20°C. During cooling, the branch pulmonary arteries are exposed from one pericardial reflection to the other. At 20°C, the aorta is cross clamped, cold cardioplegia solution is infused into the aortic root, and blood is drained into the venous reservoir. The pulmonary arteries are opened by means of a single anterior incision, which extends from the level of the right upper lobe branch (behind the right superior vena cava) across the midline to a point at or beyond the origin of the left upper lobe branch. A lateral incision is made in the right atrium from the sulcus terminalis superiorly to the right lateral insertion of the eustachian valve inferiorly. The interatrial communication is inspected to ensure that it is large and unrestrictive and is enlarged if possible. An incision is then made in the dome of the right atrium, and this is extended up into the posteromedial aspect of the right superior vena cava to a point adjacent to the furthest extent of the incision on the right pulmonary artery. At this point, the anastomosis of the pulmonary artery to the superior vena cava–right atrial junction is begun using fine running monofilament suture.

A piece of PTFE tube graft 10 mm in diameter is cut to a length that corresponds to the distance between the inferior vena cava–right atrial junction and the right superior vena cava–right atrial junction. The graft is cut in half lengthwise to be used as a baffle to channel inferior vena caval flow along the right lateral aspect of the right atrium to the superior anastomosis between the right atrium–right superior vena cava and the pulmonary arterial tree. Placement of the baffle is begun by suturing the inferior end of the graft around the orifice of the inferior vena cava, then along the right lateral floor and free wall of the right atrium up to and around the patulous orifice in the superior dome of the right atrium. This particular baffling technique was introduced to minimize complications with tricuspid prolapse or regurgitation or obstruction of pulmonary venous return to the right ventricle, which had been experienced early in this series with an alternate baffling technique. The construction of the systemic venous–pulmonary arterial system is then completed by augmenting the previously incised central pulmonary arteries with an elongated patch of cryopreserved pulmonary arterial homograft material beginning on the left pulmonary artery with a running 5–0 monofilament suture. As the suture lines approach the right pulmonary artery and adjacent right superior vena cava, the base of the triangular pulmonary artery homograft patch is sutured onto the superior lip of the right superior vena cava–right atrial incision, providing a roof for the patulous anastomosis. The initial lateral right atriotomy incision is closed with a running monofilament suture technique. This operative sequence is illustrated in Figure 14.6. Cannulae are reinserted into the aorta and right atrium, and bypass is resumed. During rewarming, an 18-gauge pressure monitoring catheter is inserted into the pulmonary arterial confluence. At 37°C, the infant is weaned from cardiopulmonary bypass and cannulae are removed. A second pressure monitoring catheter is inserted through the cannulation site in the right atrial appendage (now receiving exclusively pulmonary venous return). This modification of Fontan's procedure provides for unobstructed flow of inferior vena caval and superior vena caval blood into the pulmonary arteries, which are routinely augmented, to avoid proximal pulmonary arterial obstruction from unrecognized irregularities in size.

In the last two years, it has become apparent that mortality and morbidity may be reduced by separating Fontan's operation into two procedures by initial association of the superior vena cava with the augmented pulmonary arteries, followed in approximately 6 months by channeling the inferior vena caval return to the pulmonary arteries. The rationale for this staged approach is that some patients develop diminution in end diastolic volume rapidly after removal of the volume load associated with the previous systemic to pulmonary arterial shunt. The consequences of this process are an apparent increase in wall thickness because muscle mass does not change as rapidly, and the diastolic function of the ventricle may be impaired, resulting in an increased end diastolic pressure, increased central venous pressure, and decreased cardiac output. The preoperative physiologic

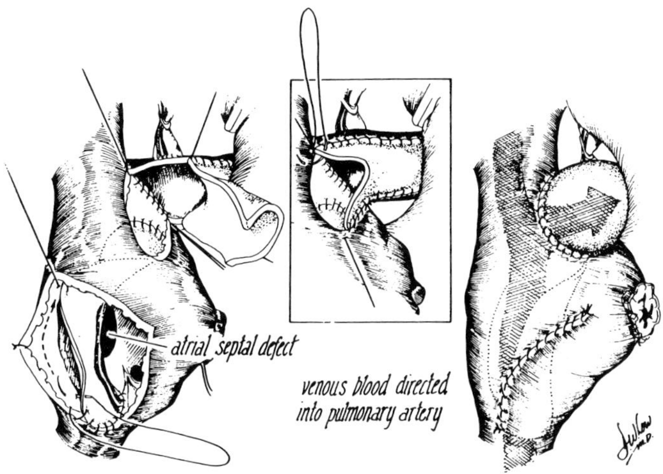

FIgure 14.6 Fontan's procedure results in separation of the previously parallel systemic and pulmonary circulations. The systemic to pulmonary artery shunt is occluded (in this case with a metallic clip). The pulmonary arteries are opened by means of a single anterior incision. An incision in the dome of the right atrium is extended into the medial aspect of the superior vena cava. The anastomosis of the pulmonary artery to the superior vena cava–right atrial junction is accomplished with fine running monofilament suture. A baffle cut from a PTFE tube graft is sutured in place within the right atrium, to direct blood from the inferior vena cava to the confluence of the superior vena cava and the pulmonary arteries. The central pulmonary arteries are augmented with a gusset of cryopreserved pulmonary artery homograft, which is also used to ensure a patulous communication between the systemic venous pathway and the pulmonary arteries.

information does not predict those patients who will develop rapid contraction of end diastolic volume. Thus, to minimize the physiologic significance of such a rapid geometrical change, the division of Fontan's procedure into two stages is postulated to allow decrease in end diastolic volume and a commensurate decrease in muscle mass, whereas only half of the systemic venous return is obligated to flow passively through the pulmonary vascular bed. Thus, although significant changes in ventricular geometry and compliance may occur following the first of these two staged procedures (the hemi-Fontan operation), it is unlikely to have a deleterious effect on cardiac output. Later, when the end diastolic volume and wall thickness ratio have normalized, completion of the Fontan procedure may be undertaken.

DISCUSSION

The results of reconstructive surgery for hypoplastic left-heart syndrome continue to improve, both for initial palliation and later reconstructive surgery, as we gain ever-increasing knowledge of the anatomy and physiology of this complex group of patients and as the surgical management evolves accordingly (Barber et al. 1988). In the 2-year period beginning January 1989, 151 newborns entered our institution for palliative surgery. There were 42 early and five late deaths among these patients. Seventy-eight of the 104 survivors have already undergone a hemi-Fontan operation (association of the superior vena cava with the augmented branch pulmonary arteries). Among the nine patients who died, five had come to hemi-Fontan operation earlier than 5 months of age because of ventricular dysfunction or shunt failure, which may have impacted unfavorably on the postoperative physiology. Of the 27 patients in this group who have so far undergone completion of the Fontan operation, there has been no mortality. Thus, our present management scheme for infants with hypoplastic left-heart syndrome includes palliation of the newborn, hemi-Fontan procedure at 6 months of age, and completion of the Fontan procedure at 12 months of age. The approach outlined here for reconstructive therapy of this malformation continues to evolve. The challenge for the future is to characterize this group of lesions better so that the preoperative, operative, and postoperative management of these and other infants with malformations characterized by the presence of a single ventricle may be further improved.

REFERENCES

Barber G, Helton JG, Aglira BA, et al. The significance of tricuspid regurgitation in hypoplastic left heart syndrome. Am Heart J 1988; 116:1563.

Barber G, Murphy JD, Pigott JD, Norwood WI. The evolving pattern of survival following palliative surgery for hypoplastic left heart syndrome. J Am Coll Cardiol 1988; 2:139A.

Fyler DC. Report of the New England Regional Infant Cardiac Program. Pediatrics 1980; 65(suppl):463.

Noonan JA, Nadas AS. The hypoplastic left heart syndrome. Pediatr Clin North Am 1958; 5:1029.

Norwood WI, Lang P, Hansen D. Physiologic repair of aortic atresia-hypoplastic left heart syndrome. N Engl J Med 1983; 308:23.

Pigott JD, Murphy JD, Barber B, Norwood WI. Palliative reconstructive surgery for hypoplastic left heart syndrome. Ann Thorac Surg 1988; 45:122.

Watson DG, Rowe RD. Aortic-valve atresia report of 43 cases. JAMA 1962; 179:14.

15

Anesthetic Techniques for Heart Surgery in Neonates

Dolly D. Hansen and Paul R. Hickey

Anesthetic techniques for neonatal cardiac surgery have developed rapidly over the last 2 decades. Before 1970, neonates with congenital cardiac defects in need of intervention were rarely considered surgical candidates. Because of prohibitive morbidity and even mortality associated with cardiopulmonary bypass in the neonatal age group, a palliative procedure would be performed, most often creation of a shunt for insufficient pulmonary blood flow or (during inflow occlusion) a valvotomy for critical pulmonic or aortic valve stenosis (Harmel and Lamont 1946; Strong et al. 1966). Before prostaglandin E_1 (PGE_1) became available, neonates with insufficient pulmonary or systemic circulation often succumbed, before diagnosis could be established and palliative or corrective surgery performed, when the ductus arteriosus (PDA) underwent physiologic closure. Even when surgical repair or palliation could be attempted, the insufficient flow in either the pulmonary or the systemic circuit produced severe metabolic abnormalities in the preoperative period, further increasing the surgical risk.

NEONATAL PHYSIOLOGY

Immediately after birth the circulation changes from the fetal parallel pattern to a transitional circulation. In the transitional circulation the obligatory increase in the systemic vascular resistance secondary to the exclusion of the low resistance placental circulation and the simultaneous fall in pulmonary vascular resistance with respiration and expansion of the lung, change the circulation from a parallel to a serial pattern. Although the right to left shunt through the foramen ovale and the ductus arteriosus decreases toward zero, progressive physiologic closure does not produce irreversible anatomic closure. For varying amounts of time, usually 24 to 72 hours, the ductus arteriosus remains physiologically open. Under pathologic conditions, this physiologic closure is prolonged, and shunting both from right to left and from left to right can occur (Hickey and Hansen 1984). Because of these potential shunts, the neonate can compensate for some congenital malformations for a limited time. However, with inappropriate anesthetic management it is possible to cause a degree of shunting that is detrimental to these neonates.

□ Temperature Regulation

Awake neonates tolerate external cold stress poorly, and they rely on nonshivering thermogenesis by burning brown fat. This temperature intolerance is not a major problem in neonatal cardiac surgery because most procedures are performed with core hypothermia either as hypothermic perfusion on cardiopulmonary bypass or under deep hypothermic circulatory arrest. Provided that induction of anesthesia and insertion of intravascular lines and the initial part of the surgical procedure are done within a short time, it is reasonable to allow the temperature to drift lower without attempting to maintain normal body temperature. As the early experience with deep hypothermia and surface cooling showed, the incidence of spontaneous ventricular fibrillation was quite low, even with temperatures as low as 28°C. The exception was in infants with borderline or insufficient coronary perfusion, in whom minimal physical or surgical stimulation could lead to ventricular fibrillation. In the majority of closed procedures, the usual maneuvers to preserve body temperature are applied. This includes the use of heating blankets, heated humidified anesthetic gases, warming lights, and room temperature as high as tolerable. This is most important in patent ductus arteriosus ligation in preterm infants.

In other closed procedures, for example, creation of shunts, moderate hypothermia to approximately 35°C might improve the tolerance to hypoxia during clamping of the pulmonary artery. Mild hypothermia may also be beneficial in reducing the risk of spinal injury in repair of preductal coarctation of the aorta.

□ Glucose Requirements

Neonates often have low glycogen storage, and they are apt to become hypoglycemic when not feeding regularly. Hyperosmotic concentrations of glucose-containing solutions are used in the neonatal nurseries, and it is rare for a baby to arrive in the operating room from the intensive care unit (ICU) without an infusion of at least 10% glucose. There is increasing evidence that high serum glucose levels may impair recovery from episodes of cerebral ischemia. Likewise, neonates exposed to operative stress, especially cardiopulmonary bypass and deep hypothermic circulatory arrest, can become significantly hyperglycemic. Our practice is to use 5% glucose in lactated Ringer's infusion for infants undergoing closed procedures and lactated Ringer's infusion for pump cases. However, this practice requires careful monitoring of serum glucose before bypass, during cooling and rewarming, and at least twice after bypass. If glucose is low, for example, less than 40 mg/dl, supplementary glucose, 500 to 1000 mg/kg, is added to the hourly maintenance infusion of lactated Ringer's solution.

PATHOPHYSIOLOGIC CONDITIONS

Most neonates who require cardiac surgery have either too little pulmonary or too little systemic blood flow.

In the first situation, shunting initially occurs from left to right through the ductus arteriosus. Sufficient pulmonary blood flow can almost always be maintained by keeping the ductus patent with an infusion of PGE_1 until palliation with a shunt or opening of the pulmonary outflow tract can be performed. In the other situation, with too little systemic flow, shunting occurs from right to left; PGE_1 can maintain systemic circulation until repair (critical coarctation, aortic valve stenosis) or palliation (hypoplastic left-heart syndrome) can be attempted (Freed et al. 1981).

In some instances, maintaining ductal patency with PGE_1 is controversial. One example is neonates with transposition of the great arteries, in which the pulmonary blood flow is sufficient but the neonate is cyanotic because of the parallel circulations and inadequate mixing between the atria. In some patients after a balloon atrial septotomy, use of PGE_1 improves mixing. In neonates with obstructed anomalous pulmonary venous connection, increasing the pulmonary blood flow with PGE_1 exacerbates the problem. That lesion remains the most urgent neonatal cardiac problem because PGE_1 worsens rather than improves the physiology, as in other life-threatening neonatal cardiac conditions.

PGE_1 is not without side effects: most prominently fever, venous vasodilatation, hypotension, jitteriness, and apneic spells (Lewis et al. 1981). All those side effects can be watched for and treated appropriately, and the benefits usually outweigh the side effects. Venous vasodilatation is uncommon when PGE_1 is given intravenously instead of in the umbilical artery. Hypotension is treated with inotropic support most often dopamine, and volume replacement. Fever requires antibiotic coverage to ensure that covert infection does not go untreated. The high incidence of apneic spells makes prophylactic intubation and ventilatory support advisable in most cases.

ANESTHETIC TECHNIQUE AND AGENTS

No surgical procedures in the sick neonate with cardiac disease should be performed without general anesthesia. Given the current knowledge about pain and stress responses in neonates, surgery without anesthesia is unacceptable (Anand et al. 1987a, 1987b; Anand and Hickey 1987a, 1987b; Anand and Aynsley-Greene 1988). A few diagnostic procedures, such as cardiac catheterization, can be performed with local anesthesia and carefully monitored sedation.

In all other cases, general endotracheal anesthesia is the method of choice. The use of inhalational agents is still the most common technique in pediatric anesthesia, but given the myocardial depressant effect of most inhalational agents on the neonatal myocardium, pure inhalational techniques are rarely used in the sick neonate (Friesen and Henry 1968; Cook et al. 1981; Friesen and Lichtor 1982).

Since the introduction of high-dose morphine anesthesia (Loewenstein et al. 1969), and later the demonstration of the safety and efficacy of high-dose synthetic opioids (fentanyl, sufentanil), narcotic–O_2–muscle relaxant anesthetic has been the most used regimen in adult cardiac surgery. The introduction of high-dose narcotic technique in pediatric cardiac surgery lagged behind in spite of the demonstration of its safety in preterm infants undergoing ligation of patent ductus arteriosus in 1981 (Robinson and Gregory 1981). In the ensuing years studies have shown the safety and efficacy of O_2-sufentanil or fentanyl-pancuronium anesthesia for cardiac surgery in infants and the safe hemodynamic effects of high-dose fentanyl on infants following cardiac surgery (Hickey and Hansen 1983; Hickey et al. 1985; Moore et al. 1985). This, combined with other studies of hemodynamic and pharmacologic effects of synthetic opioids, has led to wide use of these techniques. In most cases the synthetic opioids are preferred over morphine sulphate partly because studies suggest that fentanyl and sufentanil may protect against ventricular fibrillation (Hickey and Hansen 1991). In addition, it is seldom realistic to assume that early extubation is possible or advisable in neonates, so the prolonged effect of the narcotic anesthetic and the need for postoperative ventilation is not a practical problem. Furthermore, as the evidence for the beneficial effect of stress reduction is mounting, high-dose narcotic technique is becoming more accepted. However, if one wants to avoid the extreme of very high doses of narcotics, judicious use of low-dose inhalational agents is quite acceptable.

□ Anesthetic Systems and Technique of Ventilation

Most often neonates and young infants are ventilated using a nonrebreathing system, although a circle system can be used if care is taken to avoid unnecessary dead space. The circle system conserves heat well, especially if the gases are heated and humidified. At The Childrens Hospital in Boston, we have traditionally used a modified Mapleson D system with built-in pressure monitoring device and attachments for oxygen analyzer and mass spectrometers.

There are few reliable anesthesia ventilators capable of ventilating young infants with rapidly changing lung compliance. The Servo ventilator and Bournes ventilator are probably the most suitable for this application, but they are quite expensive. Furthermore, the need for continuously adjusting the ventilation for surgical activities in the field, for changed ventilation, and sometimes for resuscitation, makes manual ventilation our preference for the sick cardiac neonate in the operating room.

For monitoring two simultaneous ECG leads (II + V6), noninvasive blood pressure device, precordial stethoscope, pulse oximeters, and end-tidal CO_2 are used, supplemented by more extensive or invasive monitoring according to the infant's need. All patients will have an arterial line and most will have one to three transthoracic intracardiac monitoring lines (after cardiopulmonary bypass), including right and left atrial and pulmonary artery catheters. For temperature monitoring, at least two sites, a rectal or a tympanic and esophageal temperature probe are used. In cases of deep hypothermia, all three sites are monitored.

In the majority of cases, and always after deep hypothermic circulatory arrest, more than one pulse oximeter probe is used. It is important to remember that many infants with cardiac defects have very abnormal or absent pulses in upper and lower extremities or even differences from one side to the other secondary to shunts or cardiac catheterizations. During rewarming after deep hypothermic circulatory arrest, the return of pulsatile flow indicated by a pulse oximeter on the foot is a guarantee of reasonably good peripheral circulation, and by inference, an adequate cardiac output.

CLOSED PROCEDURES

With the exception of repair or preductal coarctation of the aorta, most closed procedures performed in neonates are either shunts or pulmonary artery banding. These palliative procedures are performed in neonates with lesions that are not suitable for early correction. Ligation of the ductus arteriosus in the preterm infant stands in a class by itself as a reparative procedure.

Preductal coarctation of the aorta does not become symptomatic until the ductus arteriosus undergoes normal physiologic closure 24 to 72 hours after birth. Before PGE_1 became available, preductal coarctation was a life-threatening lesion requiring emergency operation. These infants arrived in the operating room acidotic and hypotensive with extremely poor peripheral circulation. The skin was cold and mottled to the nipples. The infants were almost always anuric and hyperkalemic and had severe intractable metabolic acidosis with low pH (usually in the 7.2 range but values lower than 7.0 were not uncommon). Now the operation is no longer performed as an emergency operation but is postponed until the infant has been resuscitated with infusion of PGE_1, 0.05 to 0.1 μg/kg/min. After reopening of the ductus arteriosus has restored perfusion to the lower half of the body, the metabolic acidosis is corrected and stabilized and the renal function improves and normalizes the electrolyte status. The infants are often still quite sick and have usually required intubation and ventilatory support during the preoperative resuscitation. High afterload due to the coarctation often results in left ventricular dilatation, high filling pressure, and low cardiac output leading to hypotension. Inotropic support with dopamine or dobutamine is often necessary, in particular because PGE_1 may exacerbate the existing hypotension. Those infants who have been stressed with acidosis, electrolyte imbalance, and impending renal failure are not ready for extubation immediately after surgical repair. Furthermore, they often do not tolerate inhalational agents. Therefore, the anesthetic of choice is an intravenous high-dose narcotic (fentanyl or sufentanil) supplemented with pancuronium for muscle relaxation and controlled ventilation with an air-O_2 mixture using an FIO_2 high enough to maintain an oxygen saturation about 95%. This technique is especially advisable if the coarctation is part of a more complex defect with intracardiac shunts or transposition of the great vessels. Occasionally hypertension may have to be controlled with low concentrations of either halothane or isoflurane. Some anesthesiologists may prefer to control the hypertension with sodium nitroprusside.

To protect against spinal ischemia during cross clamping (collaterals to the lower body have not yet developed), the infant's body temperature can be allowed to drift down to 34°C simply by omitting normal procedures for keeping the infant warm: Heating the operating room and the anesthetic gases. When the aortic anastomosis is accomplished, normal heating can be resumed. In these infants, in contrast to the older child with postductal coarctation, it is often necessary to give blood transfusion. It is not infrequent that sick neonates coming to the operating room have a low platelet count and poorly defined coagulopathy. Consequently, we prefer to transfuse small infants with fresh whole blood, preferably donated by one of the parents.

□ Shunt Procedures

Neonates who come to the operating room for creation of a surgical shunt constitute a group of patients with often complex lesions all characterized by low pulmonary blood flow. These include pulmonary atresia with intact ventricular septum, tetralogy of Fallot with either prohibitively small pulmonary arteries or abnormal coronaries, single ventricle with subpulmonic stenosis, or some cases of tricuspid atresia. They are almost all treated with PGE_1 to provide pulmonary blood flow, and most are intubated and on assisted ventilation to avoid apnea. As in the former group of neonates, the preferred technique is high-dose narcotic, air-O_2, and pancuronium. Because the ductus is still open, the infants usually tolerate clamping of one pulmonary artery without pronounced hypoxemia and bradycardia, although simultaneous kinking of the contralateral pulmonary artery with positioning of clamps is not tolerated. An important point is to avoid main stem bronchus intubation, because most shunts performed are modified Blalock-Taussig shunts, so that during the procedure the neonate is dependent on the contralateral down lung for gas exchange. The aim is to keep these patients normothermic; blood transfusion is rarely necessary. Postoperatively the neonate may suffer from too much pulmonary blood flow if an excessively large shunt (4 mm Gortex [W.L.

Gore and Associates, Flagstaff, AZ] shunt or classic Waterston) has been created. This leads to a situation similar to the one seen in infants with parallel circulations: A "pulmonary steal" leads to systemic hypoperfusion with metabolic acidosis and hypotension secondary to pulmonary flooding (Hansen and Hickey 1986). Treatment is aimed at increasing pulmonary vascular resistance by decreasing FIO_2, allowing a higher PCO_2, and adding positive end-expiratory pressure. In the opposite scenario, in which shunt flow is inadequate, the systemic blood pressure must be increased with the use of inotropic pressure support, adequate blood transfused to ensure sufficient venous return, and ventilatory parameters manipulated to decrease pulmonary vascular resistance. Some surgeons prefer to anticoagulate the patient in the operating room with heparin, 0.5 mg/kg, followed postoperatively with continuous infusion of heparin.

□ Pulmonary Artery Banding

Pulmonary artery banding is a procedure that is now performed less commonly. It is applicable in cases in which the infant is suffering from excessive pulmonary blood flow, intractable cardiac failure, and failure to thrive and has a lesion not amenable to early correction. These are lesions in which correction cannot be performed in the setting of the elevated pulmonary vascular resistance of the neonate. Several formulas exist that aim at predicting the exact tightness of the band, but none are entirely satisfactory. In most cases pulmonary artery pressure is measured distal to the band and compared with the systemic arterial pressure. Another indicator of the sufficiency of the banding is the arterial oxygen saturation. Here noninvasive pulse oximeters are uniquely effective. They will detect hypoxia before bradycardia occurs and give an almost immediate warning of a excessively tight band. Because they are less effective in detecting small changes in the upper range of oxygen saturations, they are less well suited as an indicator of a loose band. In pulmonary artery banding, we prefer a high-dose narcotic technique. These infants are often hemodynamically unstable and require inotropic support, for example, dopamine 5 to 10 μg/kg/min.

A combination of shunting and banding is currently the method of choice for older neonates, who present with transposition of the great arteries and intact ventricular septum. These infants often have a left ventricular pressure less than two thirds systemic (right ventricular) pressure, and therefore the left ventricle is unprepared for the systemic afterload imposed by the arterial switch operation. To "prepare" the left ventricle for "systemic work," pulmonary artery banding and a modified Blalock Taussig (or other systemic to pulmonary artery shunt) are performed. These infants are often extremely cyanotic in spite of adequate atrial septal defects. Anesthesia is induced with ketamine, 2 to 5 mg/kg intravenously or intramuscularly, followed by pancuronium and high-dose narcotic. Because both pressure and volume loads are imposed on their left (pulmonary) ventricle, they are often quite unstable and may require days of inotropic and ventilatory support. Support may be required until the left ventricle has hypertrophied enough for the arterial switch operation to be possible, usually after 5 to 10 days.

PATENT DUCTUS ARTERIOSIS LIGATION IN THE PRETERM INFANT

With the introduction of intravenous indomethacin and improved medical management (fluid restriction), patent ductus arteriosis ligation in the tiny preterm infant has become a rare operation. Since Robinson and Gregory's description of the use of high-dose fentanyl, this has become the standard anesthetic management (Robinson and Gregory 1981). In these very small and frail infants, the importance of careful temperature control and judicious restriction of fluid simultaneous with necessary replacement of volume and fluid loss cannot be overestimated. Serum glucose should be monitored and maintenance fluid continued. The importance of low FIO_2 as a measure to prevent retinopathy of the prematurity is still debatable, and the importance of oxygen as the sole factor has been seriously questioned. Nevertheless, limited use of an increased FIO_2 during thoracotomy may be important to preserve sufficient oxygenation of brain and myocardium, kidneys, and intestines (Shohat et al. 1983; Brown et al. 1987). The debate whether to perform the operation in the operating room or in the ICU must be resolved according to local factors. One argument against transfer to the operating room for the procedure is the documented deterioration of arterial blood gases during any transfer or change from mechanical to manual ventilation.

INFLOW OCCLUSION

Inflow occlusion is a very useful technique for extremely short procedures such as pulmonary or aortic valvotomy. Lately the technique has become almost obsolete because most of the procedures requiring its use are being performed in the catheterization laboratory with balloon angioplasty. The anesthetic management of inflow occlusion does not differ from the normal anesthetic method used for neonates. High-dose narcotic technique is used, and acidosis, which might increase pulmonary artery pressure and induce right to left shunting through the foramen ovale should be avoided. Ductal patency is often maintained with PGE_1 to ensure either pulmonary or systemic circulation depending on the lesion. It is necessary to discontinue ventilation during the occlusion of the venae cava. Resuscitation of the heart is frequently necessary after circulation is restored. Usually small amounts of calcium gluconate (100 to 200 mg/kg) and bicarbonate 0.5 to 1 mEq/kg are given. Because there is a surge of endogenous catecholamine immediately after occlusion, inotropic support is rarely necessary. It is, however, important to replace the blood loss meticulously. A moderate degree of hypothermia before inflow occlusion is allowed, followed by vigorous rewarming during closure of the chest. Infants requiring this procedure are usually so critically ill that overnight ventilation is mandatory.

CARDIOPULMONARY BYPASS AND DEEP HYPOTHERMIC CIRCULATORY ARREST

Studies have shows that neonates can mount significant stress responses to anesthesia, surgery, and especially to cardiopulmonary bypass. Catecholamines and metabolic hormones show significant increases; hyperglycemia and diminished response to increased insulin levels have also been demonstrated (Anand et al. 1987a; Anand and Hickey 1987b). Suppression of these stress responses may diminish postoperative morbidity and decrease postoperative ICU stay and need for ventilatory support, although supporting data so far are only preliminary (Anand et al. 1990). There is no doubt, however, that neonates should be anesthetized, just as adults (Poland et al. 1987). For the last 10 years, our anesthetic management has consisted of high doses of fentanyl or sufentanil supplemented with low doses of inhalational agents (either halothane or more recently isoflurane), combined with muscle relaxants and ventilation with air-O_2 mixture. This regimen seems to offer the best cardiovascular stability with optimal oxygenation and balance between systemic and pulmonary circulation. Most neonates tolerate tachycardia but decrease their cardiac output somewhat with low heart rate, although the dictum that neonatal cardiac output in humans is totally rate dependent has been proved incorrect (Kenny et al. 1987). Nevertheless, pancuronium remains the drug of choice for muscle relaxation, although D-tubocurare and metocurine iodide (Metubine iodide; Eli Lilly and Co.) can also be used. Vecuronium does not seem to have any properties particularly useful in neonatal cardiac anesthesia.

Currently there is a debate over whether deep hypothermia and circulatory arrest or deep hypothermia with low flow perfusion offers the best conditions for the surgeons and has the least deleterious effect on postoperative cardiac and cerebral function. Studies of cerebral function and intellectual development in infants following deep hypothermic cardiac arrest have shown various results but are difficult to evaluate because good control groups are not available. This is a difficult issue, especially because developmental central nervous system abnormalities have been linked to congenital heart defects per se (Dickinson and Sambrooke 1979; Wright et al. 1979; Clarkson et al. 1980; Settergren et al. 1982; Newburger et al. 1984). The current consensus is that most of the children seem to function normally after deep hypothermic cardiac arrest compared with siblings but that some subtle deficits may persist, such as in language development.

To try to minimize sequelae, barbiturates 10 mg/kg are given either immediately after institution of cardiopulmonary bypass or just before deep hypothermic cardiac arrest. When deep hypothermic low flow is planned, barbiturate is administered when tympanic temperature reaches 18°C. In the early days of surface cooling followed by cooling on bypass and circulatory arrest, it was not infrequent in the early postoperative period to see either frank seizures or athetoid movements of the face and tongue. These infants usually had been in low cardiac output. Even if initial postoperative electroencephalogram was abnormal, survivors recovered normally and follow-up electroencephalogram 1 year later had become normal. This problem has not completely disappeared and may even be resurfacing. Its etiology is still not understood. Recent observations suggest that cerebral sequelae are seen more frequently in infants with extensive aortopulmonary collaterals.

Initial experience with deep hypothermic cardiac arrest and low flow perfusion suggests that the continuous low flow perfusion leads to significantly greater retention of fluid. Weight increases up to 25% in the low flow group compared with preoperative weight are frequently seen. Such fluid retention prolongs the need for ventilatory support for 1 to 2 days.

Rewarming time is considerably longer after low perfusion bypass and is associated with a tendency to appreciable decrease in temperature after bypass, necessitating specific attention to the infant's body temperature. Heating of blood products, intravenous fluids, and anesthetic gases and increasing the ambient operating room temperature are needed to partially counteract this problem.

Most often inotropic support is necessary for weaning from cardiopulmonary bypass, in most cases, dopamine, 5 to 10 μg/kg, is sufficient, but in some cases dobutamine, epinephrine, isoproterenol, or amrinone offers advantages. We have rarely found sodium nitroprusside or nitroglycerin to be of advantage. On a few occasions neonates have developed significant intrapulmonary shunting, especially with nitroglycerine.

It is critical after cardiopulmonary bypass to prevent pulmonary hypertensive crises by avoiding respiratory acidosis, hypoxia, and insufficient anesthesia. The most effective treatment, at least in the operating room, remains hyperventilation without positive end-expiratory pressure at a normal functional residual capacity. Pharmacologic treatment, apart from deepening of anesthesia, has not proved particularly useful for these problems, although infusion of PGE_1 might theoretically be of use as well as isoproterenol (Isuprel; Elkins-Sinn Inc.) for inotropic support (Hansen and Wessel 1988).

Many stressed and acidotic neonates have ill-defined coagulopathies, so use of fresh whole blood is preferable for volume replacement after cardiopulmonary bypass. Some infants have low platelet counts and need 1 to 2 units of platelets. Occasionally, especially when fresh blood is not available, cryoprecipitate may be needed. All of these concentrated blood products contain large amounts of citrate, so careful administration of calcium (gluconate) is necessary to maintain ionized calcium within normal limits. More important, these blood products contain vasoactive substances, which cause increased pulmonary vascular resistance, pulmonary artery hypertension, and subsequent right ventricular failure and secondary left ventricular dysfunction, all leading to decreased cardiac output.

Because of concern over acquired immuno-deficiency syndrome (AIDS), fresh designated blood from parents and relatives has become increasingly available and is useful for avoiding transfusion-related diseases. At least it alleviates the parents' fear thereof.

Desmopressin acetate (DDAVP) has been claimed to decrease blood loss and need for blood replacement in adults following cardiac and orthopedic surgery. Its efficacy is unproved in children, but it may be useful following protamine reversal of heparin (Seear et al. 1989). No studies of its efficacy in infants or neonates have been published.

The growing understanding of neonatal pulmonary physiology, transitional circulation, and control of pulmonary vascular resistance in infants has led to increased awareness of the entity now commonly known as postoperative pulmonary hypertensive crisis. In the 1970s, despite good intraoperative repair and a smooth intraoperative course, neonates not infrequently suddenly developed low cardiac output and deteriorating arterial blood gases in a steady downhill spiral, and they died. Some infants developed intractable bradycardia in relation to endotracheal suctioning. Various modalities for treatment of this syndrome are being used, including pharmacologic treatment with "pulmonary vasodilators," which are nonspecific. Continuation of anesthesia in the ICU using a continuous infusion of fentanyl and muscle relaxant (pancuronium or Metubine) has been used in some centers (Hickey and Hansen 1989). Unfortunately many of these infants develop tolerance, and very high doses of opioids may be required for continued effect. The long-term effects of high-dose synthetic opioids given for several days in neonates are unknown. However, there is no doubt that there is increased survival of infants, who previously would have died. In addition, the documented suppression of stress responses by high-dose narcotic anesthesia may otherwise decrease postoperative morbidity, making this form of therapy an attractive option.

REFERENCES

Anand KJS, Aynsley-Greene A. Measuring the severity of surgical stress in newborn infants. J Pediatric Surg 1988; 23:297.

Anand KJS, Carr DB, Hickey PR. Randomized trial of high dose sufentanil anesthesia in neonates undergoing cardiac surgery: Hormonal and hemodynamic stress responses [abstr]. Anesthesiology 1987a; 67:A501.

Anand KJS, Hansen DD, Hickey PR. Hormonal-metabolic stress responses in neonates undergoing cardiac surgery. Anesthesiology 1990; 73:661.

Anand KJS, Hickey PR. Pain and its effect in the human neonate. N Engl J Med 1987a; 317:1321.

Anand KJS, Hickey PR. Randomized trial high dose sufentanil anesthesia in neonates undergoing cardiac surgery: Effects on the metabolic stress responses [abstr]. Anesthesiology 1987b; 67:A502.

Anand KJS, Sippel WG, Aynsley-Greene A. Randomized trial of fentanyl anesthesia in preterm babies undergoing surgery: Effects on stress responses. Lancet 1987b; 1:243.

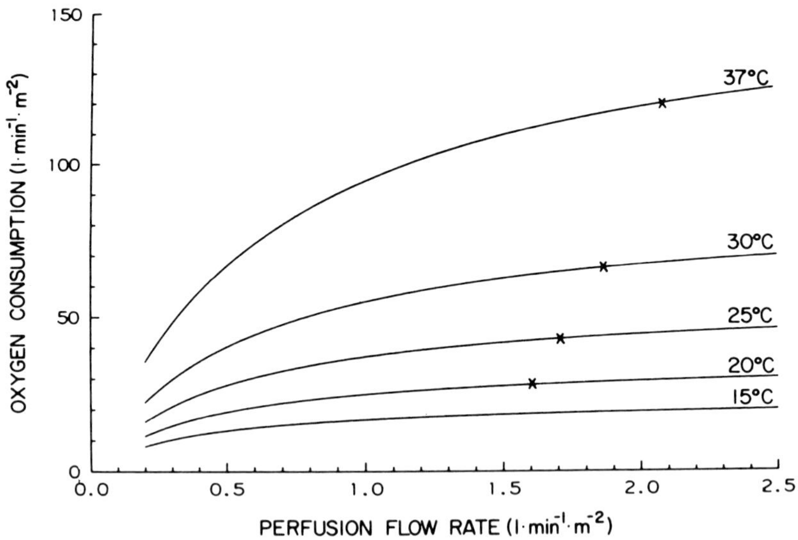

Figure 16.1 Nomogram of an equation expressing the relationship of oxygen consumption to perfusion flow rate and temperature. (Blackstone EH, Kirklin JW. In Arciniegas E, ed. Cardiac surgery. Chicago: Year Book, 1985:p 80. By permission.)

describes a nearly straight line (van't Hoff's law), which relates the logarithm of the rate directly to the temperature.

Experimental data by Horvath et al. (1953), Spurr et al. (1954), and Fairley (1961) support this exponential relationship between changes in total body oxygen consumption rate (QO_2) and temperature. The proportional increase or decrease in reaction rate in relation to an incremental temperature change of 10°C is referred to as the Q_{10}. Blackstone and Kirklin (1985) have derived a nomogram relating oxygen consumption to temperature and perfusion flow rate (Figure 16.1).

□ Metabolic Alterations

Baum, Dillard, and Porte (1968) found inhibition of insulin release in infants cooled below 30°C, despite the development of hyperglycemia due to the continued glucose infusion. This inhibition of insulin release, combined with decreased cellular glucose utilization due to hypothermia, can result in severe hyperosmolarity with intracellular dehydration and secondary dilution of extracellular electrolytes. Free fatty acids and glycerol concentrations increased during hypothermia, presumably owing to increased catecholamine levels (Brown and Cotten 1956).

□ No-Reflow Phenomenon

A microvascular occlusive lesion exists in many tissues following a period of interrupted circulation. This has been termed the no-reflow lesion, indicating incomplete reperfusion to the capillary bed when inflow is resumed. The no-reflow phenomenon has been studied most extensively in central nervous system tissue. Initially thought to be the result of perivascular edema and "extrinsic" embarrassment of the small vessels, substantial data exist to implicate several mechanisms in the genesis of the no-reflow lesion. These include postischemic hypotension, increased blood viscosity, vascular smooth muscle contraction due to increased extracellular potassium, and precapillary shunting (Ames et al. 1968; Fischer et al. 1977).

Data from Hallenbeck (1977) as well as Olsson and Hossmann (1971) indicate that the factor initiating the cascade to the no-reflow lesion is the interaction of blood components with tissues injured by hypoxia. Greely et al. (1989) at Duke, using xenon 133 clearance techniques in infants undergoing deep hypothermia and total circulatory arrest at 18°C to 22°C, found impaired cerebral perfusion following deep hypothermia and total circulatory arrest, whereas those undergoing repair with hypothermic cardiopulmonic bypass had normal cerebral reperfusion.

CHANGES IN VITAL ORGANS ASSOCIATED WITH HYPOTHERMIA

Few reports have documented morphologic alterations in the vital organs, other than the brain, following hypothermic circulatory arrest; however, the complications of renal insufficiency, necrotizing enterocolitis, liver necrosis, and atelectasis have all been described (Venugopal et al. 1973; Silane and Symchych 1977; Rein et al. 1977; Lamberti et al. 1978). Most authors have implicated low-flow postoperative states or "shunting" of splanchnic blood from visceral organs in response to elevations of circulating epinephrine and norepinephrine. Most of what is known about the morphologic organ changes due to hypothermia comes from animal research models.

Berhard, McMurrey, and Curtis (1955) demonstrated that normothermic dogs subjected to hepatic afferent circulatory occlusion for 60 minutes had a 100% mortality. With hypothermia to 25°C to 27°C by surface cooling, this fell to 7% with no hepatic necrosis seen at postmortem examination. Fisher et al. (1957) surface cooled dogs to 23°C to 24°C for periods up to 24 hours with liver sections failing to show consistently evidence of hepatocellular damage, although congestion, glycogen depletion, and slight increase in hepatic lipid were noted. Similar findings were discovered in sections taken from dogs who were rewarmed following the hypothermia.

Rabbits were cooled to 28°C for periods up to 48 hours by Hall et al. (1960), finding only hyperemia and vascular dilation and no hepatocellular damage. After combined surface cooling to 18°C to 20°C with circulatory arrest periods of up to 1½ hours in a dog model, Rittenhouse et al. (1972) found only minimal widening of centrilobular sinusoids and mild vacuolization of hepatic cell cytoplasm.

Overall, animal studies indicate that the relatively short periods of hypothermic arrest required for complete repair of congenital heart lesions are not associated with significant hepatic injury or dysfunction.

Morphologic changes in the pancreas occur infrequently following periods of hypothermia. Sano and Smith (1940) reported focal necrosis in 10% of patients with malignancies treated with hypothermia. Experimental studies by Fisher et al. (1957) confirm a 10% incidence of focal nonhemorrhagic pancreatitis with necrosis of the peripancreatic adipose tissue in dogs cooled to 23°C to 24°C. This was noted after cooling periods as short as 2 hours; however, from published clinical studies, it appears that significant pancreatitis following hypothermic arrest in infancy is rare or goes unrecognized postoperatively.

Independent studies by Rittenhouse et al. (1972) and Hall et al. (1960) on the effect of hypothermia on dog and rabbit spleens after being subjected to periods of cardiac arrest of 90 minutes showed no microscopic abnormalities except splenic congestion. Zarins and Skinner (1975) found no redistribution of blood flow away from the spleen in dogs cooled to 5°C to 10°C for up to 8 hours.

Minimal changes in adrenal structure were noted by Fisher et al. (1957), who found depletion of lipid content in the zona fasciculata and occasionally the zona glomerulosa of dogs surface cooled to 23°C to 24°C.

Silane and Symchych (1977) reported three cases of necrotizing enterocolitis in infants who underwent repair of congenital heart disease under profound hypothermia and total circulatory arrest, with arrest times of 24 to 49 minutes. They implicated physiologic shunting due to vasoconstriction as the result of marked sympathetic stimulation.

Mavroudis et al. (1984, 1985) studied the effects of surface cooling on blood flow distribution in neonatal piglets with and without left to right shunts. At normothermia, the only notable differences in distribution of blood flow was increased pulmonary flow, as expected, in the shunted group and less renal flow. With surface cooling to 28°C, a significant decrease in flow to kidneys and viscera occurred in pigs with left to right shunts but not in the group without shunts. In addition, they found that in the shunted pigs with redistribution of flow away from the visceral organs, serum amylase determinations after surface and core cooling were significantly higher ($P < 0.5$) than in those without left to right shunts who did not exhibit maldistribution of flow. Further work by Gott et al. (1987) showed that nitroprusside abolished the maldistribution of visceral flow in infants with ventricular septal defects subjected to surface cooling. It is interesting to note that all three patients with necrotizing enterocolitis reported by Silane had ventricular septal defects, presumably with left to right shunts.

Other vasoactive substances that may effect visceral perfusion are angiotensin II, vasopressin, glucagon, vasoactive intestinal polypeptide (VIP), and cholecystokinin; whether altering levels of these substances may be useful clinically remains to be examined (Parks and Jacobson 1985). In addition, evidence indicates that visceral ischemic injury from hypothermic arrest may be prevented by pretreatment with superoxide dismutase.

With current techniques producing hypothermic circulatory arrest, morphologic changes in the lung are minimal, consisting of focal atelectasis, congestion, and occasional focal alveolar hemorrhage. Examination of lung sections months after hypothermic arrest periods of up to 1½ hours shows normal microscopic architecture (Fisher et al. 1957; Rittenhouse et al. 1972; Black et al. 1976).

Earlier clinical reports documented postoperative renal insufficiency, tubular necrosis, and transient hemoglobinuria as well as death due to renal failure following hypothermic circulatory arrest. Severe renal injury appears to be largely preventable by measures insuring adequate volume loading, judicious use of diuretics, and protection of the kidney during surface cooling to avoid direct "frostbite" effects (Venugopal et al. 1973; Lamberti et al. 1978). Despite significant redistribution of blood flow away from the kidney during hypothermia, Gowing and Dexter (1956) showed that cooling to 20°C to 22°C greatly reduces the damaging effect of 1 hour of circulatory arrest. Vogt and Farber (1968) studied the metabolic effects of circulatory arrest in the rat kidney, finding an inverse correlation between return of cellular adenosine triphosphate (ATP) levels and cell death. Kramer noted a similar correlation in brain tissue, finding a threefold to fourfold increase in survival of ATP with cooling to 13°C (Kramer et al. 1968). Further histologic studies in dogs by Fisher et al. (1957) and Rittenhouse et al. (1972) show minimal changes in the kidney following extended hypothermia and circulatory arrest periods up to 90 minutes.

Earlier reports by Sarajas (Sarajas 1956; Sarajas et al. 1956) of a nearly universal incidence of myocardial cell necrosis in dogs subjected to 4 hours of hypothermia led others to investigate this more thoroughly. Johansson and Hall (1959) cooled rats, mice, guinea pigs, rabbits, dogs, and hedgehogs to 14°C to 28°C for periods up to 48 hours, noting only microscopically congestion and no necrosis. Hall et al. (1960) surface cooled rabbits to 28°C for periods up to 48 hours and found only slight dilation of the venous system and occasional cellular infiltrates, which were also noted in control animals. Fisher surface cooled dogs to 23°C to 24°C, rewarming one group after 12 hours of hypothermia and cooling one group for up to 24 hours. Subsequent microscopic analysis revealed some increase in myocardial lipid in animals cooled longer than 9 hours as well as myocardial glycogen depletion after 14 hours. No necrosis or morphologic alteration of myocardial fibers was noted (Fisher et al. 1957). Rittenhouse et al. (1972) studied the morphologic cardiac changes in dogs following cooling to 18°C to 20°C and undergoing 0, 30, 60, and 90 minutes of circulatory arrest. Focal areas of myocardial cell necrosis were noted, particularly in those animals subjected to an arrest period; however, these changes may have been secondary to defibrillation, cardiac massage, elevated catecholamines, or hypokalemia.

Impairment of the functional integrity of the brain following hypothermia and total circulatory arrest has been the focus of intensive clinical investigation since

1960, when Bjork and Hultquist (1960) issued their warning against using deep hypothermia by extracorporeal cooling in children. This early report prompted experimental animal studies to determine the structural, metabolic, and functional derangements of animals exposed to deep hypothermia and circulatory arrest. Bjork and Hultquist postulated that the microscopic brain abnormalities noted postmortem were attributable to several mechanisms, including intravascular aggregation of blood components, impairment of cellular enzyme systems, blood–brain barrier disruption, and regional blood flow derangements.

In an attempt to define the metabolic consequences of circulatory arrest with hypothermia, early investigators concentrated on measuring cerebral oxygen and glucose utilization as well as lactate and carbon dioxide production.

With the development of techniques to determine ATP levels in cerebral tissues, Kramer et al. (1968) were able to correlate irreversible brain injury with failure to recover cerebral ATP following circulatory arrest. ATP survival during circulatory arrest was prolonged by profound hypothermia (average cortical temperature 13.0°C) with a calculated half-life of 13.3 minutes, contrasting with the value of 3.8 minutes for the half-life of ATP survival in normothermic, arrested controls. Animals rewarmed after 30 minutes of hypothermic circulatory arrest recovered cerebral ATP promptly; following 60 minutes only half recovered, with no recovery of cerebral ATP noted during rewarming after 90 minutes of hypothermic circulatory arrest (Figure 16.2).

Studies by Treasure et al. (1983) confirm that functional and structural cerebral abnormalities occur with periods of hypothermia and circulatory arrest exceeding 35 to 45 minutes. Using a gerbil model, they demonstrated depressed neurologic function following 47 minutes of bilateral carotid occlusion at 18°C to 19°C as well as decreased proportions of normal neurons with occlusion times exceeding 37 minutes. Wolin et al.'s (1973) work with Rhesus monkeys further supports the contention that 30 minutes of cerebral hypothermia is "safe." The monkeys were cooled to 15°C; half then had cerebral blood flow arrest for 30 minutes; the other half were perfused by cold blood for 30 minutes. Following recovery, both groups were subjected to a battery of behavioral tasks, and none of these animals showed performance deficits.

In 1984, Molina and others published the results of work comparing structural brain abnormalities following different techniques of core hypothermia, with or without circulatory arrest (Molina et al. 1984). All dogs showed evidence of cortical, cerebellar, pontine, and medullary damage following 60 minutes at 18°C, regardless of whether circulatory arrest or pump-oxygenator perfusion was used. There was no statistical significance in the lesions noted with those animals subjected to circulatory arrest, continuous perfusion, or pulsatile perfusion. This suggests that despite provisions for maintaining cerebral circulation, some irreversible brain injury occurs with prolonged periods of cerebral hypothermia.

The concept that the rate at which cerebral hypothermia is obtained may influence the degree of brain injury is supported by the work of Almond et al. (1964). As early as 1960, Zingg and Kantor (1960) noted that with cerebral cooling to 20°C over a 20- to 30-minute period, a temperature gradient up to 7°C was noted between various parts of the brain.

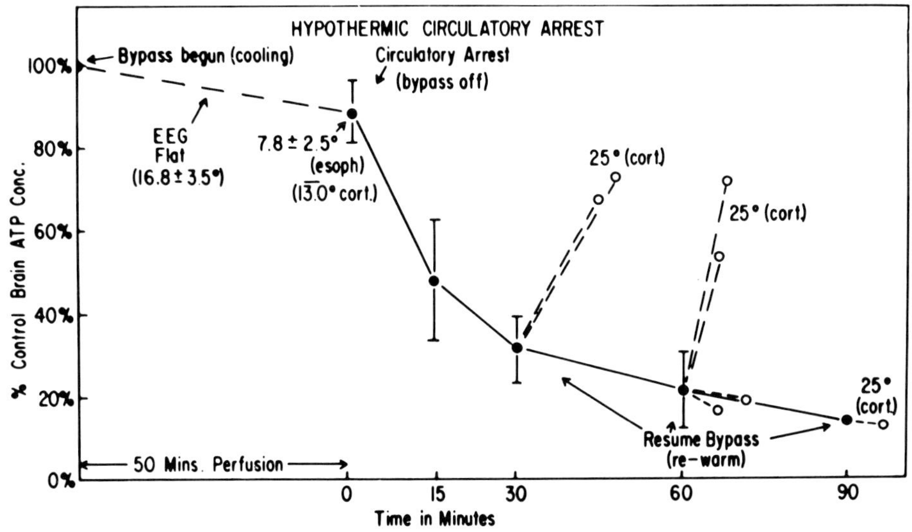

Figure 16.2 Recovery of cerebral ATP after variable periods of hypothermic circulatory arrest (open circles). Dogs rewarmed after 30 minutes of ischemia rapidly recovered brain ATP, whereas only half recovered brain ATP after 60 minutes, and no ATP recovery occurred after 90 minutes of ischemia. (Kramer R, et al. The effect of profound hypothermia on preservation of cerebral ATP content during circulatory arrest. J Thorac Cardiovasc Surg 1968; 56:699. By permission.)

Almond et al. (1964) varied the temperature gradient of mongrel dogs cooled to an esophageal temperature of 10°C, using gradients of 4°C to 6°C, 13°C to 15°C, and 20°C. After reaching esophageal temperatures of 10°C, cardiac arrest was then instituted for 30 minutes, followed by rewarming. Pathologic examination showed that the wider gradients between body temperature and perfusate correlated with increased brain cell degeneration and necrosis. It is postulated that the wide cooling gradient may cause cerebral vascular changes, resulting in early anoxic brain injury before adequate hypothermic protection. Cooling to temperatures as low as 8°C may also increase the likelihood of adverse neurologic sequelae, as suggested by Parkins et al. (1954).

Experimental animal studies thus indicate that cerebral hypothermia prolongs the appearance of but does not prevent the metabolic and structural changes that lead to functional neurologic impairment.

Early clinical reports on the adverse central nervous system consequences of deep hypothermia and total circulatory arrest have led to a concerted effort to define the neurophysiologic changes associated with postoperative functional central nervous system impairment as well as to ascertain clinically the incidence of immediate and remote neurologic and physiologic abnormalities. Cardiac surgeons, neurologists, pediatricians, psychologists, and neurophysiologists are charged with the difficult task of correlating intraoperative central nervous system physiologic derangements with subsequent cognitive and motor dysfunction in infants subjected to early repair of congenital heart disease. Hypoxia, electrolyte abnormalities, hemodynamic instabilities, infections, and concomitant congenital anomalies are but a few of the variables that make a comprehensive analysis of causal relationships difficult.

Adverse neurologic sequelae that have been observed during periods of deep hypothermia and total circulatory arrest in infants include seizures, choreoathetosis, paresis, rigidity, muscular hypotonia, intellectual impairment, coma, and death.

The reported incidence of postoperative seizures varies from 4% to 14%. Ehyai et al. (1984) at Vanderbilt University noted 15 of 165 infants and children developed seizure activity following deep hypothermia and total circulatory arrest. Five of these patients had demonstrable causes for seizures other than hypothermic arrest, including cerebral ischemia from cardiac arrest, brain edema secondary to renal failure, and marked hypocalcemia and hypoglycemia. The remaining 10 developed seizures in a time period from 25 to 48 hours postoperatively; all had complete control of seizure activity, and at a mean follow-up of 36 months, none had seizures or required anticonvulsants. There was no correlation between the type of cardiac abnormality (cyanotic versus acyanotic) or the duration of hypothermic arrest and the development of seizures.

Choreoathetoid movements have been noted in infants following deep hypothermia and total circulatory arrest. In a collected series of 413 patients, 6% developed postoperative choreoathetosis, most commonly diagnosed 2 to 6 days following deep hypothermia and total circulatory arrest (Bergouignan et al. 1961; Castaneda et al. 1974; Brunberg et al. 1974; Clarkson et al. 1980; Stuart 1988). Although the movements usually gradually abate, persistent choreiform movements have been noted. From the early clinical data, it appears that choreoathetosis appears with increasing frequency when circulatory arrest times approach 45 minutes.

The occurrence of severe brain damage or brain death attributable solely to a period of hypothermic circulatory arrest in infancy appears to be very low. Poor neurologic outcome, as reported by Bjork and Hultquist (1960) and Egerton et al. (1963) with deep hypothermia and total circulatory arrest in operations on adults and children over 3, is rarely noted with repairs performed in infancy and early childhood. This is illustrated with data from the University of Alabama at Birmingham (Figure 16.3), which relates the probability of major adverse neurologic events to total circulatory arrest duration. No major postoperative neurologic events occurred in those whose arrest times were less than 45 minutes. Of interest also, no major neurologic events were noted in those surface cooled to 20°C before core cooling. This may be explained by different perfusate to brain temperature gradients, resulting in inadequate protection for those with core cooling alone.

A nomogram can be used to estimate the probability of a "safe" circulatory arrest period at various nasopharyngeal temperatures (Figure 16.4).

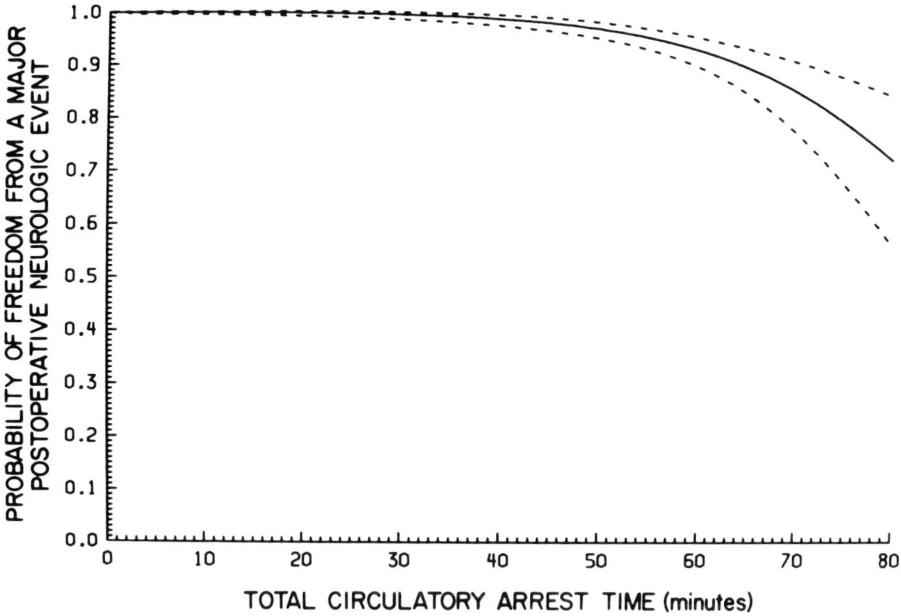

Figure 16.3 Relationship between the probability of the occurrence of a major neurologic event postoperatively and the total circulatory arrest time in patients undergoing open intracardiac operations. (Kirklin JW. Hypothermia, circulatory arrest, cardiopulmonary bypass. In Kirklin JW, Barratt-Boyes BG, eds. Cardiac surgery. New York: John Wiley & Sons, 1986:p 39. By permission.)

EFFECT OF HYPOTHERMIA ON INTELLECTUAL DEVELOPMENT

Despite 30 years of clinical application of profound hypothermia and total circulatory arrest techniques in infancy, no uniform conclusions can be made regarding the effects of the technique on later intellectual development. Infants and young children undergoing correction of cardiac defect with profound hypothermia and total circulatory arrest often are critically ill, are moribund, or have concomitant illnesses that preclude accurate preoperative assessment of intellectal or psychomotor development. Variations in arrest temperatures and cooling techniques, degrees of cyanosis, complexity of repair, and perioperative complications are some of the factors that obviate collection of a "standard" study group. Selection of a "control" group for comparison is a subject of controversy as well. Siblings

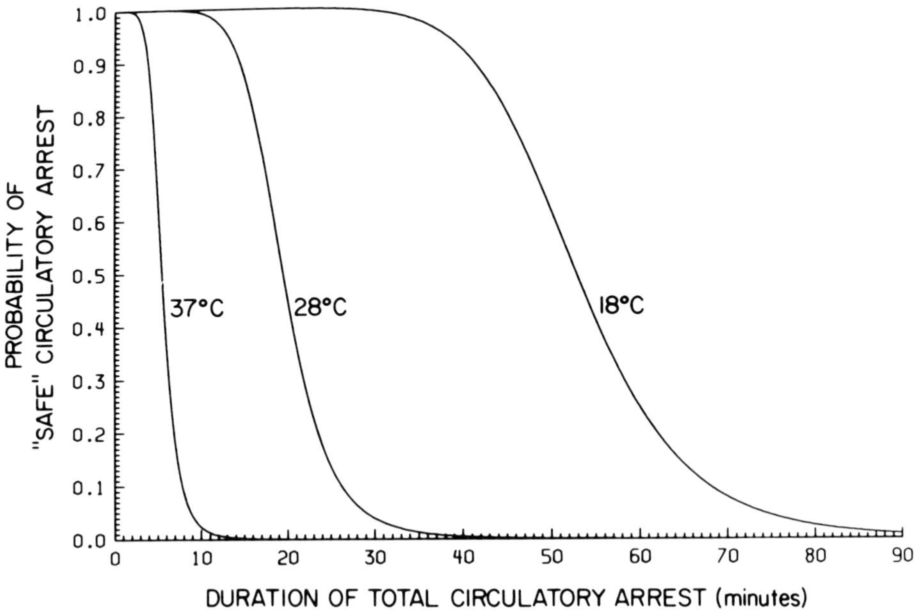

Figure 16.4 Nomogram of an estimate of the probability of "safe" total circulatory arrest at various nasopharyngeal temperatures. (Kirklin JW. Hypothermia, circulatory arrest, cardiopulmonary bypass. In Kirklin JW, Barratt-Boyes BG, eds. Cardiac surgery. New York: John Wiley & Sons, 1986:p 41. By permission.)

of circulatory arrest patients, patients with similar anomalies operated on with cardiopulmonary bypass perfusion, patients with severe noncardiac illnesses in infancy, and "normal" healthy children have all been compared with the study group, but disputes still exist as to which provide the most accurate comparison of psychomotor development.

The largest study series to date was published by Clarkson et al. (1980), in which 72 patients (ages 11 days to 26 months) had surgical repair using profound hypothermia and circulatory arrest, most with surface cooling alone, to an esophageal temperature of 22°C. Formal psychometric testing carried out at a mean age of 4 years yielded a mean IQ of 92.9 ± 16.5. A control group of 69 children taking the Stanford-Binet IQ test at 57 months was used for comparison. These were singleton caucasian births with 38- to 42-week gestational ages, birth weights 3 to 4 kg, with no evidence of congenital malformation or perinatal illnesses. The mean IQ of the control group was 106.2 ± 11.6 and was significantly different from the study group of patients ($P = 0.0001$).

A critical analysis of the study group of patients showed that only 25 of the 72 patients were similar to the control group in all respects except for the presence of congenital heart disease; these 25 had a mean IQ of 101.4 ± 15.0, which was not significantly different from those of the control group. The authors concluded that postoperative IQ scores reflected the characteristics of individual patients, and no significant deleterious effect on subsequent intellectual development could be attributable to the surgical methods of profound hypothermia and total circulatory arrest.

Support for Clarkson's conclusion can be obtained by examining the work of Stevenson et al. (1974) at the University of Washington. Formal psychometric testing was performed on 21 children who underwent surface cooling to 14.5 °C to 21.8°C and circulatory arrest times of 20 to 58 minutes. Using multiple psychometric tests, they found a mean postoperative IQ of 103. Seven children fell below the normal range, explainable perhaps by severe postoperative complications, familial retardation, language barriers, and uncooperative behavior during testing.

Messmer and colleagues at the University of Zurich reported on 11 patients who underwent total correction of congenital cardiac anomalies in infancy, using surface cooling to 20°C to 25°C in an average duration of circulatory arrest of 23.5 minutes (Messmer et al. 1976). When compared with a normal control population, the average nonverbal IQ measurements (Snijders-Oomens nonverbal) and average verbal IQ measurements (Hamburg-Weschler) were not statistically different; however, the range of scores were different, with three of the 11 patients exhibiting retardation. Poor scores in these three patients were explained by postoperative complications, genetic origins, and unstable scoring; Messmer concluded that deep hypothermia and circulatory arrest did not cause harm to somatic, psychomotor, or intellectual development.

Dickinson and Sambrooks (1979) used core cooling to arrest temperature 18°C to 19°C with average circulatory arrest time 47 minutes in 38 children (average age of operation 9 months). At an average age of 50 months, psychometric testing revealed a mean IQ of 99.2 ± 19.5. As in Messmer's study, there was no significant difference in a mean IQ compared with a normal population; however, the range of IQ about the mean in the patient population was wide, with seven children (18%) scoring at least 1 standard deviation below the mean. If three children known to have preoperative neurologic abnormalities were excluded, the distribution of IQ scores did not vary significantly compared with the normal population. This suggests that hypothermia arrest, achieved with core cooling, does not in itself adversely influence subsequent intellectual development.

Wright et al. (1979) compared intellectual development among two groups of patients who underwent repair of ventricular septal defect: One group (N = 15) had continuous perfusion by cardiopulmonary bypass, and one group (N = 17) had repair under deep hypothermic arrest. They reported abnormal intellectual development of 20% of the cardiopulmonary bypass group and 47% of the hypothermic arrest group. A critical point in evaluating these data is that development assessment was based on observations rather than formal testing; whether this would be reproducible by objective testing is conjectural.

Haka-Ikse, Blackwood, and Steward (1978) combined observations of patients with the revised Yale developmental scale to measure the developmental quotient (developmental age to chronologic age ratio) of 17 patients arrested after combined surface and core cooling. Seven siblings were used as a control for comparison. The mean developmental quotient of the patients was 92.5, significantly lower than that of the control group, which was 103. They surmised that performance on the developmental tasks was lower; however, birth problems and other complications could account for the retarded development rather than implicating the "insult" of hypothermic arrest.

In 1983 Wells and others published data that conflict with previous works by other authors. A comparison between total circulatory arrest patients and their siblings and cardiopulmonary bypass patients and their siblings was carried out (Wells et al. 1983). The baseline characteristics of circulatory arrest and cardiopulmonary bypass groups were similar, a lower mean weight in the total circulatory arrest group being the exception. Thirty-one patients with profound hypothermia and total circulatory arrest scored a mean IQ of 91 ± 4.0. Eighteen patients operated on with cardiopulmonary bypass technique achieved a mean IQ score of 103 ± 5.2. Comparing these two groups yields a significance level of $P = 0.09$. Further comparison of the total circulatory arrest group versus the cardiopulmonary bypass group, with their respective siblings, shows the total circulatory arrest mean IQ scores to be significantly lower than the siblings' ($P > 0.05$), but no statistically significant scores were noted between the cardiopulmonary bypass patients' mean IQ and their siblings'. Wells also noted a significant mean IQ score difference for those whose arrest times exceeded 50 minutes (IQ 83 versus 100 if less than 50 minutes). This observation is not supported by others who found no definite relationship of IQ scores to the duration of circulatory arrest.

Conflict in clinical data exists as to the impact of profound hypothermic circulatory arrest on subsequent intellectual and psychomotor function. Further studies are needed, particularly emphasizing objective preoperative and postoperative testing as well as selection of ideal control groups. As noted by Kirklin and Barratt-Boyes (1988), no data exist at present on late intellectual development following operations in infants using profound hypothermia with continuous perfusion, nor are there data following intermittent hypothermic perfusion interrupted by periods of circulatory arrest.

INTRAOPERATIVE CEREBRAL MONITORING

The functional state of the brain during profound hypothermia and total circulatory arrest has traditionally been monitored by electroencephalogram (EEG) (Cohen et al. 1977) and more recently by auditory evoked response, visual evoked potentials, and somatosensory evoked potentials.

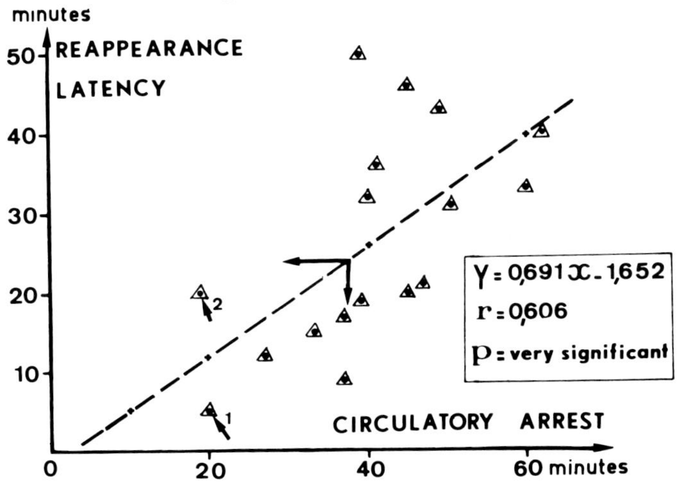

Figure 16.5 Correlation between duration of circulatory arrest and EEG reappearance latency. (Weiss M, et al. A study of the electroencephalogram during surgery with deep hypothermia and circulatory arrest in infants. J Thorac Cardiovasc Surg 1975; 70:316. By permission.)

At the time of circulatory arrest, brain waves undergo progressive slowing until they disappear completely. This time interval between circulatory arrest and EEG equipotentiality (EEG survival time) is prolonged when arrest occurs at cooler temperatures, indicating a reduction in metabolic demand to supply ratio at lower temperatures (Harden et al. 1966). Reappearance latency is the time from the start of extracorporeal circulation rewarming until the first wave appears on the EEG and is thought to be related to the metabolic "debt" incurred during arrest (Figure 16.5). Weiss et al. (1975) found a correlation between duration of arrest and the length of reappearance latency. In 1978, Reilly stated that the EEG amplification used by Hardin and Weiss was unable to demonstrate persistent low voltage activity during deep hypothermia (Reilly et al. 1978). These 1- to 2-microvolt discharges may reflect cortical activity; therefore, Reilly believed loss of visual evoked potentials may be a more sensitive indicator of early impairment of cerebral function. Coles and others compared return of somatosensory evoked potentials to duration of total circulatory arrest as well as temperature and pH at arrest. The time required for the recovery of cortical evoked response on reperfusion was a linear function of the time-temperature integral of the arrest period as well as the pH at the onset of circulatory arrest (Coles et al. 1984). The pH range associated with most rapid recovery of neurophysiologic function was pH 7.6 to 7.8. That this may be the optimal pH for cerebral flow was suggested by the animal studies by Becker et al. (1982) as well as by Reeves (1977).

POSTOPERATIVE CARE

Routine postoperative care following cardiopulmonary bypass and total circulatory arrest with hypothermia in infants emphasized maintenance of oxygenation, ventilation, and adequate volume loading. In addition, attention should be directed at assessing for postoperative neurologic dysfunction, renal insufficiency, and other organ dysfunctions resulting from the period of altered blood flow.

REFERENCES

Almond C, Jones J, Synder H, Grant S, Meyer B. Cooling gradience and brain damage with deep hypothermia. J Thorac Cardiovasc Surg 1964; 48:890.

Ames III A, Wright L, Kowada M, Thurston J, Majno G. Cerebral ischemia. II. The no-reflow phenomenon. Am J Pathol 1968; 152:437.

Barratt-Boyes BG, Neutze J, Seelye E, Simpson M. Complete correction of cardiovascular malformations in the first year of life. Progr Cardiovasc Dis 1972; 15:229.

Baum D, Dillard D, Porte Jr D. Inhabitation of insulin release in infants undergoing deep hypothermic cardiovascular surgery. N Engl J Med 1968; 279:1309.

Becker H, Lazar H, Manganaro A, Buckberg. Pathophysiology and techniques of cardiopulmonary bypass. In Utley JR, ed. Hypothermia: Lessons from comparative physiology, vol 1. p 154.

Bergouignan M, Fontan F, Trarieux M, Julien J. L'enfant au decours d'interventions cardiochirurgicales sous hypothermie profonde. Revue Neurologique (Paris) 1961; 105:48.

Bernhard W, McMurrey J, Curtis G. Feasibility of partial hepatic resection under hypothermia. N Engl J Med 1955; 253:159.

Bigelow WG, Lindsay WK, Greenwood WF. Hypothermia; its possible role in cardiac surgery; and investigation of factors governing survival of dogs at low body temperatures. Ann Surg 1950; 32:849.

Bjork V, Hultquist G. Brain damage in children after deep hypothermia for open heart surgery. Thorax 1960; 15:284.

Black P, VanDevanter S, Cohns L. Effects of hypothermia on systemic and organ system metabolism function. J Surg Res 1976; 20:49.

Blackstone EH, Kirklin JW. Dr. Mavroudis is citing fig 8-2, Nomogram of an equation expressing the relation of oxygen consumption to perfusion flow rate and temperature, an equation derived by EEH Blackstone and JW Kirklin. This figure appeared in: Kirklin JK, Kirklin JW, Pacifico AD. Deep hypothermia and total circulatory arrest. In Arciniegas E, ed. Pediatric cardiac surgery. Chicago: Year Book, 1985:p 80.

Brown T, Cotten, M. Evaluation of factors enhancing cardiac force during hypothermia. Pharmacol Exper Therapeut 1956; 15:405.

Brunberg J, Doty D, Reilly E. Choreoathetosis in infants following cardiac surgery with deep hypothermia and circulatory arrest. J Pediatrics 1974; 84:232.

Castaneda A, Lamberti J, Sade R, Williams R, Nadas A. Open heart surgery during the first three months of life. J Thorac Cardiovasc Surg 1974; 68:719.

Clarkson P, McArthur B, Barratt-Boyes B, Witlock R, Neutze J. Developmental progress after cardiac surgery in infancy utilizing hypothermia and circulatory arrest. Circulation 1980; 62:855.

Cohen M, Olszowka J, Subramanian S. Electroencephalographic and neurological corrolets of deep hypothermia and circulatory arrest in infants. Ann Thorac Surg 1977; 23:238.

Coles J, Taylor M, Pearce J, et al. Cerebral monitoring of somatosensory evoked potentials during profoundly hypothermic circulatory arrest. Circulation 1984; 70(1):96.

Dickinson D, Sambrooks J. Intellectual performance in children after circulatory arrest with profound hypothermia in infancy. Arch Dis Child 1979; 54:1.

Dillard D, Mohri H, Hessel E, et al. Correction of total anomalous pulmonary venous drainage in infancy utilizing deep hypothermia and total circulatory arrest. Circulation 1967; 35, 36(I):105.

Egerton N, Egerton W, Kay J. Neurologic changes following profound hypothermia. Ann Surg 1963; 157:366.

Ehyai A, Fenichel G, Bender Jr H. Incidence and prognosis of seizures in infants after cardiac surgery with profound hypothermia and circulatory arrest. JAMA 1984; 252:3165.

Fairley HB. Metabolism in hypothermia. Br Med Bull 1961; 17:52.

Fischer E, Ames III A, Hadley-Whyte E, O'Gorman S. Reassessment of cerebral capillary changes in acute global ischemia and their relationship to the "no-reflow phenomenon." Stroke 1977; 8:36.

Fisher E, Fedor E, Fisher B. Pathologic and histochemical observations in experimental hypothermia. Arch Surg 1957; 75:817.

Fuhrman GJ, Fuhrman FA. Oxygen consumption of animals and tissues as a function of temperatures. J Gen Physiol 1959; 42:715.

Gollan F, Blos P, Schuman H. Exclusion of heart and lungs from circulation in the hypothermic, closed-chest dog by means of a pump oxygenator. J Applied Physiol 1952; 5:180.

Gott J, Cox S, Mavroudis C. Nitroprusside abolishes the deleterious effects of surface-induced hypothermia on immature pigs with ventricular septal defects. J Thorac Cardiovasc Surg 1987; 93:647.

Gowing N, Dexter D. The effects of temporary renal ischemia in normal and hypothermic rats. J Pathol Bacteriol 1956; 72:519.

Greeley W, Ungerleider R, Smith L, Reves J. The effects of deep hypothermic cardiopulmonary bypass and total circulatory arrest on cerebral blood flow in infants and children. J Thorac Cardiovasc Surg 1989; 97:737.

Haka-Ikse K, Blackwood M, Steward D. Psychomotor development in infants and children after profound hypothermia during surgery for congenital heart disease. Devel Med Child Neurol 1978; 20:62.

Hall P, Bjorkman G, Johansson B, Juhlin L, Tibblin G. The influence of hypothermia on the microscopical picture of different organs in rabbits. Acta Pathol Microbiol Scand 1960; 49:151.

Hallenbeck J. Prevention of postischemic impairment of microvascular perfusion. Neurology 1977; 27:3.

Harden A, Pampiglione G, Waterston D. Circulatory arrest during hypothermia in cardiac surgery: An EEG study in children. Br Med J 1966; 5:1105.

Horiuchi T, Koyamada K, Matano I, et al. Radical operations for ventricular septal defect in infancy. J Thorac Cardiovasc Surg 1963; 46:180.

Horvath S, Hutt B, Spurr G, Stevens G. Some metabolic responses of dogs having low body temperature. Science 1953; 118:100.

Johansson B, Hall P. Electrocardiographical and microscopical heart studies in hypothermic rats, mice, rabbits, guinea pigs, dogs, and hedgehogs. Cardiologia 1959; 35:171.

Kirklin JW. Hypothermia, circulatory arrest, and cardiopulmonary bypass. In Kirklin JW, Barratt-Boyes BG, eds. Cardiac surgery. New York: John Wiley & Sons, 1986:p 41.

Kirklin JW, Dawson B, Devloo RA, Theye RA. Open intracardiac operations: Use of circulatory arrest during hypothermia induced by blood cooling. Ann Surg 1961; 154:769.

Kramer R, Sanders A, Lesage A, Woodhall B, Sealy W. The effect of profound hypothermia on preservation of cerebral ATP content during circulatory arrest. J Thorac Cardiovasc Surg 1968; 56:699.

Kunkel R, Hagl S, Richter J, Habermeyer P, Sebening F. The effects of deep hypothermia and circulatory arrest on systemic metabolic state of infants undergoing corrective open heart surgery: A comparison of two methods. Thorac Cardiovasc Surg 1979; 27:168.

Lamberti J, Hartley-Winkler M, Waldman JD, Waldman J. Cardiopulmonary bypass and deep hypothermia with circulatory arrest in infants. In Utley JR, ed. Textbook pathophysiology and techniques of cardiopulmonary bypass, vol 1. Baltimore: Williams & Wilkins, 1982:p 166.

Lamberti J, Lin C, Cutilletta A, et al. Surface cooling (20°C) and circulatory arrest in infants undergoing cardiac surgery. Arch Surg 1978; 113:822.

Lewis FJ, Taufic M. Closure of atrial septal defect with the aid of hypothermia; experimental accomplishments and the report of one successful case. Surgery 1953; 33:52.

Mavroudis C, Brown G, Katzmark S, Howe W, Gray Jr L. Blood flow distribution in infant pigs subjected to surface cooling, deep hypothermia, and circulatory arrest. J Thorac Cardiovasc Surg 1984; 87:665.

Mavroudis C, Gott J, Katzmark S. The effect of surface cooling on blood flow distribution in infant pigs with mature left-to-right shunts. Cryobiology 1985; 22:243.

Messmer B, Schallberger U, Gattiker R, Senning A. Psychomotor and intellectual development after deep hypothermia and circulatory arrest in early infancy. J Thorac Cardiovasc Surg 1976; 72:495.

Mohri H, Hessell E, Nelson R, et al. Use of Rheomacrodex and hyperventilation in prolonged circulatory arrest under deep hypothermia induced by surface cooling. Am J Surg 1966; 112:241.

Molina J, Einzig S, Mastri A, et al. Brain damage in profound hypothermia. J Thorac Cardiovasc Surg 1984; 87:596.

Olsson Y, Hossmann K. The effect of intravascular saline perfusion on the sequelae of transient cerebral ischemia—light and electron microscopical observations. Acta Neurol Pathol 1971; 17:68.

Parkins W, Jensen J, Vars H. Brain cooling and the prevention of brain damage during the periods of circulatory occlusion in dogs. Ann Surg 1954; 140:284.

Parks D, Bukley G, Granger D. Ischemic injury in the cat small intestine; role of superoxide radicals. Gastroenterology 1982; 82:9.

Parks D, Jacobson E. Physiology of the splanchnic circulation. Arch Intern Med 1985; 145:1278.

Pembrey MS, White WH. The regulation of temperature in hibernating animals. J Physiol 1895; 19:477.

Reeves R. The interaction of body temperature and acid based balance in ectothermic vertebras. Ann Rev Physiol 1977; 39:559.

Reilly E, Kondo C, Brunberg J, Doty D. Visual evoked potentials during hypothermia and prolonged circulatory arrest. EEG Clin Neurophysiol 1978; 45:100.

Rein J, Freed M, Norwood W, Castaneda A. Early and late results of closure of ventricular septal defect in infancy. Ann Thorac Surg 1977; 24:19.

Rittenhouse E, Mohri H, Reichenbach D, Merendino K. Morphological alterations in vital organs after prolonged cardiac arrest at low body temperature. Ann Thorac Surg 1972; 13:564.

Sano M, Smith L. A critical histopathologic study: Fifty postmortem patients with cancer subjected to local or generalized refrigeration compared to a similar controlled group of thirty-seven nonrefrigerated patients. J Lab Clin Med 1940; 26:443.

Sarajas H. Evidence for heart damage association with systemic hypothermia in dogs. Am Heart J 1956; 51:298.

Sarajas H, Senning A, Kaplan J. Heart damage in dogs subjected to hypothermia, circulatory arrest, and cardiac surgery. Am Heart J 1956; 52:836.

Sealy WC, Brown Jr IW, Young Jr WG, et al. Hypothermia, low flow extra corporeal circulation and controlled cardiac arrest for open heart surgery. Surg Gyn Obstet 1957; 104:441.

Silane M, Symchych P. Necrotizing enterocolitis after cardiac surgery. Am J Surg 1977; 133:373.

Spurr G, Hutt B, Horvath S. Responses of dogs to hypothermia. Am J Physiol 1954; 179:139.

Stevenson J, Stone E, Dillard D, Morgan B. Intellectual development of children subjected to prolonged circulatory arrest during hypothermic open heart surgery in infancy. Circulation 1974; 49, 50(2):54.

Stewart RW. In Kirklin JW, Barratt-Boyes BG, eds. Cardiac surgery. New York: Churchill Livingstone 1986.p 38.

Tharion J, Johnson D, Celermaier J, et al. Profound hypothermia with circulatory arrest; nine years clinical experience. J Thorac Cardiovasc Surg 1982; 84:66.

Treasure T, Naftel D, Conger K, et al. The effect of hypothermic circulatory arrest time on cerebral function, morphology, and biochemistry. J Thorac Cardiovasc Surg 1983; 86:761.

Venugopal P, Olszowka J, Whener H, et al. Early correction of congenital heart disease with surface deep hypothermia and circulatory arrest. J Thorac Cardiovasc Surg 1973; 66:375.

Vogt M, Farber E. On the molecular pathology of ischemic renal cell death. Am J Pathol 1968; 53:1.

Weiss M, Weiss J, Cotton J, Nicolas F, Binet J. A study of the electroencephalogram during surgery with deep hypothermia and circulatory arrest in infants. J Thorac Cardiovasc Surg 1975; 70:316.

Wells F, Coghill S, Caplan H, Lincoln C. Duration of circulatory arrest does influence the psychologic development of children after cardiac operation in early life. J Thorac Cardiovasc Surg 1983; 86:823.

Wolin L, Massopust Jr L, White R. Behavioral effects of autocerebral perfusion, hypothermia and arrest of cerebral blood flow in the rhesus monkey. Exper Neurol 1973; 39:336.

Wright J, Hicks R, Newman D. Deep hypothermic arrest: Observations on later development of children. J Thorac Cardiovasc Surg 1979; 77:466.

Zarins C, Skinner D. Hemodynamics and blood flow distribution following prolonged circulation at 5°C. Am J Physiol 1975; 229:275.

Zingg W, Kantor S. Observations of the temperatures in the brain during extracorporeal differential hypothermia. Surg Forum 1960; 11:192.

17

Myocardial Preservation in the Newborn

Mark D. Iannettoni and Edward L. Bove

□

The ability to perform definitive repair in the infant with complex congenital cardiac malformations has resulted in an increased interest in the neonatal myocardial response to ischemia. The knowledge that the neonate responds differently than the adult to ischemia requires a search for both experimental and clinical methods of improved myocardial preservation. A thorough understanding of the differences in histology, physiology, and biochemistry between the neonate and adult is required.

HISTOLOGIC DIFFERENCES

Although the right and left ventricles at birth are of almost equivalent thickness and mass, the fall in pressure of the right side of the heart and increase in pressure requirements for the left side of the heart result in changes in these ventricular chambers. The size of the heart itself undergoes dramatic changes: The newborn heart increases to twice its birth size by 6 months of age and three times its birth size by 1 year of age (Stammers and Bove 1986). Force generation is determined mainly by the amount of contractile proteins available and the cellular machinery needed to activate and use these proteins. In comparison to the adult, the neonate has less contractile mass per unit tissue, and the cellular organelles and their enzymes required for contraction are significantly reduced (Friedman 1972; Kirkpatrick et al. 1976; Legato 1979; Langer and Jarmakani 1984; Nakanishi and Jarmakani 1986; Nassar et al. 1987).

Significant ultrastructural differences are found in the neonatal heart at the level of the subcellular organelles. The immature myocyte has nuclei and mitochondria that are centrally located in the cell, resulting in its characteristic rounded appearance. This shape has two distinct disadvantages. The first is that this central location of the cellular organelles creates a greater internal load against which the cell must contract, thereby limiting the amount of shortening available to generate tension (Lakatta 1987; Nassar et al. 1987). The relocation of these organelles to the periphery in an organized fashion occurs with cellular maturation, resulting in an increase in developed tension as well as increase in the velocity of sarcomere shortening. The second disadvantage is that this more spherical shape results in a less densely packed and a more random arrangement of myocytes with a decreased amount of contractile elements per unit area (Friedman 1972; Legato 1979).

The cellular machinery responsible for contraction, mitochondria, T tubules, sarcolemma, nerves, vasculature, and cell membrane, all have varying stages of development that contribute to differences in the response to contraction and intervention in the neonate. The most notable deficiencies in cellular organelles are found in the sarcoplasmic reticulum, not only in the cell membrane but in the mitochondria as well. The sarcoplasmic reticulum, including T tubules and plasma membrane–bound sarcolemma, control the major determinant of impulse production: calcium. The amount of calcium liberated and presented to the cell by the sarcoplasmic reticulum is responsible for force and velocity of contraction by initiating the excitation contraction coupling of the sarcomere (Lakatta 1987). However, the neonate lacks diadic junctions and T tubules, resulting in a decreased amount of calcium presented to the cell (Legato 1979). In addition, the reaccumulation and storage of calcium is extremely limited owing to the immaturity of the sarcoplasmic reticulum (Langer and Jarmakani 1984; Nakanishi and Jarmakani 1986).

Important differences in cellular organelles are also seen in the mitochondria, which are fewer in number and arranged randomly within the cell (Legato 1979; Nakanishi and Jarmakani 1986). The internal structure of the mitochondria is less convoluted, resulting in less available surface area for oxidative phosphorylation and a decrease in the ability to convert creatine to adenosine triphosphate (ATP) (Ingwall et al. 1981).

The neonatal heart lacks a mature sympathetic nervous system. The paucity of nerve endings found in the myocardium limits the ability to break down norepinephrine and may account for the hypersensitivity to exogenous catecholamines (Friedman 1972). In addition, a significant difference is seen in the quantity and structure of the neonatal vasculature. The normal adult capillary to fiber ratio is 1:1, but in the neonate it is 6:1. This may account for the increased tissue perfusion in the neonate and the ability to deliver more substrate to the cells (Roberts and Wearn 1941). The vasculature in the neonate has thicker walls, which resist leakage to a greater extent than the adult. The neonate also has a lower coronary resistance and perfusion pressure than the adult, which aids in preventing tissue edema due to capillary leakage (Parrish et al. 1986).

PHYSIOLOGIC DIFFERENCES

The physiologic expression of these histologic changes results in a higher resting pressure in the neonatal myocardium. The increased internal load results in a decreased amount of force that the neonatal heart can exert for external work (Nassar et al. 1987). Before the development of external force, the cell must generate enough tension to overcome this internal load. Several reasons account for these differences in contractile function. Since the neonatal heart has the same intracellular and extracellular volumes by weight as the adult (80% and 20%, respectively) organizational changes must occur to increase the force of contraction during maturation. Friedman (1972) has shown that the contractile mass of the neonatal heart is 30%, compared with 60% in the adult. This decrease in contractile mass is due to less collagen and a higher water content as well as an increased amount of noncontractile proteins (Parrish et al. 1986). The increase in internal loading in addition to the higher water content makes the neonatal heart less compliant.

A basic concept of all muscle is the length/tension curve of force generation. For cardiac muscle, this has been expressed in terms of the Frank-Starling relationship. A major determinant of contractile force is the resting fiber length, or preload (Lakatta 1987). Preload is altered not only internally, but by stroke volume, which determines end diastolic fiber length. Although the adult and neonatal heart respond in a similar fashion to changes made in response to stroke volume, the neonatal heart is already operating at the peak of the Frank-Starling curve. The isometric force developed in the neonate is less in both extent and velocity when compared with the adult. However, when the velocity and extent of shortening are normalized for the ratio of noncontractile to contractile mass differences in the neonate and adult, the differences are not significant (Figure 17.1). Friedman (1972) has demonstrated that the sarcomeres in the neonate and the adult have the same individual speed and strength, but it is these noncontractile mass differences that account for the decrease in force generation in the neonate.

The lack of T tubules and sarcoplasmic reticulum in the immature heart results in a decreased ability to deliver and store calcium. The newborn is therefore reliant on extracellular calcium for contraction (Langer and Jarmakani 1984). The delivery of this extracellular calcium is at a much lower concentration than that stored by the sarcoplasmic reticulum of the adult cell, allowing the neonate to function at lower calcium levels. The calcium paradox that results from the removal of calcium in the extracellular milieu and its sudden return causes severe contracture and cellular damage, with the majority of the disruption at the intercalated discs and junctions of the T tubules. This disruption leads to a rapid influx of calcium, leading to further cellular disruption. Because the neonate has a relatively immature sarcoplasmic reticulum and few intercellular connections, this disruption in the neonate is limited. The ability of the neonate to operate at lower levels

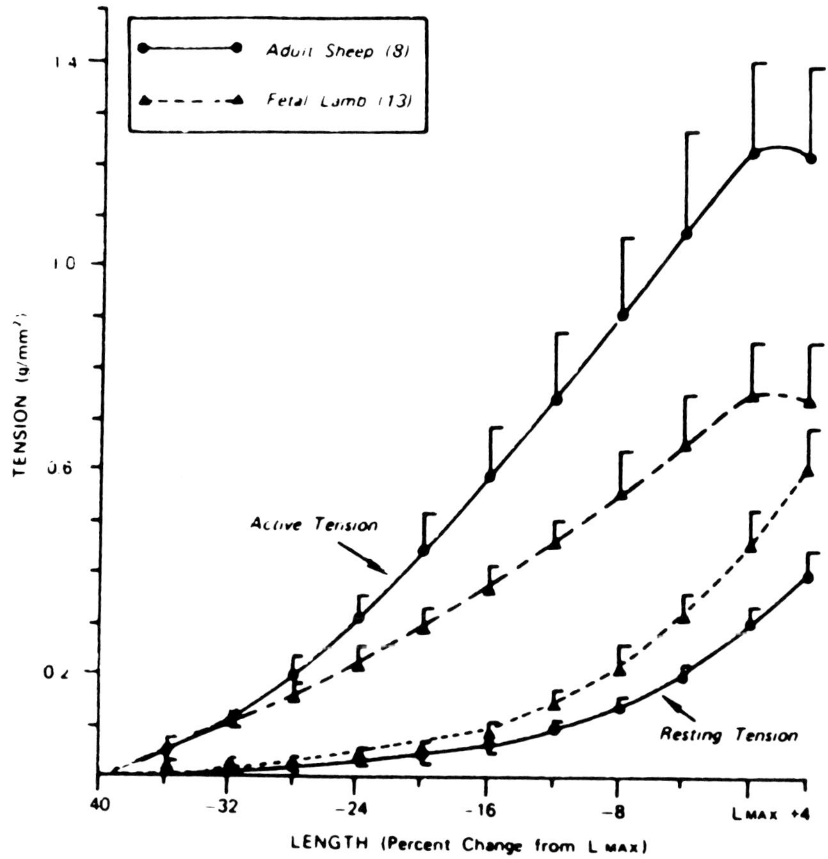

Figure 17.1 Example of the difference in isometric passive and active length-tension curves for fetal and adult sheep. This demonstrates the greater resting tension as well as the limited active tension development of the neonate compared with the adult in percent change in length. (Friedman WF. The intrinsic physiologic properties of the developing heart. Prog Cardiovasc Dis 1972; 15:87. By permission.)

of calcium also make it relatively insensitive to its depletion, thereby eliminating the effects of the calcium paradox in myocardial tissue less than 15 days of age (Chizzonite and Zak 1981).

Force generation consists of two calcium dependent phases: contraction and relaxation. The inability to exchange calcium rapidly in the neonate results not only in a decreased velocity of contraction, but also in a longer duration of contraction. Relaxation of the myocyte is dependent on the removal of calcium from the cytosol, which is modulated by a sodium-potassium–dependent ATPase pump.

In the neonate, this pump is still relatively immature and results in a prolonged contracture state (Reder et al. 1981).

The increased time required for diastolic relaxation results in an abbreviated period available for diastolic filling. Appleton demonstrated by echocardiography that the velocity of lengthening increased dramatically with age, allowing a more rapid determination of preload during diastole. This increase in the rate of relaxation increases filling time and improves systolic function by increasing the velocity of shortening. This improvement was independent of preload, afterload, or heart rate (Appleton et al. 1987).

METABOLISM AND BIOCHEMISTRY

There are three major areas in which the neonate and the adult differ with respect to metabolic and biochemical function: calcium exchange, metabolic processing, and enzyme activity. In mature myocytes, 80% of the rapidly exchangeable calcium is bound to the sarcoplasmic reticulum (Burt and Langer 1982). Because the neonate has a relatively immature sarcoplasmic reticulum, another source of calcium must be available for contraction. The alternative source is extracellular calcium through transsarcolemmal influx controlled by voltage-dependent calcium ion channels (Boucek et al. 1985). This unbound calcium is seen in relatively low concentrations in the extracellular fluid. Another important difference in the neonate relates to the activation of calcium-sensitive ATPases in the cell. These enzymes, which are responsible for the breakdown of ATP stores, are found at decreased concentrations in the neonate (Ingwall et al. 1981).

An important metabolic difference between the neonate and the adult is the use of different energy sources for ATP production. The major substrate for the adult is fat, which provides 129 moles of ATP when the free fatty acid palmitate is used. In comparison, the neonate uses primarily glucose as a substrate, producing only 38 moles of ATP when 1 mole of glucose is completely metabolized (Wittels and Bressler 1965). The inability of the neonate to use fat is due to an immaturity of the enzyme acyl CoA in the mitochondrion (Veerkamp et al. 1985). However, the relatively low levels of ATP production from glycolysis are compensated for in the neonate by higher oxygen delivery to the mitochondria, resulting in higher levels of oxidative respiration. This higher tissue presentation of oxygen is achieved by the increased capillary to fiber ratio in the neonate (Rakusan 1980; Veerkamp et al. 1985). This finding is also responsible for the increase in substrate presentation to the cell and the more rapid removal of metabolic wastes.

The neonatal heart has the ability to store high levels of glycogen in the myocardial tissue (Clarke 1973). These higher tissue levels as well as the metabolic machinery needed to increase glycogenolysis are lost as the ability to use fats increases (Clarke 1973). The major advantage of this enhanced glucose metabolism is seen with the shift from aerobic to anaerobic metabolism in the face of ischemia.

Finally, the neonate possesses enhanced enzymatic function in the anaerobic pathway of glycolysis. To compensate for the lower level of ATP production from glycolysis, the neonate has an increased activity of several enzymes responsible for enhancing the rate of glycolysis. The first of these is the increase in hexokinase, which facilitates the rapid conversion of glucose to glucose-6-phosphate. This also stimulates glycolysis by a positive feedback mechanism. The enhanced ability to cleave glucose is especially evident when the cell is deprived of oxygen, as the neonatal myocyte is then able to shift in the Embden-Meyerhof pathway for ATP production more rapidly than the adult (Hoerter and Opie 1978). This pathway results in the formation of pyruvate, which is shuttled to the mitochondria for additional high energy phosphates in the tricarboxylic acid cycle. When oxygen is present, the lactate formed by glycolysis is converted to pyruvate by lactate dehydrogenase (LDH), which results in further production of high energy phosphates. The LDH seen in the neonate functions at an enhanced level and removes lactate more efficiently than in the adult (Coles et al. 1987). However, with anaerobic conditions this lactate overload results in intracellular acidosis. The neonate combats this higher hydrogen ion load by a greater ability to buffer its own milieu (Parrish et al. 1987). As tissue acidosis increases, the neonate has acid-sensitive ATPases, which are inactivated, enhancing ATP production from glycolysis under anaerobic conditions, which continues at levels that permit normal maintenance of cellular function.

The last important enzymatic difference in the neonate is the relative immaturity of purine nucleotide metabolism and cellular transport of the degradation products of these metabolites. The breakdown of ATP results in adenosine diphosphate (ADP), adenosine monophosphate (AMP) and inorganic phosphorus, all of which are potent stimulators of the glycolytic pathway. AMP, in particular, is a potent stimulator of phosphofructokinase, which is the rate-limiting step of glycolysis. In the adult, adenine nucleotides leak from the cell because anaerobic metabolism is unable to maintain membrane integrity. Further breakdown to inosine allows increased leakage from the cell. In the neonate, the enzyme responsible for the breakdown of AMP, 5′nucleotidase, is still relatively immature, resulting in higher levels of AMP and ADP to act as high energy phosphate precursors after reperfusion (Abd-Elfattah et al. 1986; Chui and Bindon 1987).

MYOCARDIAL RESPONSE TO ISCHEMIA

Ischemia results in a shift from aerobic to anaerobic metabolism, and free fatty acid utilization is quickly replaced by glycolysis. The eventual depletion of glycogen results in the loss of membrane integrity in the mitochondria as well as the cell itself. The two major effects of this loss of membrane integrity are (1) abnormal ionic fluxes in the cytosol and (2) leakage of adenine nucleotide precursors from the cell.

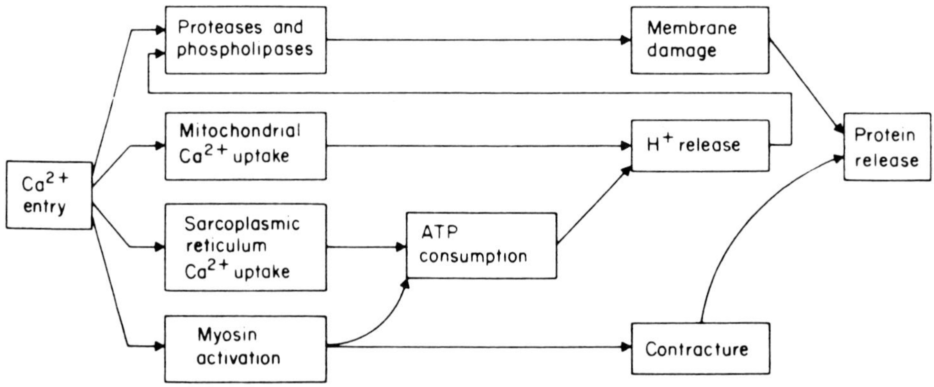

Figure 17.2 Possible pathways for calcium-induced reperfusion injury associated with the calcium paradox as well as damage from calcium entry associated with ischemia. (Grinwald PM, Nayler WG. Calcium entry in the calcium paradox. J Mol Cell Cardiol 1981; 13:8670. By permission.)

The ionic alterations seen with ischemic membrane damage are closely related to changes in calcium homeostasis. The inability of the cell to maintain the sodium-potassium-ATPase pump results in calcium influx and the inhibition of calcium reflux. Lack of sufficient ATP production results in ineffective removal of calcium from the cytosol by the sarcoplasmic reticulum (Shamoo and Ambudkar 1984). This increase in cytoplasmic calcium leads to the activation of calcium-sensitive ATPases, proteases, and lipases, resulting in further membrane damage. This elevation in solute load from calcium, sodium, and chloride causes increased osmolarity with a net influx of water. The cellular swelling leads to further membrane disruption (Figure 17.2).

The increase in ADP, AMP, and inorganic phosphorus results in increased levels of glycolysis, eventually using all available substrate for ATP production. When all available ATP is used, contracture ensues. There is some protection from this ischemic contracture since the acid-sensitive ATPases are inhibited, preventing further breakdown of ATP stores. These ischemic intervals are tolerated to a large extent through the high concentration of ATP stores in the adult and the high levels of glycogen in the neonate.

□ Reperfusion Injury

The most vulnerable period for the myocardium occurs during the period of reperfusion. Reperfusion injury has two major sources: calcium and oxygen free radicals. The calcium paradox results from the sudden influx of calcium and the utilization of all available ATP, leading to sustained contracture. As stated previously, this effect is not seen in the newborn until 15 days after birth (Chizzonite and Zak 1981). This may be due to the relatively low levels of calcium required for function in the neonatal heart, allowing a greater tolerance to the absence of calcium and less response to its sudden appearance in the reperfusion phase. In a study comparing the neonatal heart to the adult, Pridjian et al. (1987) found no change in intracellular sodium or calcium after 40 minutes of ischemia in the neonate. An increase in intracellular calcium was seen in the adult, however, and was associated with a significantly worse functional recovery. It has been demonstrated that there is an inverse relationship between the amount of calcium in the reperfusate and the level of functional recovery after ischemia. Additionally, the lower the level of ATP in the cell, the greater the sensitivity of that cell to damage by calcium on reperfusion (Neely and Grotyohann 1984).

The source and mechanism by which oxygen free radicals are formed are still undetermined. Xanthine dehydrogenase, which is responsible for the conversion of hypoxanthine and xanthine to uric acid, is converted to xanthine oxidase by the action of intracellular proteases during ischemia. This new enzyme converts xanthine and hypoxanthine to uric acid but also has the ability to form toxic oxygen radicals on reperfusion. The effects of the oxygen radicals are that of vacuolization and edema seen in the cellular membrane and in the mitochondria. These effects are aggravated in the presence of acidosis. This membrane disruption alters the ability of the sarcoplasmic reticulum to remove calcium from the cytosol, causing an increase in resting tension and decreased functional recovery. The formation of the hydroxide radical (OH^-) is another consequence of oxygen free radical formation. This OH^- radical reacts with fats, especially those found in the membranes of the cell and cellular organelles, leading to the breakdown of these membranes.

MYOCARDIAL PROTECTION

Decreasing the oxygen requirements with hypothermia and elective mechanical arrest remains the mainstay of myocardial protection. The techniques used to protect the adult myocardium are frequently adopted for the neonate. However, the ability of the neonate to recover from these stresses may simply be a reflection of the superior tolerance of the immature myocardium to ischemia. Although the debate as to whether the neonatal myocardium is more or less resistant to ischemia continues, there is general agreement that when functional recovery is used as the indicator of resistance to ischemia, the neonate recovers significantly better than the adult (Bove and Stammers 1986; Grice et al. 1987; Pridjian et al. 1987; Baker et al. 1988).

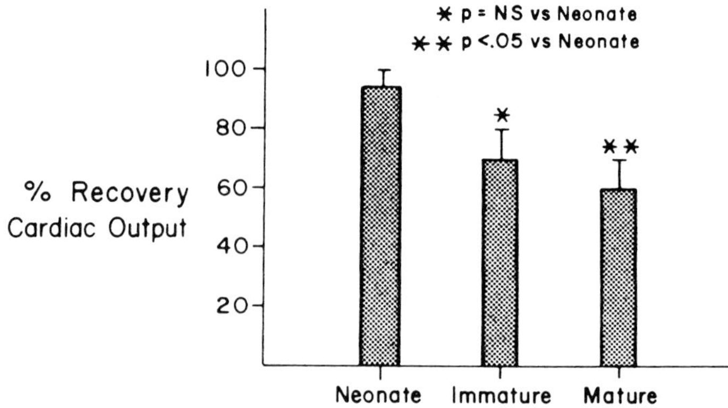

Figure 17.3 Percent recovery of cardiac output after 30 minutes of ischemia at 20°C in the isolated working heart. The neonate shows significantly better myocardial function than the adult. (Bove EL, Stammers AH. Recovery of left ventricular function after hypothermic global ischemia: Age related differences in the isolated working rabbit heart. J Thorac Cardiovasc Surg 1986; 91:115. By permission.)

□ Hypothermia

The use of topical and systemic hypothermia remains one of the major advances in myocardial protection for cardiac surgery. Topical hypothermia for cardiac arrest was first described by Shumway in 1959 for the repair of tetralogy of Fallot. This method of protection is frequently combined with systemic hypothermia and cardioplegia to achieve rapid myocardial cooling and arrest. It appears particularly beneficial in the small heart of the neonate, in which myocardial hypothermia has been shown to be of great importance (Figure 17.3) (Bove et al. 1988). When compared with mature rabbits, the neonatal heart is more resistant to ischemia during both normothermic and hypothermic conditions (Sawa et al. 1989). Although it is well accepted that the effects of hypothermia when combined with cardioplegia are additive in protecting the adult myocardium (Hearse et al. 1980), the results for the neonate are less clear (Bove and Stammers 1986; Baker et al. 1988; Aukiran and Hearse 1989; Sawa et al. 1989).

□ Elective Myocardial Arrest

A cardioplegic solution should provide complete and rapid electromechanical arrest, maintain the electrolyte milieu, deliver substrates, wash out metabolites, prevent cellular swelling, adjust cellular pH to a protective level, and allow a bloodless field. The search continues for the perfect cardioplegic solution, and many solutions with different additives are used in cardiac surgery today.

Blood cardioplegia was thought to be able to deliver oxygen and substrates to the tissues during the induction of arrest. However, when crystalloid solutions containing comparable ionic and osmotic ingredients are compared with blood cardioplegia at low temperatures (5°C), the crystalloid solutions appear superior in their delivery of oxygen (Magovern et al. 1982). Our group failed to demonstrate any additional benefit when oxygen was added to crystalloid cardioplegic solutions used for the protection of the neonatal rabbit heart (Lynch et al. 1988). However, it is possible that the rheologic properties of dilute blood solutions may make it superior to crystalloid solutions. Clinical studies have demonstrated superior protection of the right atrium and ventricle with blood cardioplegia, resulting in significantly less postoperative supraventricular arrhythmias than in hearts protected with crystalloid cardioplegia alone.

The most frequently used crystalloid cardioplegia in clinical practice today is a modified St. Thomas' solution, a form of extracellular cardioplegia. Extracellular solutions use constituents found in concentrations which approximate the extracellular fluid with large amounts of potassium to induce diastolic arrest. Potassium depolarizes the membrane and prevents impulse transmission by inhibiting the action potential. This high level of potassium also prevents calcium influx.

Magnesium, a major component of St. Thomas' solution, has the ability to induce myocardial arrest by inhibiting calcium influx. Magnesium is known to inhibit the release of calcium from the sarcoplasmic reticulum, reduce mitochondrial uptake of calcium, and reduce the influx of calcium into the cell.

An acalcemic cardioplegia solution may render the heart more susceptible to reperfusion damage secondary to the calcium paradox. Although hypothermia protects against this calcium reperfusion injury, damage may occur as temperature increases. Hearse has demonstrated that the optimal calcium concentration in cardioplegia solutions used to protect the adult rat heart is 1.2 mM/L (Yamamoto et al. 1984). In our laboratory, we have shown that this concentration is optimal for the neonate as well (Zweng et al. 1990).

The majority of research on myocardial protection provided by cardioplegia has been done in the adult and extrapolated to the neonate. Akvian and Hearse (1989) have reported that not only is the neonatal myocardium inherently more resistant to ischemia than the adult, but that cardioplegia was indeed protective under conditions of normothermic ischemia. Kempsford and Hearse (1989) subjected the neonatal heart to normothermic ischemia to evaluate the effects of four different cardioplegia solutions and found that good functional recovery was obtained with the use of cardioplegia and that the best overall results were obtained with the use of St. Thomas' and Tyers solutions. Additionally, they found that while the Bretschneider and Roe solutions may be effective in the adult, these acalcemic solutions caused marked deterioration in the neonatal heart preparations.

Published reports have suggested that the standard St. Thomas' solution may not provide the same protection in the neonate as seen in the adult (Baker et al. 1988; Sawa et al. 1989). In studies by Sawa et al. (1989), multidose cold cardioplegia combined with topical hypothermia was not as effective as single-dose cardioplegia or hypothermia alone in protecting the neonatal myocardium (Figure 17.4). These results were confirmed by Watanabe, who showed that although the neonate

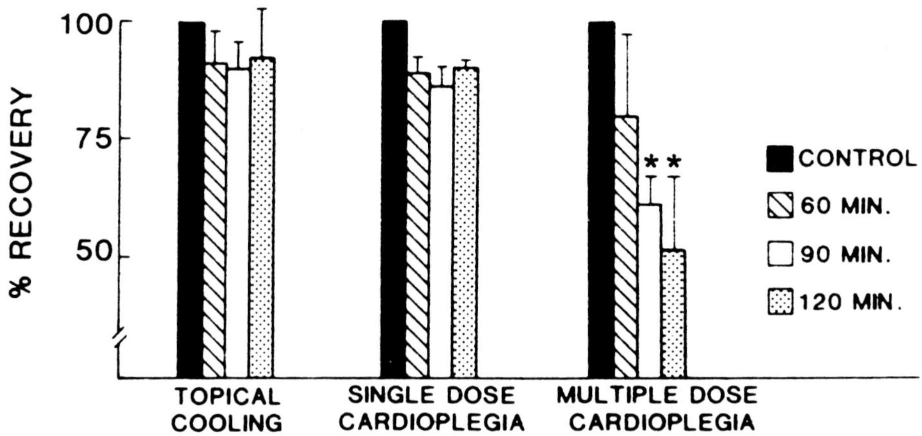

Figure 17.4 Effect of topical cooling, single-dose cardioplegia, or multiple-dose cardioplegia on recovery of aortic flow after 60, 90, and 120 minutes of ischemia in the isolated neonatal heart. Recovery was significantly worse after 90 and 120 minutes of ischemia when multiple-dose cardioplegia was administered. (Magovern JA, et al. Protection of the immature myocardium: An experimental evaluation of topical cooling, single-dose, and multiple-dose administration of St. Thomas' Hospital cardioplegic solution. J Thorac Cardiovasc Surg 1988; 96:408. By permission.)

recovered significantly better than the adult from ischemia, recovery was not as good with St. Thomas' cardioplegia. This group further showed that contracture was seen in the neonate with administration of St. Thomas' cardioplegia but not in the adult. This resulted in a greater resting tension and decreased myocardial function in the reperfusion period (Watanabe et al. 1989). Baker et al. (1988) combined hypothermia and cardioplegia to evaluate the neonatal and adult response to ischemia and confirmed greater tolerance to ischemia by the neonate. However, they found that multidose St. Thomas' cardioplegia administered to the neonate during ischemia caused a "decremental loss of postischemic function in contrast to incremental protection with multidose cardioplegia in the mature heart." When the neonate was given washouts during ischemia with Krebs solution, myocardial recovery was improved, leading to the conclusion that St. Thomas' cardioplegia is not protective in the neonatal heart (Baker et al. 1988). Lofland et al. (1989) demonstrated both clinically and experimentally that current methods of neonatal myocardial protection using hypothermia and St. Thomas' cardioplegia were inadequate to preserve the preischemic ATP pools of patients undergoing open-heart surgery.

The studies showing a decrease in functional recovery of the neonatal heart when exposed to St. Thomas' cardioplegia have used an alkalotic cardioplegia, as originally advocated for the adult. We evaluated the functional recovery of the neonatal myocardium following normothermic ischemia at various pH ranges (Iannettoni et al., in press). Maximal functional recovery was obtained when the myocardial pH during ischemia was maintained in an acidic range (pH = 6.33). When the pH of the cardioplegic solution was raised (7.4 to 8.2), the functional recovery was substantially worse. This inverse relationship between pH and functional recovery may, in part, be due to inactivation of acid-sensitive ATPases, preventing further depletion of ATP stores during ischemia.

DISCUSSION

The ideal method of neonatal myocardial protection has not yet been determined. There is general agreement that hypothermia is an integral part of preventing ischemic damage. Present evidence does provide support for additional protection with cardioplegia in the immature heart. Further studies are needed to determine the components needed to achieve optimal functional recovery both experimentally and clinically. It has become clear in our limited knowledge of neonatal myocardial protection that the neonate can no longer simply be assigned the methods used for adult myocardial protection with the expectation of similar results.

REFERENCES

Abd-Elfattah ASA, Murphy CE, Salter DR, et al. Developmental role of myocardial 5′-nucleotidase and AMP-deaminase isoenzymes in the increased tolerance of immature hearts to ischemic injury [abstr]. Circulation 1986; 74(suppl II):492.

Appleton RS, Graham TP Jr, Cotton RB, Morceau GA, Boucek RJ Jr. Altered early left ventricular diastolic cardiac function in the premature infant. Am J Cardiol 1987; 59:1391.

Akvian M, Hearse DJ. Protection of the myocardium during global ischemia: Is crystalloid cardioplegia effective in the immature myocardium? J Thorac Cardiovasc Surg 1989; 97:220.

Baker JE, Boerboom LE, Olinger GN. Age-related changes in the ability of hypothermia and cardioplegia to protect ischemic rabbit myocardium. J Thorac Cardiovasc Surg 1988; 96:717.

Boucek RJ Jr, Shelton M, Artman M, Landon E. Myocellular calcium regulation by the sarcolemmal membrane in the adult and immature rabbit heart. Basic Res Cardiol 1985; 80:316.

Bove EL, Gallagher KP, Drake DH, et al. The effect of hypothermic ischemia on recovery of left ventricular function and preload reserve in the neonatal heart. J Thorac Cardiovasc Surg 1988; 95:814.

Bove EL, Stammers AH. Recovery of left ventricular function after hypothermic global